MEAT, MEDICINE AND HUMAN HEALTH
IN THE TWENTIETH CENTURY

STUDIES FOR THE SOCIETY FOR THE SOCIAL HISTORY OF MEDICINE

Series Editors: *David Cantor*
Keir Waddington

MEAT, MEDICINE AND HUMAN HEALTH IN THE TWENTIETH CENTURY

EDITED BY

David Cantor, Christian Bonah and Matthias Dörries

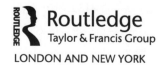

Routledge
Taylor & Francis Group

LONDON AND NEW YORK

First published 2010 by Pickering & Chatto (Publishers) Limited

Published 2016 by Routledge
2 Park Square, Milton Park, Abingdon, Oxfordshire OX14 4RN
711 Third Avenue, New York, NY 10017, USA

First issued in paperback 2015

Routledge is an imprint of the Taylor & Francis Group, an informa business

© Taylor & Francis 2010
© David Cantor, Christian Bonah and Matthias Dörries 2010

BRITISH LIBRARY CATALOGUING IN PUBLICATION DATA

Meat, medicine and human health in the twentieth century. – (Studies for the Society for the Social History of Medicine)
1. Meat – Health aspects – Europe – History – 20th century. 2. Meat – Health aspects – North America – History – 20th century. 3. Meat industry and trade – Health aspects – Europe – History – 20th century. 4. Meat industry and trade – Health aspects – North America – History – 20th century.
I. Series II. Cantor, David, 1957– III. Bonah, Christian. IV. Dorries, Matthias.
641.3'6-dc22

ISBN-13: 978-1-138-66442-5 (pbk)
ISBN-13: 978-1-8489-3103-9 (hbk)

Typeset by Pickering & Chatto (Publishers) Limited

CONTENTS

ACKNOWLEDGEMENTS

The original workshop on which this book is based was sponsored by the U.S. National Library of Medicine; the Institut de Recherche sur les Sciences et la Technologie (IRIST, EA 3424) at the University of Strasbourg; the Medical Faculty at the University of Strasbourg; and the Maison InterUniversitaire des Sciences de l'Homme-Alsace (MISHA). The editors would like to thank these organizations for their assistance; the conference and this book would not have happened without their support. At the Library we particularly thank Donald Lindberg, Elizabeth Fee, and Paul Theerman for their support of the workshop and book. We would also like to thank Carine de Sagazan and Catherine Douvier at Strasbourg for their assistance with the organization of the workshop. The anonymous referee of this book provided invaluable help to the editors in shaping the volume.

LIST OF CONTRIBUTORS

Rima D. Apple is Professor Emerita at the University of Wisconsin-Madison. She has published extensively in women's history, the history of medicine, and the history of nutrition. Among her books are *Perfect Motherhood: Science and Childrearing in America* (New Brunswick, NJ: Rutgers University Press, 2006) and *Vitamania: Vitamins in American Culture* (New Brunswick, NJ: Rutgers University Press, 1996) which received the Kremers Award, 1998, from the American Institute of the History of Pharmacy.

Christian Bonah is Professor for the History of Medical and Health Sciences at the University of Strasbourg and holds at present a research professorship at the Institut Universitaire de France (IUF). He has worked on comparative history of medical education, the history of medicaments and vaccines, and the history of human experimentation. Recent work includes research on risk perception and management in drug scandals and courtroom trials as well as studies on medical film. Recent publications include: *L'expérimentation humaine. Discours et pratiques en France, 1900–1940* (Paris: Les Belles Lettres, 2007); 'Packaging BCG: Standardizing an Anti-Tuberculosis Vaccine in Interwar Europe', *Science in Context*, 21:2 (2008), pp. 279–310. He has co-edited volumes on *Harmonizing 20th Century drugs: Standards in pharmaceutical history* (Paris: Glyphe, 2009); *Histoire et médicament au XIXe et XXe siècle* (Paris : Glyphe, 2005) and *Nazisme, science et médecine* (Paris: Glyphe, 2006).

Michael Broadway is Professor of Geography and Interim Dean of Arts & Sciences at Northern Michigan University where he teaches a course on Food and Society. His research expertise focuses on the meatpacking industry's community impacts. He has studied small towns with packing plants across the Great Plains and Prairies and published over thirty articles and book chapters on the topic. In 2006 he was a visiting Fulbright Research Chair in the Department of Rural Economy at the University of Alberta where he studied the impact of the province's outbreak of 'mad cow' disease on a rural community. He is a co-author with Donald Stull of *Slaughterhouse Blues: The Meat and Poultry Industry in North America* (2004 Wadsworth).

David Cantor is Deputy Director of the Office of History, National Institutes of Health, Bethesda, Maryland. His scholarly work focuses on the twentieth-century history of medicine, most recently the histories of cancer and medical film. He is the editor of *Reinventing Hippocrates* (Aldershot: Ashgate, 2002) and *Cancer in the Twentieth Century* (Baltimore, MD: Johns Hopkins University Press, 2008), and series editor (edited collections) of the series in which this book appears: *Studies for the Society of the Social History of Medicine* published by Pickering and Chatto.

Matthias Dörries is Professor for History of science at the University of Strasbourg, France. His research and interests focus on the geophysical sciences and most recently climate change with an interest in linking these issues with health, medicine and the health sciences at large. His most recent research includes articles on the history of volcanism and climate change, and the nuclear winter theory

Jean-Paul Gaudillière is a senior researcher at Le Centre de Recherche Médicale et Sanitaire and l'Institut National de la Santé et de la Recherche Médicale (CERMES-INSERM) in Paris. His work addresses many aspects of the history and sociology of the biomedical sciences during the twentieth century, particularly molecular biology and medicaments. His present research focuses on the history of biologicals as drugs, ways of regulating medicaments, and pharmaceutical innovation between the North and the South. Amongst others, he has edited, 'Drug Trajectories', a special issue of *Studies in the History and Philosophy of the Biological and Biomedical Sciences*, 36:4 (2005) and 'How Pharmaceuticals Became Patentable in the Twentieth Century', a special issue of *History and Technology*, 24:2 (2008); he has co-edited, with Volker Hess, *Ways of Regulating: Therapeutic Agents Between Plants, Shops and Consulting Rooms* (Max-Planck Institut für Wissenschaftgeschichte, Preprint Series, 363, 2009) and is the author of *Inventer la biomédecine. La France, l'Amérique et la production des savoirs du vivant (1945–1965)* (La Découverte, 2002).

Susan E. Lederer is the Robert Turell Professor of the History of Medicine and Bioethics at the University of Wisconsin School of Medicine and Public Health. A historian of medicine and biomedical ethics, she has published extensively on the history of both human and animal experimentation. Her books include *Subjected to Science: Human Experimentation in America Before the Second World War* (Baltimore, MD: Johns Hopkins University Press, 1995); *Frankenstein: Penetrating the Secrets of Nature* (New Brunswick, NJ: Rutgers University Press, 2002), and *Flesh and Blood: A Cultural History of Transplantation and Transfusion in Twentieth-Century America* (New York: Oxford University Press, 2008).

Ilana Löwy is a historian of science and medicine at Le Centre de Recherche Médecine, sciences, santé et société (CERMES – INSERM, CNRS, EHESS) in Paris. She is interested in the history of bacteriology, immunology, tropical medicine and oncology, and in the relations between the laboratory and the clinic, and the intersections between biomedicine and gender. She has published, among other things, *Between Bench and Bedside: Science, Healing and Interleukin-2 in a Cancer Ward* (Cambridge, MA: Harvard University Press, 1996) and *L'emprise du genre. Masculinité, féminité, inégalité* (La Dispute, 2005). Her latest book is *Preventive Strikes: Women, Precancer and Prophylactic Surgery*, (Johns Hopkins University Press, 2009).

Naomi Pfeffer is an Honorary Fellow at the Department of Science and Technology Studies, University College London. Her current research focuses on how human tissue is collected for medical purposes at the beginning and end of life. Her latest publication *Insider Trading: a Comparative History of Cadaver Tissue Banking in the United States of America and the United Kingdom* is forthcoming from Yale University Press.

Jeffrey M. Pilcher is Professor of History at the University of Minnesota. He has written a history of the modernization of Mexico's meatpacking industry, *The Sausage Rebellion: Public Health, Private Enterprise, and Meat in Mexico City, 1890-1917* (2006). His other works include *¡Que vivan los tamales! Food and the Making of Mexican Identity* (1998), *Food in World History* (2006), and a forthcoming book on the globalization of Mexican food entitled, *Planet Taco*.

Donald D. Stull is Professor of Anthropology at the University of Kansas, where he teaches graduate seminars on Doing Ethnography and Meat and Drink in America. His research and writing focus on the meat and poultry industry in North America, rural industrialization and rapid growth communities, industrial agriculture's impact on farmers and rural communities, and food. His writings include *Doing Team Ethnography: Warnings and Advice* (Thousand Oaks, CA: Sage, 1998), written with Ken Erickson; and *Slaughterhouse Blues: The Meat and Poultry Industry of North America*, written with Michael Broadway (Wadsworth, 2004). Don has been coeditor of *Culture & Agriculture* (1996–7), editor-in-chief of *Human Organization* (1999–2004), and president of the Society for Applied Anthropology (2005–7). He is the 2009 recipient of the Society for Applied Anthropology's Sol Tax Distinguished Service Award.

Ulrike Thoms, of Charité-Universitätsmedizin Berlin, works on the history of science and medicine and its intersections with economic and social history. Her dissertation on the diet in hospitals and prisons was the beginning of a long term interest in the histories of diet and the nutritional sciences, and of obesity on which she has published numerous articles. Her other areas of research are the histories of biomedicine and pharmaceuticals. She is involved in a French–German collaborative project on the history of pharmaceutical marketing.

Keir Waddington is a Reader in History and head of History in the Cardiff School of History and Archaeology, Cardiff University. His primary research interests are in the history of hospitals, public and rural health, the history of food, and urban history. He is co-author with Andrews, Briggs, Porter and Tucker of *The History of Bethlem 1247–1995* (London: Routledge, 1997) and author of *Charity and the London Hospitals 1850–1898* (Woodbridge and New York: Royal Historical Society, 2000), *Medical Education at St Bartholomew's Hospital* (Woodbridge and Rochester, NY: Boydell Press, 2003) and *The Bovine Scourge* (Woodbridge: Boydell Press, 2006), along with numerous articles on hospital charity, the medical profession, nursing, diseased meat and public health, bovine TB, and Victorian benevolence. He has recently completed *An Introduction to the History of Medicine, 1500 to the present* (Palgrave) as well as articles on sausages and is currently undertaking a study of public health in rural Wales.

LIST OF FIGURES AND TABLES

INTRODUCTION: MEAT, MEDICINE, AND HUMAN HEALTH IN THE TWENTIETH CENTURY

David Cantor and Christian Bonah

In July 2008, the United States Department of Agriculture (USDA) announced that it would make public the names of retail stores that received tainted products. Coming soon after the Hallmark/Westland Meat Packing Co. recalled 143 million lbs of meat, then the largest meat recall in United States history, the USDA's plan was to name retail stores only when there was a good chance a person would become ill or die by consuming the meat or poultry product – so-called Class I recalls. Other recall classes, in which there was little or no chance of illness, would not be covered. Richard Raymond, the agriculture undersecretary who oversaw the USDA's Food Safety and Inspection Service, noted: 'We need this rule to reinstall confidence in the American public that we are in control here'.[1]

For many critics, the USDA's ruling had less to do with public health than with restoring confidence in a meat industry shaken by a variety of health crises, in retailers anxious to avoid a reputation for carrying tainted meat, and in a Department caught unawares. While some lawmakers and consumer groups welcomed the new USDA ruling, many criticized it, claiming that, because it did not include all meat and poultry recalls, it failed to fully protect the public. As the debate spread across the internet and other media, the issues became more confused and complex. Responses to the ruling and the recall were intertwined with concerns about the appropriate treatment of animals, the morality of meat eating, anxieties about modern farming, processing and preservation methods, and worries about the influence of commercial, advocacy and political interests on nutrition policy and dietary habits. Vegetarians, health activists, animal activists, the meat industry, policymakers, lawmakers and regulators all drew very different conclusions as to the meaning of the USDA's action.

I.

The USDA's ruling and the responses to it capture an issue central to this volume: the diversity of public health messages about the healthiness of meat. This volume explores such diversity in a variety of historical contexts, and seeks to embed it in broader cultural, social and economic interests and agendas around meat during the twentieth century. Its focus is less on whether meat is truly healthful or otherwise, than on the changing historical meanings and uses of claims about the health benefits or dangers of meat and meat products, and on the many different efforts to control and regulate these hazards. As the 2008 example above suggests, different groups and individuals have drawn very different lessons from efforts to protect the public health.

This volume not only highlights the diversity of public health messages about meat, but also the diversity of players involved in debates about meat. We focus on four players: the meat industry, government, consumers, and the medical sciences, and especially on the confusion of messages about their role in promoting health or illness.[2] Thus, in the case of the meat industry, the papers in this collection show that it has both been blamed for many of the untoward effects of rising meat production and consumption, and has been credited with improvements in health. On the one hand, articles demonstrate that modern methods of meat processing, the sheer quantities of meat available in modern societies, and the ways in which the industry has promoted meat and meat products to the public have all been variously blamed for health problems that are characteristic of modernity. On the other hand, they also show that these same factors have also been promoted as causes of improvements in the health of the population: policymakers, scientists and others have argued that the widespread availability of meat – together with other foods – has led to healthy, productive and fit populations, and that the modern meat industry has been a precondition for the development of a range of new medicines, including beef extracts in the nineteenth century, and hormones such as cortisone in the twentieth century.[3]

In the case of government, there is a similar confusion of perspectives on its role in promoting health. On the one hand, the papers show that governments encouraged meat consumption to promote a healthy population, increase economic productivity, advance military readiness and ensure national survival. On the other hand, they also show that the close association that developed between government and the meat industry came to be seen by some critics as a cause of ill health associated with meat consumption.[4] Critics of the meat industry blamed governments for reluctance to impose and enforce regulation and reform on the meat industry. Thus, while in the early twentieth century the meat industry experienced an increase in new government-imposed health and veterinary regulations, critics often attacked these as insufficient to address the harmful consequences of meat consumption. For its part, the meat industry tended to criticize such regulations as overly restrictive.

The volume also highlights the confusion of perspectives on the role of consumers.[5] For critics, consumers of meat have themselves contributed to the growing public health crises associated with the production and consumption of meat, the inhumane treatment of animals destined for slaughter, and the ecological impact of the meat industry on the environment. For others, consumers of meat were the dupes of the meat industry and its allies in government, easily swayed by the industry's efforts to advertise its products, the confusion of messages coming from government, and the efforts of the meat industry to create uncertainty about the harmful effects of meat or components. Thus, the focus on consumers raised questions about who could speak for consumers, and whether it was possible to disassociate 'real' consumers from the organizations that purported to speak for them.

Finally, the papers in this volume explore contradictory perceptions of science: science has been portrayed both as a solution to the health issues raised by meat, and as a cause of these problems. Two sets of contradictions are of concern here. First, on the one hand, science and medicine have been credited as means of counteracting the health problems associated with modern methods of meat production, and of contributing to the invention and improvement of drugs and other medications that rely on the meat industry for their development. On the other hand, their role in the development of modern food processing industry has been portrayed as contributing to the very health problems that consumption of excessive, tainted or the wrong sorts of meat (or its components) generate. The second set of contradictions focuses on the values embedded in scientific knowledge. While, on the one hand, scientific knowledge about the healthiness or otherwise of meat has been promoted as an objective, value-free means of maintaining human health, on the other hand it has also increasingly come to be seen as shaped by either the meat industry or by its critics. Either way, claims that scientific knowledge is less than objective – informed by industrial interests, or the pre-existing concerns of those who are critical of the industry or of meat-eating in general – have become powerful ways of undermining its credibility. Public health messages about meat are increasingly confusing not only because these messages are often contradictory, but also because it is difficult to disentangle the interests and agendas behind the various health claims, including those based in science.[6]

II.

This book can be set against a growing body of historical literature that traces the dramatic transformation in European and American eating habits during the nineteenth century.[7] This literature has shown that the lower classes and parts of the middle class shifted from a largely cereal and undiversified diet to one that increasingly included meat, in addition to vegetables, fruits and dairy products. Many historians argue that this change meant an improvement after centuries of protein deprivation: larger quantities of amino acids were added to the general diet, and contributed to a more than doubling of the European population by the turn of the twentieth century.[8] Anthropometric studies highlight a general improvement of the nutritional status of the general population in France during the long nineteenth century as measured by the increasing height of military recruits. Nevertheless, the immediate consequence of industrialization and urbanization was a worsening of working-class malnutrition, before the beginnings of improvement two or three decades later.[9]

A standard story goes that this transformation in eating habits was made possible by the agricultural and industrial revolutions of the latter half of the eighteenth century and the first part of the nineteenth. These permitted an unprecedented increase in the supply of meat, along with other protein-rich products such as milk and eggs. New technologies such as canning and refrigeration, developments in fodder production and animal husbandry, and the introduction of new methods of animal slaughter and transportation by railroads and steamship, all made meat and protein more widely available.[10] Protein consumption is said to have risen at all levels of society, helped by the fact that over time some incomes rose, while the price of meat either held steady or declined, and public authorities came to see meat consumption as essential for population growth and military and industrial efficiency. By the eve of World War I, many commentators appear to have forgotten that there had been a time in the past when the vast majority of Europeans and Americans had to do without meat.

This is not to say that everyone had equal access to meat. A common argument is that many of the poor continued to survive on a diet of white bread, tea, sugar, gin, beer and porridge, and those of the working class with access to meat were often restricted to the more fatty cuts. Women often ate less meat than their fathers, husbands and brothers, sometimes denying themselves to provide for their men. Meat was more available in some geographical areas than others: some meats were more easily obtained by the rural than the urban poor, and some countries and regions seem to have solved problems of supply better than others. Nineteenth-century European visitors to the United States commented on the vast quantities of meat consumed by even the poorest of Americans; quantities unimaginable at home.[11] At the same time, American commentators, such as Catherine Beecher and Harriet Beecher Stowe, suggested that American housewives follow their French and English counterparts and properly prepare meat in small quantities.[12]

The existence of national differences in meat consumption was regularly commented on by contemporary physicians. For example, Michel Lévy, consulting physician to the French Emperor and director of the Military Academy of Val de Grâce,[13] noted that while the average consumption of bread was more or less identical for inhabitants of London and Paris in the 1860s, this was not the case for meat. If the average Parisian consumed 207 grams of meat per day, inhabitants of London consumed 25 per cent more meat per capita per day.[14] Lévy noted that regional eating habits depended on traditional agriculture practices, but also blamed the variations on 'civilization': 'civilization, multiplying means of viability and exchange between nations modified the diet of people and social classes'.[15] In the case of meat, figures for France indicated that consumption was primarily a matter of money and social class. Those with higher incomes and higher social standing had greater access to and better cuts of meat. Lévy also highlighted several other aspects of the differential consumption of meat. Thus, he noted that between 1816 and 1833 urban meat consumption apparently did not change much in France, though it decreased for the overall population by 50 per cent between 1789 and 1836. By the mid-nineteenth century meat consumption had not attained the level that existed before the French Revolution, and it would not return to its pre-Revolutionary levels for a further two decades. Most important for Lévy were regional disparities: of the 500,000 cattle slaughtered in the 1860s annually in France, 140,000 – that is 28 per cent – went to Paris while the capital only accounted for 3 per cent of the French population. In the countryside, meat consumption could be as low as $^1/_{30}$ of that of major cities though eating habits changed there as well – albeit more slowly – as cattle breeding became more common.[16]

Rising consumption of meat had mixed consequences for human health. On the one hand, historians have argued that the increasing availability of meat resulted in a decline of illnesses associated with protein deficiencies. Before the nineteenth century protein starvation was commonplace, especially among artisans, factory workers and peasants, who did not consistently get fifty to seventy grams of protein a day. The consequence was that infants and children were more likely to experience stunted growth and the general population to be susceptible to viral and bacterial diseases. As meat consumption rose, these conditions did not disappear, but they were less likely the result of poor protein consumption. Moreover, rising meat consumption, in combination with a more varied diet, may have helped contribute to the decline in mortality from acute infectious diseases. From Arthur Newsholme in 1908 to Thomas McKeown in the 1960s, public health officials and epidemiologists have argued that the rise and fall of infectious diseases, such as tuberculosis, could be positively correlated to food prices in modern and contemporary Western societies.[17]

On the other hand, historians have also highlighted a variety of downsides to rising meat consumption. From this perspective, the increasing availability of meat and the resulting consumption of excessive or the wrong sorts of meat (or its components) resulted in a number of ills, including heart disease and obesity. New methods of livestock farming, slaughter, and food preservation led to illnesses associated with tainted meat and the presence of contaminants (such as hormones in the twentieth century).[18] The new meat processing industries also resulted in a range of injuries and illnesses associated with the working conditions specific to those industries, vividly captured in Upton Sinclair's *The Jungle* (1906)[19] and in the contemporary work of Jeremy Rifkin (1992), Eric Schlosser (2001) and Steve Striffler (2005), among others.[20] More recently, there has also been concern about the environmental consequences of mass meat production, and its impact on the availability of staple foods for the World's poor and developing nations. Increasingly meat consumption has become central to debates about the future of food and the capacity of humans to feed themselves. In Frances Moore Lappé's evocative phrase, a factory animal is sometimes seen as 'a protein factory in reverse'.[21] Writing in the 1970s, Lappé argued that American and Western consumption of meat literally starved the developing world. In her view a meat diet was unfair, unhealthy and unsustainable.

III.

While this collection of papers traces some of the dramatic consequences for workers' health of the industrialization of meat production, it does not discuss the 'real' health consequences of rising meat consumption.[22] Instead, this volume shifts attention to the meanings and uses of such consequences: how these meanings and uses were embedded in broader transformations in the meat industry, in the emergence of the state, in the mobilization of consumers, and in how people evaluated the nutritional value of meat, especially by means of the new sciences of nutrition that emerged from the 1840s.[23] Our point is not that these sciences provided a better way of understanding how meat influenced human health, but to explore how they were deployed as authoritative arguments by both advocates and critics of meat consumption. Moreover, we also suggest that meat provides a valuable window on the changing boundaries between the categories of food and drug. Thus, papers in this collection show how the nutritional consequences of consuming meat could be portrayed as form of therapy, and how extracts of meat came to be considered as drugs. They also trace a variety of political and cultural responses to meat, from efforts to regulate it, to efforts to undermine claims about its nutritional or healthful qualities. In short, this book explores the meanings and uses of claims about the health consequences of meat for a variety of different groups, at different times within the twentieth century, and in different social, economic and institutional contexts.

These groups can broadly be divided into two categories – those who advocated meat production or consumption on the grounds that it improved health, and those who were critical of such claims: The former included meat producers themselves – farmers, meat processors, butchers and retailers – as well as their allies in government, the media, medicine and science; the latter included vegetarians, animal-rights activists, and other critics of the meat industry, together with their allies in government, the media, medicine and science. Both categories – advocates and critics – included a broad, shifting range of groups and individuals, sometimes with competing agendas and interests, who might disagree on what made meat healthy or unhealthy, and who might move from one category to another depending on the issue. For example, public health activists might promote meat eating as a means of improving the health of the population, but differ with the meat producers and retailers about how much or what types or preparations of meat were healthful. Workers in the slaughterhouses might join with the owners to promote consumption of meat as part of a healthy diet, but disagree with them on the healthiness of working conditions. Thus advocates and critics could blur into one another, distinct at times, but shading into one another as debates and issues changed.

***

In the United States, the emergence of the meat processing industry in the Midwest, from its initial stages as a part-time activity of merchants in the 1840s, to a major industry characterized by large-scale, specialized plants in the 1870s, meant that farmers, butchers, and merchants, operating in regional and local markets, gave way to large, efficiently organized corporations whose relentless efforts to control the national food chain – aided by the development of new technologies of transportation and food preservation – helped to make the United States into a vast consumer of meat and meat products. The new corporations vigorously promoted meat as a crucial part of a healthy diet, and forcefully challenged suggestions that their product might be a cause of ill-health.

It is commonly assumed that beef packing dominated the Chicago meatpacking industry. But in fact beef accounted for only for 30 per cent of meat shipped from the Union Stockyards in 1890. Nineteenth-century Americans tended to consume cured and salted pork throughout, in part because of fears of food contamination. This began to change during the Civil War, when the War Department demanded that the Chicago meatpackers supply fresh beef to troops along the Mississippi. Large numbers of men were consequently introduced to fresh beef, and came to acquire a taste for it. This helped to prompt meatpackers to develop facilities to ship fresh meat, and commercial meatpackers, and later home meatpackers, subsequently turned to fresh meat production. Gradually consumption of fresh beef and pork came to challenge consumption of salted meats.[24]

A central development was the factory slaughterhouse, which, during the nineteenth century, came to replace the hand-slaughter of livestock by individual butchers. According to Paula Young Lee, the centralized slaughterhouse emerged as a political response to the public's increasing lack of tolerance for 'dirty' butchering practices, as defined by changing norms of social hygiene and fear of meat-borne disease.[25] Located first in major urban centres such as Chicago, and by the late twentieth century in rural locations nearer livestock farms, the slaughterhouse rationalized animal slaughter according to capitalist imperatives. It aimed to transform living animals into a relatively standardized product that might be easily transported and sold, and slaughterhouse owners relied for this task on unskilled, usually immigrant labour, often working under dangerous conditions. Upton Sinclair's (1906) exposé might have highlighted the terrible conditions under which workers worked, and the 1906 Pure Food and Drug Act might have sought to ensure that no meat sold as human food consisted of 'filthy, putrid or decayed animal', but it was economic interests that drove support for government regulation. The industry's low standards of hygiene had severely undermined sales of meat, and the dreadful conditions under which workers worked and animals died were not the major factors in the political calculations.

If efforts to promote and protect the healthiness of meat came to be linked to efforts to maintain the profitability of the modern meat industry, they also came to be linked to other concerns. As meat production became an increasingly important export commodity, claims that meat might be tainted came to pose a threat to efforts to promote these exports, and the industry vigorously campaigned to counter such threats. In addition, against a backdrop of concerns about immigration, the meat industry sought to portray meat eating as a defining characteristic of what it was to be an American and to be modern, though regional and ethnic patterns of meat consumption persisted and thrived. Meat became the centrepiece of the American dinner table, paradoxically a marker of American, ethic and regional identity, and suggestions that it might be unhealthy or tainted posed a significant threat to such claims. For such reasons, the meat industry increasingly promoted meat as part of a healthy diet in advertising and in educational programmes, often invoking nutritional research in support of such claims. Not that such nutritional research was always independent of the industry. Meat producers also sought to shape public knowledge about meat by financing research on the role of meat in nutrition and health, to promote a view of meat as part of a healthy diet, and to discredit suggestions that it might be a cause of ill health.[26]

Not all meats were equal. Beef consumption came to match that of pork during World War I, and consumption of the two meats remained equivalent until the 1950s, when pork began a relative decline. The decline coincided with purchase by Ray Kroc of the McDonald's franchise and the appearance of Burger King. The emergence of thousands of small, brightly lit restaurants scattered across the suburbs, supplying cheap meat (and French fries and soda) were popular among suburban children and their parents. The restaurants sponsored numerous children's sports leagues, and became a destination for parents who increasingly shuttled their children from one organized activity to another. Changes in family life, with millions of middle-class women increasingly balancing work and family, and the shift from unstructured play to organized leisure activities for children, combined with the popularity of convenience foods, made the owners of fast food restaurants into millionaires, and helped solidify the shift towards beef. At the same time, chicken consumption rose, stimulated perhaps by the shortages of beef and pork during the war, by transformations in chicken production that allowed producers to grow chickens faster, by the creation in the 1950s of fast food outlets such as Colonel Sanders Kentucky Fried Chicken franchise and by the emergence in the 1960s of concerns about the healthiness of beef and pork. Consumption of the latter two meats declined since the 1970s, and was surpassed by chicken in the 1990s. [27]

In some ways the situation in Europe was similar to that in the United States. Meat producers and their allies on both sides of the Atlantic promoted meat as a central part of national diets, a defining part of national identities: think of John Bull, the portly personification of England, whose surname echoes the alleged fondness of the English for beef, or the French nickname for the English: 'les rosbifs', the 'Roast Beefs'[28] As in the United States, European producers and their allies also promoted meat as crucial to national and military efficiency and effectiveness. They also sought to protect sales by challenging suggestions that their product might be unhealthy, strategies that often went in tandem in the early twentieth century with new government regulations on commercial marketing methods, the abandonment of free trade and introduction of tariff controls and quotas.[29]

In other ways, however, the European situation was quite different to that in North America. For example in contrast to the United States, the nineteenth-century ownership of the British meat trade tended to be concentrated in the hands of individual farmers and butchers who might kill three or four animals each week in time to meet peak demand for meat for the Sunday roast. These animals were killed in what civil servants called 'private premises', a make-shift place on a farm, an inner-city cellar, a corner of a side street, or the yard at the back of a butcher's shop. The farmer or butcher often killed the animals themselves, or hired a man to do the job for them by the hour. The situation would change in the second half of the nineteenth century, but an economic incentive to modernize in the American way was largely absent in Britain because the price of meat was held down by cheap imports.[30] New techniques of chilling and freezing allowed vast quantities of meat to be imported – beef from Ireland, Argentina and the United States of America, lamb from Australia and New Zealand and bacon from Denmark. Evidence given before the Departmental Committee on Combinations in the Meat Trade (which reported to Parliament in 1909) showed that most of the meat sold in major British cities was imported. In Smithfield Market in London more than 80 per cent of meat sold came from abroad. In Manchester half the meat was imported.[31]

This is not to say that local supplies disappeared. In some places they remained plentiful, and foreign imports did not overwhelm the market. Indeed, home-produced meat sometimes commanded a premium because it was fresh. But, much of the 'roast beef of olde England' was rotten, and outbreaks of food poisoning were not uncommon.[32] Most butchers' shops lacked refrigeration and, when meat was past its best, its price would be reduced. The cheapest bits of animals – heads, tails, kidneys, tongues, hearts, livers and skirt – were found on market stalls or on a street seller's pitch. The 1875 Public Health Act allowed local authorities to intervene in order to prevent the sale of rotten meat.[33] And some authorities built large public slaughterhouses where, for a small fee, farmers, butchers and private individuals could have their animals killed. By the 1930s, 115 had been built and one in every four animals slaughtered abandoned its life in one of them.[34] However, some of the older ones were little more than a collection of small killing stalls where the standard of hygiene was not much better than that found in many private premises. In the mid-1930s, the government decided to industrialize livestock slaughtering, and in 1937, it set up the Livestock Commission whose responsibilities included building three industrial slaughterhouses. In its view, modern abattoirs were better for animals, workers and meat eaters. These plans were disrupted by the war, but over course of the twentieth century the public abattoir came to replace the private abattoir, and eventually large centralized slaughterhouses emerged in Britain as they had in the United States. Yet the change happened more slowly in Britain than across the Atlantic, and the range of groups promoting change in Britain was also quite different.[35]

In many Continental countries, including France and Germany, the production of meat and meat products remained an artisan trade for much of the twentieth century.[36] The killing and preparation of fresh meat was dominated by local butchers, and marketing strategies of the sort seen in the USA were not developed until the widespread emergence of brand-name packaged meats (such as Wiesenhof poultry and packaged sausage) in the 1950s in Germany and later and to a lesser extent in France. Indeed, in contrast to the United States (and to some extent Britain), artisans continued to dominate the Continental European food industry as a whole until well after World War II, and industrial food preparation only started in the 1950s and 60s, often in response to specific national and regional developments.[37] In Germany, for example, the impetus for the industrialization of meat production emerged not with fresh packaged meat but rather canned sausages, such as the 'Frankfurter Würstchen'.[38] This is not to say that there was no marketing of meat and meat products in Europe: as we discuss later the marketing of meat products in Europe can be traced back to Liebig in the 1840s, and one might also cite the example of canned pâté de foie gras which commercialized in Alsace from the mid-nineteenth century onward.[39] But in general in Germany marketing strategies for individual food products were initiated not in the area of 'Nahrungsmittel' (literally food substances) but in the area of 'Genussmittel' (literally substances ingested for pleasure and taste such as alcoholic drinks, tobacco and spices).[40] Early market strategies thus focused on pleasure and taste rather than nutritional value or healthiness.[41] 'Genussmittel' tended to be industrialized and commercialized earlier that 'Nahrungsmittel', eventually paving the way for food advertisement for basic foods when the latter came to be attached to brand names. Central professional agencies for butchers and meat processing were only created after 1945 in major European countries, initiating marketing strategies to enhance consumers' trust and the professions general image as well as that of their specific product, mcat.

***

As meat consumption rose in the late eighteenth and nineteenth centuries so did anxieties about its ill effects. Such anxieties can be traced to antiquity, but they gained particular attention in the late eighteenth century when attention focused on the role of an increase in luxury and excess – including immoderate meat eating – in the emergence of a variety of 'new diseases,' including gout, constipation, nervous diseases and cancer. Historians have associated anxieties about luxury and excess with the emergence of a consumer society, the expansion of international trade, the introduction of 'ardent' liquors, and cultural anxieties about the moral and spiritual effects of intemperance, all expressed through discourses on bodily ill health. Anxieties about meat and its effects on the body and health were part of this larger critique of emergent consumer culture.[42]

Anxieties about meat reflected a variety of other concerns. First, in the late eighteenth and early nineteenth centuries they reflected growing concerns about animal welfare among evangelicals. Inspired by John Wesley's promotion of the 'social gospel' of Christianity, British evangelicals petitioned Parliament to legislate against many injustices including the slave trade, child labour, the harsh penal code and the mistreatment of animals used for labour or sport. In 1822, the British Parliament passed the first animal welfare legislation to protect work animals from abuse.[43] The new interest in animal protection helped set the stage for a revitalized vegetarianism. Numbers of vegetarians seem to have increased, and what was once a trickle of vegetarian publications turned, if not into a flood, certainly into a steady stream that often mixed abhorrence of meat and animal cruelty with Romantic appreciation of the beauty and innocence of nature. By the 1840s, the first vegetarian societies had been formed, first in Great Britain (1847), followed by the United States (1850), Germany (1867) and France (1878) among other countries.[44] Thus as meat production began to industrialize, there emerged a vibrant vegetarian movement, and though it remained numerically small and marginal to the mainstream, it gained sustenance from transformations in meat production. For example, from the mid-nineteenth century, critics attacked the cruelty of shipping vast numbers of animals in crowded boxcars and ship holds. By the 1870s, vegetarian restaurants began to appear – London had at least a dozen by the end of the century. The first international organization was established in 1908 – the International Vegetarian Union.[45]

Second, anxieties about meat also reflected broader concerns about emergent urban-industrial society. Thus, for example, from the 1820s, organized vegetarian movements increasingly linked the consumption of meat to a range of ills, often associated with urban industrial conditions. Vegetarian critics looked back to an allegedly golden rural age before industrialization and urbanization, in which so-called 'primitive' peoples tended to eat a diet relatively low in meat. In their view, such low-meat diets meant that diseases associated with modernity were also relatively rare in pre-industrial society – a point supported later in the century by anthropological evidence that looked at the low rate of modern diseases among contemporary 'primitive' peoples, statistical studies that linked rising meat consumption with a variety of modern ills, and evolutionary studies that identified the physiological and anatomical reasons for humans to eat vegetarian diets. In the view of some vegetarians, humans were either evolutionarily more adapted to vegetarian diets, or their sedentary lifestyle in modern urban industrial societies made consumption of meat more potentially hazardous than in earlier times when life was more physically strenuous.

Vegetarians were not the only ones to be concerned that rising consumption of meat was producing a range of new ills that were characteristic of modernity. For example, during the nineteenth and twentieth centuries, health reformers repeatedly criticized the tendency within modern societies to over-indulge in meat and meat products, and they sought new ways to maintain health by urging people to limit or eliminate meat consumption. Such self-restraint allowed people not only to maintain health, they argued, but also a sense of moral equilibrium in a world that encouraged uncontrolled consumption. For some critics of meat eating, the rejection or reduction of meat consumption could be portrayed as a return to primitive, pre-industrial conditions. For feminists, the rejection of meat could be portrayed as a way to usher in a new society which gave greater significance to women's values, a return for some to pre-industrial gender relations. Thus, some feminists came to invert meat's association with maleness in an approved sense: strength and power became cruelty and aggression; masculine vigour became violence, and forces of human destructiveness. Even meat's life-giving qualities could also be inverted: it came to be seen as 'dead' food, symbolic of decay at both a physical and moral level. By contrast fruits, nuts, grains and vegetables came to be re-conceptualized as pure and full of the essence of life, and of worldly salvation.[46]

If critics came to associate meat eating with the problems of modernity, this did not mean that they necessarily rejected everything about modernity. While a few may have pressed for a return to nature – the abandonment of cities and modern industry – most wanted to inject into modern urban-industrial society something of an older 'primitive' world, and a rejection or reduction of meat consumption provided one way of doing this, and so of counteracting the ill-effects of modernity. Such arguments were reinforced by science – we have already noted how evolutionary theory, anthropology, statistics and clinical observations provided scientific foundations for critics of meat eating. In addition, early nineteenth-century understandings of the role of diet in ill health were often discussed in terms of understandings of human physiology that stressed the need for moderation in diet to maintain the health of the organism. By the end of the century, such thinking was joined by newer knowledge that stressed the role of proteins, calories and, in the twentieth century, vitamins in maintaining health and inducing illness.[47]

IV.

This last point highlights a final issue that this book seeks to address: the emergence of science as an arbiter of the healthiness or otherwise of meat, and its intersection with the politics around meat.[48]

Although an interest in the relationship between nutrition and health can be traced back to the ancient world, it was only from the early nineteenth century and especially the 1840s that physiologists and chemists began to transform nutrition into a science by relating the chemistry of foods to animal physiology.[49] In this process, the nutritional value of meat came to be understood in terms of the precise composition of aliments, such as the chemist, Justus Liebig's, distinction between carbohydrates, fats and proteins. More importantly for the history of meat, Liebig labelled foodstuffs rich in nitrogen 'plastic' materials: materials, he claimed, that produced muscle tissue and at the same time provided the energy for work force that could be stored and released for later use.[50] Thus, Liebig and others came increasingly to take an interest in what the body did with meat when consumed. In sum, as Michel Lévy put it in 1869, meat 'developed organic force, increased resistance to working fatigue ... and thus its presence or absence in the working class diet conditioned numbers of sick and death'.[51]

More broadly, the new nutritional science helped to turn the relationship between what the body consumed as meat (or more specifically its component chemicals) and what the body produced as work into a scientific and economic calculus. As Jakob Tanner puts it, the new nutritional science, combined with work physiology and labour economics and industrial hygiene helped to reconceptualize the worker's body.[52] Workers came to have essentially two bodies: an individual one which was fundamentally a nutritional industrial plant that turned food into work force, and a collective one that transformed food into the health and wealth of the nation.[53] Thus, where protein metabolism became a key to the individual worker's capacity to work, meat consumption by the collective body of workers became a key to solving industrial, social and economic problems. At the same time, a lack of meat came to be framed as a 'protein gap', which at times became the focus of national attention as a social issue.[54]

The emergence of modern nutrition science coincided not only with the emergence of industrial hygiene and work physiology but also with the development of the modern meat industry in its various national forms. Indeed, the latter increasingly turned to the new sciences to promote and explain the nutritional and health benefits of its products. The point can be made by a focus on the development from the 1840s of commodities such Liebig's extract of meat and later other extracts such as Bovinine, Bovril, Valentines, and Richet's Zomine.[55] Liebig,

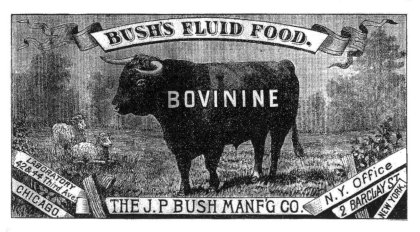

Figure I.1: Bush's Fluid Food, Bovinine.

for example, used physiological chemistry to support claims that the product which made him a household name improved muscle power and was generally invigorating.[56] Whatever the truth of such statements – they were later disputed – they helped to stimulate huge demand for the product, to promote the creation of a new industry, and to transform farming practices as farmers sought to meet the new demand for the product. Physiological chemistry was thus crucially tied to the nineteenth-century transformations in meat processing and farming discussed above.[57] It also helped to reshape the changing dividing line between the categories of food and drug. While this dividing line had been blurred before the 1840s, the growing interest in scientific understanding of the precise composition of aliments and their transformation when absorbed by the human body provided new ways of thinking about this dividing line. Physiological chemistry provided a rationale for the therapeutic value of Liebig's and similar extracts, and was also helped to explain the value of numerous restorative therapeutic regimens.[58] One of the aims of this collection is to highlight the connections between medical therapeutics and the meat industry. The story of extracts illuminates only part of this connection. As other papers show, the consumption of (raw) meat became a therapy for conditions such as tuberculosis and pernicious anaemia, and waste products of the meat industry provided ingredients for the modern pharmaceutical industry.[59]

By the 1890s a focus on the consumption of specific components of meat – such as proteins –was increasingly displaced by an 'energetic' approach that focused on calorimetric analysis.[60] Increasingly, meat and other foodstuffs were translated into calories, a move that shifted attention from particular constituents of food to the energy produced by food, and so also allowed the possibility of substituting different components of food for one another. Tanner argues that nutritional scientists were increasingly less concerned with the role of chemical supplies in nutrition than with questions of energy transformation and balances; questions that brought together the contemporary sciences of thermodynamics and work physiology.[61] In this process, the human body came to be portrayed as an 'engine'[62] that burned calories no matter what substance they were derived from.[63] Between 1890 and 1950 the 'human motor' was the dominant metaphor for the body in European industrial societies, shaping the understanding of both industrial work and economic growth.[64]

The new focus on the energy produced by food could have undermined the place of meat as the 'superior food stuff'[65] for workers. After all, if different components of food could be substituted for one another, then protein derived from meat no longer had any greater importance to nutrition than protein from any other source. Yet, in fact, meat remained highly valued and lost little of its reputation. In the first place, the new interest in the energy produced by food did little to undermine the high cultural value assigned to meat and its older associations with physical strength, masculinity, social power and status.[66] In the second place, the interest in food energy was challenged, with the identification by World War I of vitamins and other micronutrients that were defined as essential accessory food factors, and which shifted attention back to the composition of foods.[67]

Until the discovery of these of hitherto unsuspected components it had generally been agreed that health depended on the caloric content of the diet. From this perspective, it was suggested that the three major components of diet – carbohydrates, fats and proteins – could replace one another in proportion to their calorific content. Some protein, it was suggested, was required to provide nitrogen, and different proteins had equivalent nutritive value. In the early twentieth century, however, the idea that all proteins were nutritionally equivalent began to break down when animal experiments revealed that certain amino acids were needed for growth and survival, and that different proteins had different amino acid contents, and hence different nutritive values, and that these amino acids could not be synthesized by the body, but had to be supplied via the diet. A diet of carbohydrates, fats and proteins – combined with water and minerals – was insufficient to sustain life. A new focus on and what came to be known as essential amino acids and especially on vitamins shifted attention away from the energy content of the diet and undermined the idea that carbohydrates, fats, and proteins could replace one another.[68] It also shifted attention away from chemical physiology towards a new upcoming field of biochemistry – which like its predecessor was appropriated by various groups debating the health value of meat in the diet, albeit at different times in different countries.[69]

In this move the composition and quality of foods came to be rehabilitated and has remained a permanent factor for nutrition science ever since. This did not mean that the interest in calories disappeared. On the contrary, the economic calculus of calorie input increasingly came to be combined with estimates of nutritional quality and with a growing interest in how cooking procedures and kitchen techniques might prevent vitamin loss. Food preparation and cooking thus became key issues for the nutritional sciences. Thus, this new nutritional science increasingly came to be seen a crucial way of improving domestic cooking practices. Women on both sides of the Atlantic were routinely encouraged to turn to these new sciences to understand how techniques of food preparation and cooking affected the nutritional value of the meals they prepared.[70] The new nutritional science also came to inform the emergent Life Reform movement of the early twentieth century by stressing the role of naturally occurring micronutrients and vitamins in fruits and vegetables. Greens and grains were symbols of the alternative way of life the movement promoted.

This is not the place to review the complex history of nutrition in the twentieth century.[71] But the story of the emergence of biochemistry and vitamins shows that science was not a monolithic entity.[72] Many different sciences contributed to knowledge about the nutritional and health value of meats – including chemistry, physiology, physiological chemistry, biochemistry, the clinical sciences and epidemiology, and social sciences such as anthropology and sociology – and their results could sometimes be contradictory.[73] Such contradictions posed a problem for advocates of the health benefits of meat, and also an opportunity. While contradictory findings could raise questions about the claims of advertisers and marketers, they also provided an opportunity for the selective presentation of favourable findings, and also an opportunity to create uncertainty about claims that meat might be a cause of ill health. During the twentieth century, it came to be assumed that men and women needed to learn the latest scientific knowledge about nutrition to be good workers, mothers and soldiers. But such knowledge could be a problem for advertisers and marketers, and they also sought to shape public perceptions of what constituted good science and, at times, to undermine those sciences that posed a threat.

So far we have explored how the emergence of modern nutrition science coincided with the development of industrial hygiene, work physiology and the modern meat industry in its various national forms. It also coincided with the rise of the modern nation state. Increasingly, European and North American state institutions turned to the new sciences of nutrition to regulate and intervene in the diet of their populations. Over the course of the nineteenth century, state organizations in both continents came to inquire into what constituted an adequate diet for different groups of citizens – mothers, soldiers, workers and so on – an interest that spurred significant research in chemistry, physiology and physiological chemistry in state-sponsored university laboratories, research institutes and elsewhere. Research was often stimulated by war when attention came to focus on the nutritional adequacy of the rations of the armed forces and civilians.[74] In combination with other foods and nutritional components, meat and meat products came to be seen as crucial to improving the health of the population, and so of improving military and national efficiency.[75]

It should, however, be pointed out that issues of human health were not always at the top of the states' agendas.[76] From the mid-nineteenth century, initiatives for state intervention and regulation were often framed more as problems of animal health than of human health. From this perspective, government policymakers paid considerable attention to questions of meat availability and affordability. Issues of the quality of meat often had less to do with human health than economic concerns. Farmers and meat producers and suppliers increasingly worried that anxieties about animal health would undermine their economic interests, especially where people worried that animal diseases might be transmitted to humans. As Delphine Berdah notes in her recent PhD thesis, efforts to address such issues between 1866 and 1915 played out in different ways in Britain and France, albeit that officials in both countries had similar concerns about the impact of animal health on the growing international trade in meat and livestock.[77] Efforts to regulate the trade in meat and livestock thus oscillated between efforts to contain animal diseases and zoonoses at the national borders, and efforts to eradicate animal diseases in order to be able to export, and different countries adopted different strategies at different times. Inevitably such strategies were entangled with their utilitarian use as tools of economic regulating of nation states, and nineteenth-century struggles between laissez-faire and protectionist economic politics.

A new professional group – veterinarians – were central to these efforts to regulate animal diseases and the trade in meat.[78] Indeed, not only were veterinarians crucial to efforts to protect the trade in meat, but efforts to protect the trade were themselves crucial to the professionalization of veterinarians. Veterinarians successfully sought to represent their knowledge of animal diseases as critical to the development and implementation of regulations designed to protect the trade in meat: they defined the nature of animal diseases, and used this knowledge to help shape and put into practice policies – such as 'stamping out' in the UK – for controlling them, and these efforts to design and implement regulations consequently became crucial to the construction of veterinarians' special expertise. By developing such expertise, and by allying themselves with farmers and meat producers, veterinarians were able to demark themselves from physicians and public health officials more concerned with human health.

V.

If the new knowledge of nutrition came to be exploited by proponents of meat, it also came to be exploited by its critics.[79] Early nineteenth-century criticism of meat relied for much of its appeal on what its advocates saw as the moral abhorrence of killing animals for food, and the physical repugnance of eating meat. The problem these critics faced was that people generally believed that because it was closer chemically to human muscles, meat must be more easily digested and assimilated than plants. Thus, vegetable diets were often regarded as debilitating, while meat provided greater strength and endurance. The moral imperative was thus not as clear as the vegetarians liked to assert: did care of other species really trump human health and self-preservation? In such a context, vegetarians increasingly turned to science and medicine, to show that an alternative diet could be healthful and that meat could be harmful.

In the eighteenth and early nineteenth centuries English physicians such as George Cheyne and William Lambe provided medical evidence that a vegetarian diet could promote physical well-being, and that meat eating was responsible – among other things – for many ills association with indulgence. Lambe, for example, used his medical notes on patients to argue for a long tradition of medical vegetarianism that included Cheyne. He explained that because the natural physiological state of all animals was health, disease must be a result of unnatural habits. Many ills, including cancer, could be prevented by avoiding meat and other dietary impurities. Indeed, he claimed that people returning to a natural diet might experience an increase life-expectancy – perhaps double the norm – and he found support for his view in statistical evidence that abstinent monks had a longer than average life expectancy.[80]

Other scientific evidence was also used to support vegetarian arguments. For example, in the 1840s, Liebig's assertion that there was no difference between plant and animal protein, and that plants were the primary source of protein provided scientific support for vegetarian arguments that plant-based foods could substitute for meat. By mid-century they also turned to anthropology and statistics. Advocates of vegetarianism pointed to the predominantly vegetable diets of 'primitives' and pre-industrial populations as evidence of their natural-ness, and healthful qualities.[81] From this perspective, many of the ills of modern urban industrial society could be blamed on the increasing quantity of meat in the human diet, brought about by the transformations in farming, meat produc-tion, transportation and preservation. Nineteenth-century physicians provided scientific evidence that human teeth and intestines were more similar to those of herbivores than of carnivores. During the late nineteenth and twentieth centuries innumerable statistical studies linked the rise of modern diseases of civilization to rising meat consumption.

Critics attacked meat for of its unhealthful qualities; but health was only part of the picture. In his wide-ranging account of vegetarianism, Tristram Stuart describes vegetarianism as a 'counter-cultural critique' advocated in the eighteenth century by 'medical lecturers, moral philosophers, sentimental writ-ers and political activists.'[82] Stuart shows how thinkers such as Francis Bacon and Thomas Bushell claimed that a vegetarian diet not only provided a means of attained longevity but also spiritual perfection.[83] In their view, God had permit-ted Adam and Eve to eat only plants, fruits and seeds, and a return to such a diet would also return humanity to the harmony with nature that had existed before the Fall. Stuart also shows how seventeenth- and eighteenth-century travellers to India introduced the Hindu idea of *ahimsa* (the preservation of all life) as an ideal for a society that would no longer kill animals, and so provoked a crisis in European thinking about diet. In all these approaches to diet, scientific ration-ales for vegetarianism (the effect of meat eating on human health and character) were mixed with religious and philosophical arguments – the implications of Scripture for human diet; debates about the proper relationship between man and other animals, what it is to be human, and the relationship between killing and violence – a mix that can be found in Romantic proponents such as Shelley and Rousseau. Indeed, later nineteenth-writers added their own mixtures of religion, philosophy and science to justify a vegetarian diet. For example, the health reformer Sylvester Graham, from the 1820s to the 1850s argued that physiology had to be in harmony with morality: any behaviour that stained the soul also injured the body, and meat eating (along with extramarital sex, and many other practices) was harmful to both: an argument based, in part, on Broussaisian pathology that saw ill health as the consequence of over-stimulation of the body tissues, especially those of the digestive tract.

This countercultural mix of morality and science persisted among twentieth-century vegetarians and health reformers, though the scientific evidence changed, as did some of the moral justifications.[84] John Harvey Kellogg, Alexander Haig and many other early twentieth-century health reformers mixed science and moral reasoning to justify their critiques of meat, yet their prominence was not matched by popular support for vegetarianism. Later in the twentieth century vegetarian attempts to turn to the newer knowledge of nutrition based on biochemistry, for example, were equally ineffective in helping to encourage significant support for their movement. While the discovery of vitamins promoted a new appreciation of the importance of vegetables in the diet[85] and criticism of the dominance of meat, white bread and butter, potatoes, sugar, tea and coffee in the diet, this did not result in a significant move towards vegetarianism among the bulk of the population. Nor did the discovery of appalling conditions in the meat-processing plants in the early twentieth century; rather than promote vegetarianism, this tended to push for greater state regulation of meat production. As previously mentioned, the state tended to promote meat as part of a healthy diet, to maintain a strong workforce and military, and to ensure that mothers brought strong healthy children into the world, and raised them in a healthy manner.[86]

Thus until the 1960s and 70s, scientific evidence critical of the healthfulness of meat did not result in greater public support for vegetarianism. Such evidence was unpersuasive to many, and did little to counter the cultural and societal forces promoting meat eating. Numbers of vegetarians remained small, and the movement remained marginal to the mainstream. Despite efforts to link criticism of meat eating with criticism of animal experimentation, and feminist criticism of male cruelty, meat came to be a central part of European and North American diets. Vegetarians were often regarded as a minor sect, though one that may have had more support among women than men given the associations drawn between the exploitation of women and animals. Nor did vegetarian efforts to appeal to scientific and other evidence help significantly in changing this situation. Vegetarianism seemed doomed by its countercultural origins. It bore the mark of dissent, and consequently the mark of marginality.

This began to change in the 1960s. The debate over the morality of eating meat changed – from a focus on the morality of slaughter to a focus on the conditions under which animals lived and were transported and killed. Stimulated by the transformation of farming into an agribusiness, and by the development of factory farming, there emerged a growing concern about the environmental consequences of animal farming, revulsion at what many saw as the cruelty of mass production and slaughter, and the rise of the animal rights organizations. This is not to say that vegetarianism's triumph is preordained. It remains unclear whether distaste of factory farming will lead more people towards vegetarianism. On the one hand, criticism of factory farming has gone hand-in-hand with the expansion since the 1960s of McDonald's and its competitors across the globe, despite being haunted by criticism that it helps to promote obesity, destroys the rainforests, promotes factory farming and undermines indigenous cultural food traditions.[87] On the other hand, criticism of factory farming has also led to pressure for more sustainably produced, healthier and tastier meat. For example, contemporary Argentine beef connoisseurs argue that the introduction of American style feedlots to Argentina has resulted in a different quality of meat – more marbled, more American, less healthy and less tasty.[88]

Environmental vegetarianism has a long history that goes back at least to the late eighteenth century. The Reverend William Paley argued that the main aim of politics was to encourage the growth of a nation's population, and that this raised a problem as regards the consumption of meat. A piece of ground given over to 'grain, roots, and milk',[89] he argued, could support twice the population as that given over to animals to be killed for food. Adam Smith made a similar point in *The Wealth of Nations* (1776), arguing that a cornfield of moderate fertility produced a greater quantity of food than the best pasture of equal extent.[90] It was a small step from here to link utilitarian political economy to efforts to promote the health and strength of the nation, and vegetarian environmentalism continued to make this link through to the twentieth century – a valuable counter to the arguments discussed above that represented meat as a key to national, industrial and military survival. Thus, during the food shortages of the 1930s and 1940s, Nazi leaders attacked farmers who gave to animals grain which could have been used to feed Germans. Today, environmental arguments focus as much on sustaining the environment as on sustaining human populations. We are asked to calculate whether eating vegetables uses less fossil fuels than eating meat, how much tropical forest is destroyed to graze cattle, and how much biodiversity will disappear with the livestock, and the corn and soybeans grown to feed them. In all these calculations, science, philosophy, religion and morality coexist, sometimes uneasily. Human health has sometimes been displaced, and sometimes linked, to the health of the planet.

VI.

It should be clear by now that the story of meat, medicine and human health in the twentieth century is part of a longer tale that goes back at least to the late eighteenth century, if not before. It is a story of how, in the last 200 years, concerns about the impact of meat and meat products on human health have intersected with transformations in dietary practices, the emergence of the modern meat industry, the development of a variety of critiques of meat eating, the growing use of science (and a variety of sciences) to justify and attack meat and meat products, and the beginnings of efforts to regulate their safety. All these themes can be found in the essays that follow, but they also show that twentieth-century attitudes towards meat and human health cannot be entirely reduced to these longer-term trends. In what follows we explore the continuities and discontinuities between twentieth-century and earlier developments. The discussion is in three parts: I. Meat and Therapeutics, II. Meat, Politics and Culture and III. Meat, Risk and Regulation.

Part I explores the relations between meat and therapeutics, especially the vast, constantly shifting borderline between the categories of food and drug. Meat and meat products have long been seen as therapeutic and preventive agents; if not drugs, then something close to them. Physicians often regarded consuming meat or meat extracts as ways of fortifying the constitution, and extracts such as beef tea were popularly used as stimulants. They could maintain health, fend off illness, help revive an invalid, and sustain a patient during and after the rigours of surgery. Yet, they had to be used cautiously if they were not to undermine efforts at restoring or healing a patient: too much stimulation could be bad for a weak constitution. In such cases, strong meats or an excess of beef tea could do more harm than good. Yet, during the nineteenth and especially the twentieth centuries the relationship between meat and therapeutics began to change. While meat and meat extracts continued to be used to bolster the constitution, scientists also began to identify and collect therapeutically active components from them. In so doing they transformed them into pharmaceutical commodities that had very different cultural and social meanings to the meat products from which they had been derived. The papers in this section illustrate various aspects of this transformation.

Ilana Löwy looks at the work of the French physiologist Charles Richet, who developed a raw meat diet to treat tuberculosis patients, following successful experiments with dogs infected with the disease. However, the therapeutic use of raw meat – or more specifically the meat juice – in humans turned out to have some important limitations: it only seemed to work on patients with less severe forms of the disease and did not cure them. Löwy shows, however, that these limitations did not daunt the entrepreneur within Richet. On the contrary, he promoted his therapy as a means to improving military efficiency and as a cost-saving device for the state. It provided a way of getting sick soldiers back to the Front, and of helping sick workers get back to work. The military would retain an efficient fighting force; the state would avoid the expense of providing workers with an invalidity pension.

Löwy's account is also a story of the intersection of therapeutics and so-called food idiosyncrasies, allergic reactions to animal products. Löwy shows how Richet's belief in the therapeutic virtues of meat was linked to his interpretation of anaphylaxis (for which he received the Nobel Prize): Given that raw meat was extracted from living cells and was close in structure to the human body, it was for Richet the 'most easily assimilated aliment'. For Löwy, Richet's raw meat extract can be classed as neither a food nor a drug. Instead, she argues, it constituted a historical *sui generis* entity, albeit one whose status was constantly changing. Inspired by the rise of the chemical and pharmaceutical industry in Germany, Richet went on to develop a standardized commercial, industrially produced preparation based on the original treatment – a lyophilized extract in the form of a powder. What had once been a meat product had been transformed into a pharmaceutical product, however one that was not a success, in part because it was expensive.

Cost issues are also important to Susan Lederer's story about the work during the 1920s of the Boston physicians George R. Minot and William P. Murphy. Following a series of experiments on dogs, the two men developed a successful liver treatment for pernicious anaemia. Patients fed with large amounts of raw liver experienced rapid improvement; their life expectancy would have been much less before the treatment, perhaps seven years at most. Like Richet, the two doctors promoted their therapy as cost-effective – though for patients and their families rather than the state – since patients were able to return to work after treatment. At first the treatment itself was inexpensive because organ meats such as liver were generally cheap and abundantly available. But part of the reason for the low cost of liver was a problem for the therapy, that is that most Americans regarded organ meats as distasteful. So while Minot and Murphy had little problem in obtaining supplies of liver for their patients, patients found the meat unappetizing, if not repulsive, especially as they had to eat vast quantities of the offal for the therapy to work. Thus, the issue of palatability came to be central to the success of the treatment. Physicians found themselves working hard to make the meat acceptable to patients, even experimenting with new recipes, such as liver ice cream, to tempt their sick charges to swallow more. Ironically, the success of liver therapy was followed by an increase in liver prices. The combining of growing costliness and palatability forced Minot and Murphy to look for alternative means of administration in a more concentrated form, such as extracts and injections. But it provided a boon to the meat industry, which found a new market for a part of the animal that was hitherto among the cheaper cuts.

Naomi Pfeffer looks at a different relationship between the meat and therapeutics. Her focus is the work of the Berkeley professor of anatomy Herbert McLean Evans, who did experimental work with the pituitary gland, a small gland at the base of the brain which produces hormones that affect many functions of the body, including growth. Evans succeeded in producing rats of unusual size by injecting them daily with a soup of beef cattle pituitary glands, and Pfeffer traces the supply line back to explore where Evans got his glands, and what it tells us about the relations between the meat industry and the experimental endocrinology. Pfeffer shows that, given the small size of the pituitary gland and the difficulty of accessing it, the extraction of the gland from cows was economically feasible only where vast numbers of animals were killed in enormous, highly centralized meat-processing centres. For this reason, studies such as Evans's that required large numbers of pituitary glands happened in America, rather than (for example) England which, as we have seen above, had a more decentralized system of meat production. Glands and hormones provided a welcome opportunity for the meat industry to turn a former waste product into a profitable drug, thereby transforming the industry itself into a supplier of raw materials for drug production. For medical researchers, the American meat market offered exciting new possibilities for studying hormones, and contributed to the emerging field of endocrinology. However, access to large amounts of glands was never easy or cheap, and required excellent negotiating skills on the researcher's side.

Pfeffer's story is less about turning a food into a drug than about the food industry turning into a supplier of raw materials for the drug industry. The large-scale industrialization of meat opened the possibility of obtaining hormones in substantial quantities, which could subsequently be studied in long-term experimental or clinical studies. Virtually every scientist working in endocrinology during the interwar years was dependent on abattoirs for research material. Endocrinology therefore emerged to a large extent as an American science, and the commercialization of endocrine products was eagerly pursued by a meat industry that was able to deliver the raw material using large-scale industrialized and standardized procedures. Like Lederer, Pfeffer shows how economic market forces transformed meat production into a search for optimizing the marketability of the animal corpse, and how the production of potentially powerful drugs based on animal byproducts opened new areas of profitability. The growing involvement of meat producers in the pharmaceutical trade also fitted nicely into the industry's promotion of meat as good for health. In the end, unfortunately for Evans and the meat industry, his attempts to apply his findings on rats to human beings was not successful.

Part II of this volume explores the complex political and cultural intersections of meat and human health and disease, and how they played out in a variety
of different sites – the workplace, the disease campaign, the advice book and the
local community – and in different geographical and political contexts. In part,
it is a story of how a variety of twentieth-century developments – the relocation of North American meat production away from urban environments, the
introduction of American-produced meat to other countries and cultures, the
twentieth-century phenomenon of the cancer campaign, the development of
dietary advice in the twentieth century, and the rise of Nazism – transformed
the relations between meat and human health in a variety of different ways.

In the first essay in this section, Donald Stull and Michael Broadway explore
the impact of industrialized meat production on contemporary communities
situated in small American and Canadian towns. Where historically North
American meat processing was based in large conurbations such as Chicago, in
recent years processing has shifted closer to the farms and feedlots where the
livestock are raised. The result has been the sudden arrival in small, remote towns
of large processing plants, and an influx of large numbers of unskilled, often Hispanic, workers and their families into these communities. As Stull and Broadway
show, this influx has strained and on occasion overwhelmed social and health
services, and sometimes led to problems with the original inhabitants of these
rural areas. In short, their point is that a focus on the working conditions in the
factories alone does not do justice to the broader impacts of meat production
on human health. Theirs is a story of the complex intersection of the politics of
health, meat and immigration.

Where Stull and Broadway focus on the health implications of meat production for local communities, Jeffrey Pilcher's paper shows how the introduction
of American-style meat production into Mexico was shaped in part by local con-
ceptions of what constituted healthy meat: anxieties about the healthiness of
refrigerated meat tipped the balance against the introduction of industrialized
meat production into Mexico, at least for a while. Pilcher's story is thus, in part,
a tale of the intersection of cultural perceptions of taste and healthfulness. For
him the marketing of refrigerated American meat in Mexico was mediated by
Mexican preferences for fresh meat, by local politics and by the economic and
financial status of slaughterhouses in the early twentieth century. Mexican anxieties about the healthiness of refrigerated meat undermined the consumption of
American meat and efforts to introduce new methods of meat processing and
distribution.

David Cantor's paper shifts the focus to the emergence of the twentieth-century American campaigns against cancer. He shows how scientific and medical
evidence suggesting that meat consumption caused cancer threatened campaigns
to promote programmes of cancer control based on early detection and treat-

ment, and so were sidelined by the American Society for the Control of Cancer (ASCC) in the 1920s and 30s. For the ASCC, scientific evidence that meat caused cancer was not only often quite unpersuasive, it was also uncomfortably close to the claims made by those they labelled 'quacks' that reducing meat consumption would help prevent cancer. The risk was that people who reduced their consumption of meat so as to prevent cancer would be lulled into complacency about the disease, drawn into the arms of quacks and other alternative healers, or tempted to ignore the early warning signs of the disease. The result, the ASCC claimed, could be deadly to patients who would wait too long to seek qualified medical attention, and could also be deadly to the Society's efforts to develop programmes of early detection and treatment. Yet the organization often felt overwhelmed by the vast public interest in the role of meat as a cause of cancer, threatened by the confusion of medical and scientific messages about the subject, and frustrated by its inability to present a consistent message. In the end, it opted for a policy of undermining public faith in the relationship between diet and cancer by raising questions about the scientific validity of causal connection. This was in contrast to its policy towards public belief in the hereditary nature of cancer. To the ASCC/ACS such beliefs were as threatening to its programme of early detection and treatment as public beliefs in a dietary cause of cancer. But whereas it tended to attack public beliefs about diet by raising questions, it tended to attack public beliefs about heredity by outright rejection of them. Thus, this paper highlights a range of attempts by the ASCC to manage popular beliefs about cancer that threatened their policy of cancer control. At one end of the spectrum was blunt rejection of popular beliefs; at the other end was a policy of raising doubts through questions.

Rima Apple's paper shows what happened when scientific ideas about the relation of meat to human health got into the public sphere. Apple argues that during the early decades of the twentieth century there was a veritable explosion of nutrition research in the United States. These scientists looked beyond their laboratories to bring the new knowledge of nutrition into the home, to inform women how best to feed their families. Women's magazines and newspapers of the period eagerly published the latest breakthroughs for the benefit of their readers. Nutritionists travelled around the country offering lectures to interested audiences and created textbooks for home economics classes in state-run schools. In addition, food companies, both manufacturers and distributors, employed contemporary discoveries in their promotions to persuade home-makers to purchase their products. Their advertisements filled a significant portion of the periodical literature.

Apple's chapter examines the nutrition information about meat disseminated through American magazines, newspapers and home-economics instruction. Her story is part a story of anxieties about meat consumption, and she traces concerns that Americans ate too much, poorly prepared or the wrong sorts of meat. She also traces calls for people to reduce their consumption, advice on safe food preparation, and recommendations as to what sorts of meats were healthy and what sorts were not. Yet, despite anxieties about meat, Apple notes that meat remained a centrepiece of the American dinner table, nutritional scientists urged people to eat meat for their physical and mental health, and meat producers hyped the advantages of meat in the diet. The drive to educate Americans, primarily female consumers, about the place of meat in a healthful diet often portrayed the food as a means of producing healthy and economically productive (often male) bodies, a good thing for the country in two ways – it produced economically productive citizens, and it produced an economically successful meat industry. Despite the fact that in the second half of the twentieth century these arguments were challenged by growing questioning of the healthiness of consuming large quantities of meat, by the emergence of a revitalized vegetarian movement, by growing concerns about the ecological harm created by the meat industry and by national and economic crises, meat was not dislodged from its central place in the American diet. On the contrary, the search for meat substitutes during periods of crisis, Apple argues, confirms the continued centrality of meat to American culinary culture.

Finally, Ulrike Thoms shows what happened to vegetarian critiques of meat in the 1930s and 40s under the National Socialist regime in Germany. She argues that vegetarianism had its roots in earlier Life Reform moments, and Life Reformers and vegetarians generally welcomed Hitler's rise to power – he was, after all, a vegetarian himself. Yet, Thoms argues, once in power National Socialists had a very ambiguous relationship with vegetarians and Life Reformers: they selected those elements of their philosophies that suited their agendas, and that fitted with nutritional policies focused on National Socialist goals of human performance and economic autarchy. What this meant in effect was that vegetarian policies tended to lose out whenever there was a conflict with National Socialist goals of improving human performance and economic autarchy. In practice, the regime was ideologically inconsistent, adopting elements of vegetarian and Life Reform philosophies in piecemeal fashion wherever it supported or did not challenge its broader goals, and rejecting vegetarianism and Life Reform whenever they posed a problem.

Part III of this volume explores the ideas of 'risk' and 'regulation' in relation to meat and human health. Hitherto, most historical attention has focused on the role of the state in the development of efforts to regulate meat production and consumption, generally to counteract the worst effects of the transformations in meat production and consumption described earlier in this introduction. As such, it is also a story of how in the nineteenth and early twentieth centuries regulation was part of a broader effort by the state to improve industrial, military and national efficiency, and to promote and protect the national and international trade in meat and meat products. As we've already noted, responses to scandals and scares such as Upton Sinclair's 1906 revelations about Chicago meatpackers were probably more about their costs to the meat industry than about the conditions under which workers worked and animals died.

As the recent crises over Bovine Spongiform Encephalopathy (BSE) illustrate, critics continue to argue that late twentieth-century state policy is primarily about protecting the meat industry. But efforts to protect the meat industry were joined by another concern. As the state became increasingly involved in the provision of health and welfare services, costs to these services – for example from caring for people with Creutzfeldt–Jakob disease (CJD) or with any of the other conditions associated with the consumption of too much or the wrong sorts of meat (obesity, stomach cancer or colon cancer, for example) – came to be a further factor in state interest in meat production and consumption. Even in countries where the taxpayer is not automatically expected to pick up the bill for healthcare, the state has taken a role in helping to control the costs of such conditions to the health industry and to welfare services. On the one hand, the state having done this reflected a concern that the problems associated with meat eating often unduly affected the poor and disadvantaged who ate cheaper, less nutritious and overly fatty cuts of meat or meat products; people who were most likely to end up as a cost to the local or national taxpayers or to charitable services. On the other hand, this also reflected the growing attempts by health advocacy groups, the health insurance industry, hospitals, physicians, charities, environmental groups and public health officials (and perhaps less influential groups such as animal rights groups or vegetarians) to lobby for state support for efforts to reduce meat consumption or to protect the public from diseased meat. As such the story of twentieth-century state regulation is of a growing tension between regulatory efforts designed to promote and protect the meat industry, and regulatory efforts designed to protect the public health. The state often seems divided in its loyalties between the people and industry.

These tensions are highlighted by the regulatory regime in the United States, which is run through US Department of Agriculture (USDA, founded in 1862): the Food and Drug Administration (FDA) regulates the majority of foods, but it does not regulate most meat and poultry products. The point is illustrated by the Hallmark/Westland recall described at the start of this chapter which, to critics of the USDA, demonstrated the divided loyalties of the Federal regulatory agency. How, they asked, can a government department that aims to promote and protect the agricultural industry also protect the public's health? Is it more susceptible to industrial or to consumer influences? Indeed, in this controversy the categories of 'industry' and 'consumer' become problematic. Could a Department that aimed to protect the farming and meat industry also serve to protect the health industry from the consequences of eating tainted meat? And how could a Department that failed to protect consumers of meat hope to protect consumers of healthcare who might be affected by tainted meat? As Keir Waddington's paper suggests, similar tensions can be described in other countries.

Keir Waddington's paper explores British government responses to bovine tuberculosis and BSE, and their relations to the ways in which the risks to humans from animal diseases have been understood. Waddington argues that bovine tuberculosis and later BSE were both framed initially as animal health issues, and that officials interpreted preliminary scientific evidence as indicating that consumption of diseased meat had negligible risks for human health. The consequence, he claims, was that government responses in both cases initially focused mainly on efforts to halt the spread of the disease in cattle – stamping out the disease by killing or isolating infected animals or animals deemed at risk of infection, and compensating farmers for their economic loss.

Much as in the case of American responses to the 1906 revelations about Chicago meatpackers, British responses to BSE were probably more about their costs to the meat and farming industry than about the health of consumers. But, at least in the case of BSE, these responses seem to have backfired. As the possibility that animal-to-human transmission of the causative agent of BSE came to gain scientific credibility, the government's initial policy of focusing on efforts to halt the spread of the disease in cattle came into question. The policy increasingly threatened the British beef industry with the loss of consumer confidence and of international exports. It also raised questions about the adequacy of government scientific advice, and generated criticism of the power of Ministers and the farming lobby to quash scientific evidence that suggested a link between BSE and CJD. In this case, the situation was further complicated by the discovery of a novel agent of disease transmission – the prion. Scientific uncertainty about the nature of this entity, and what it meant for animal to human transmission, fed into an already fraught political and commercial environment, and confused efforts to develop policies designed to combat the possibilities of animal to human transmission. Waddington also highlights the changing role of the media in the last 100 years. Whereas, he argues, the media played a relatively minor role in the case of bovine tuberculosis, in the case of BSE the media served to transform the internal policy debates. Politicians, government officials and the meat industry found themselves constantly wrong-footed by public reports on the outbreak, and forced to respond to revelations that raised serious questions about policy decisions.

The second and final contribution to this section, Jean-Paul Gaudillière's study of the DES scandal, broadens the focus of regulation away from the state. According to Gaudillière, there were historically at least four different 'ways of regulating' in the twentieth century. These 'ways' were all individually motivated by different imperatives, employed different forms of science, and used different strategies of enforcement. The four ways were 1) professional regulation (driven by the interests and agendas of professional and scientific organizations), 2) administrative regulation (driven by the interests and agendas of government and other state agencies), 3) industrial regulation (driven by the interests of commercial firms) and 4) consumer regulation (driven by consumers' interests, or at least those who purport to represent them).

While most historical attention has focused on the role of the state in regulating meat and other products, Gaudillière's point is that the state has not been the only institutional player involved in regulation, or even always the main one. Professional organizations and industrial organizations have also argued that they have important roles in regulation: the former arguing that professional norms should be the motor behind regulation, the latter arguing that the market should be the primary regulator, and the state has sometimes been willing to farm out regulation to these different groups. More recently, as Gaudillière shows in the 'meat and DES affair' consumer and advocacy groups have increasingly sought to intervene in regulation, mistrustful of what they see as the paternalism of professional regulation, the self-interest of industrial regulation, and the divided loyalties of state regulation. Gaudillière's focus is on the tensions between all four ways of regulating, as their advocates jostle for power in changing political, economic, scientific and medical environments. This, in short, is a story of displacement rather than replacement, as the influence of particular ways of regulating have waxed and waned. His specific case also shows how the growing use of hormones in meat production transformed approaches to the public health risks of meat, from infectious to toxicological models, and at the same time reconfigured the animal health/human health relationship.

Gaudillière's point about the multiple ways of regulating brings us back to the main point of this volume – the diversity of public health messages about the healthiness or otherwise of meat. In their different ways, the essays in this volume seek to embed such diversity in broader cultural, social and economic interests and agendas, and to show how these interests and agendas reflect the many different perspectives of the various players involved in debates about the health consequences of consuming meat and meat products. If Gaudillière highlights diverse ways of regulating the health consequences of meat consumption, others highlight the diversity of sciences brought to the problem of the consequences for human health of meat consumption, their impact on the workplace, the hospital, or the dinner table, and of the complex ranges of groups and interests involved in this. This diversity is the meat of our book.

Acknowledgements

This introduction has benefited from the ideas and suggestions of many people, including the anonymous referee of this volume, and the commentators at the workshop, 'Meat, Medicine, and Human Health in the Twentieth Century' held at the National Institutes of Health, Bethesda, Maryland, 14–15 November 2006, especially Rima D. Apple, Toine Pieters, and Volker Hess. Matthias Dörries was involved in the early planning for this introduction, and provided helpful editorial comment. Finally, we thank Janelle Winters for her research assistance as a 2008 Summer Intern in the Office of History at the National Institutes of Health.

1 ZOMINE: A TALE OF RAW MEAT, TUBERCULOSIS, INDUSTRY AND WAR IN EARLY TWENTIETH CENTURY FRANCE

Ilana Löwy

In 1900 the French physiologist Charles Richet published a short paper which reported that a raw meat diet could cure tuberculosis.[1] The paper originated in a semi-accidental observation: a rapid improvement in the health of tuberculosis-infected dogs, fed with a large quantity of uncooked meat. Since the 1890s, Richet and his colleague, Jules Héricourt had tried to cure tuberculosis with a wide range of antiseptics and other substances. These experiments, conducted in a rather chaotic way, did not produce results, until Richet and Héricourt's tuberculosis-infected dogs recovered. This was the starting point for Richet's attempts to develop a raw-meat-based treatment against tuberculosis and related pathological conditions.[2]

In developing his 'meat therapy', Richet followed the steps of an earlier famous scientist, the German chemist and physiologist, Justus von Liebig (1803–73), one of the pioneers of modern theories of nutrition. In 1840, Liebig had developed a beef extract marketed under his name, building on a longer tradition which viewed meat as a major strength-providing substance, able to restore health. At least since the work of the French inventor, Denis Papin in the 1680s, physicians had proposed using meat extracts to increase the health of the working classes. Liebig added his scientific authority to this view, and his meat extract came to be considered a borderline product, part food and part drug. What Liebig proposed was that it should be given to soldiers to improve their resilience and fighting capacity, and to sick people to help their recovery. From 1865 onwards, the extract was produced on a large scale by the Liebig Extract Meat Company (Lemco). The enterprise was London-based, but the meat extract itself was manufactured in South America (mainly in the company's Fray Bentos plant in Uruguay). In the late nineteenth century the company diversified its products adding a preparation of tinned corned beef, a cheaper version of Liebig extract named Oxo, and Oxo bouillon cubes – all substances used for cooking, but also to 'restore forces' to people weakened by illness or hardship.[3]

In some ways, Richet's story seems to mirror that of Liebig. Like Liebig's tale, Richet's endeavour was in part a story of the intersection of science and commerce; how science was used to rationalize the medical uses of a meat product, and to promote its commercial exploitation (albeit without the success that Liebig enjoyed.) As with Liebig, Richet established his product at the intersection of meat and the military: the former promising to restore sick servicemen to the front; the latter providing a controlled population on which Richet could experiment. And, like Liebig, Richet situated his meat commodity at the blurry boundary between foods and drugs: Richet strongly argued that his preparation was neither a mere foodstuff, nor was it purely a drug – rather it was something that occupied a space somewhere between the two. Yet Richet's story differs from that of Liebig in one significant point. As the paper will highlight, Richet not only considered that his 'raw meat juice' was something distinct from meat the food, but he also devoted considerable energy to distinguishing it from meat the restorative, including restoratives such as Liebig's extract and Oxo. To understand why it was distinct, I suggest, we have to explore how it was embedded in a web of meaning that derived from Richet's particular understanding of how his raw meat preparation worked in the body.

Charles Richet's Raw Meat Therapy

Richet's interest in a topic that linked food, physiology, healing and commerce is not surprising. Charles Richet (1850–1935) was a true polymath. Trained as physician and physiologist, he combined scientific activities with numerous cultural and political interests. Early in his medical career Richet became interested in phenomena at the boundary of physiology and psychology and he wrote his doctoral thesis on somnambulism. Working as a young researcher at the College de France, he collaborated with Jules Etienne Marey (1830–1904) and was influenced by Marey's experimental approach. Thanks partly to his family connections (he was the son of a famous surgeon, Alfred Richet), Charles Richet had rapidly climbed the academic career ladder, and at the age of thirty-seven he was appointed to the chair of physiology at the Paris Medical School. In following years he became a member of the French Academy of Medicine and of the Academy of Sciences, president of the Society for Biology, and eventually Nobel Prize Laureate (he received the 1913 Prize in Medicine and Physiology for his studies of anaphylaxis). Richet was furthermore interested in socialism, pacifism and eugenics, promoted the development of aviation, and had a long-time interest in psychic phenomena and the paranormal. In his youth he pursued a literary career, writing numerous novels and plays. Abandoning his playwright activities in the 1890s, he nevertheless continued to write essays, popular scientific works and popular historical studies.[4]

Through one of his teachers, the physiologist Alfred Vulpian (1826–87), Richet became close to the founding group of the Pasteur Institute, and developed a lifelong interest in bacteriology and immunology. In late 1880s, he attempted to cure infectious diseases through transfusion of blood from immunized animals, an approach he named 'hemotherapy'. Richet claimed that such transfusions protected sheep from anthrax and rabbits from sepsis through the transfer of 'immune blood'. He tried then to apply this method to the cure of tuberculosis. His failed attempts to treat tuberculosis shortly preceded Behring's and Kitasato's successful serotherapy of diphtheria. While Richet – regretfully – acknowledged that, unlike Behring, he failed to grasp the general principle of the therapeutic use of immune sera, he viewed his 'hemotherapy' studies as his most important contribution to medical science. Until the end of his life he continued to claim priority for the discovery of the principals of serotherapy.[5]

An enthusiastic supporter of the 'Pasteurian revolution' in medicine, Richet never became a true follower of the Pasteurian method, and remained faithful to a more physiological way of thinking.[6] Trained in the tradition of French physiology shaped by Claude Bernard, Richet combined an organicist point of view, focused on the understanding of the living organism as a whole, with a reductionist aspiration to uncover physical and chemical mechanisms that govern the basic phenomena of living entities. He was a dedicated experimentalist, an attitude that was not shared by the majority of his colleagues at the Medical Faculty in Paris.

Richet and Héricourt first observed a quasi-miraculous cure of a single tuberculosis-infected dog fed on an exclusive diet of raw meat in 1897. Richet explained later that the decision to feed dogs with great quantity of raw meat was inspired by the observation that tuberculosis is rare in people who suffer from gout. A diet rich in raw meat increased the concentration of uric acid in the blood and may, Richet speculated, hamper the growth of Koch's bacillus.[7] They confirmed this result on a few other dogs, and then rapidly started experiments on humans. In the mid-1880s Richet complained that he could not keep more than six or seven dogs at the tiny laboratory allocated to him at the Medical Faculty's building. He decided therefore to rent, at his own expense, facilities in Jointville le Pont, near Paris, where he was able to keep over forty dogs at a time. This increase in laboratory space opened new possibilities for his studies on treatments for tuberculosis, including by changing the dog's diet.[8]

The results obtained with TB patients fed raw meat extract were less spectacular than those seen in dogs. Nevertheless, Richet and Héricourt claimed that their method was efficient. The 'zomotherapy', as they had called the new approach (from 'zomos', meat broth in Greek) improved the health of patients with less severe forms of tuberculosis, although, alas, it did not help those with a more advanced disease.[9] Richet and Héricourt described zomotherapy as a 'specific treatment' referring to specificity as an essential characteristic of a drug. Even if their notion of specificity remained vague in relation to their meat extracts, this qualification was intended to move their status from food to drug. Scientific explanations mentioned by Héricourt included the possibility that the meat juice neutralized bacterial toxins, favoured phagocytosis or, alternatively, was a 'specific tonic for the nervous system' strengthening the organism's defence mechanisms indirectly, by stimulating the nerves.[10] Richet proposed that substances present in meat juice fought infection either directly, through the neutralization of microbial secretions, or indirectly, through the induction of a 'post alimentary leucosis' leading to an improvement of ingestion of bacteria by white blood cells.[11]

If Richet and Héricourt were not sure how exactly the ingestion of raw meat juice helped to fight an infection with Koch's bacillus; they were persuaded that zomotherapy was a specific therapy which differed from general food products. In later years Richet acknowledged that zomotherapy was less specific in humans than in dogs and attributed this difference to the fact that dogs suffered nearly always from a 'closed' tuberculosis (the pulmonary lesions were delimited by a granuloma and thus circumscribed) while human tuberculosis was usually characterized by 'open' lesions (lesions without encapsulation from which tubercle bacilli were discharged out of the body). Nevertheless, he claimed that in patients with a 'closed' tuberculosis, zomotherapy was almost specific.[12] However, Richet's claim did not settle the issue as other researchers in Richet's laboratory, Albert Josias and Jean Charles Roux, questioned the treatment's specificity. Following an attempt to cure tuberculous children with raw meat juice, Josias and Roux found that some of their young patients regained strength, but, rather than attribute these observed changes to the specificity of the treatment, they attributed them to a general improvement in the child's nutritional status.[13] Around 1902, Richet codified the regimen and dosing of zomotherapy, setting the daily ration of extract as at least one kilogram of crude meat and, in more severe cases, up to two kilos.[14] Patients were expected to drink extract preparations equalling between 500 and 800ml of meat juice several times a day. Aware of the difficulty of making patients drink a large quantity of fresh meat juice, Richet proposed to aromatize it with bouillon or to mix it with a thick soup.[15]

In 1901 Richet gave a talk on therapeutic virtues of zomotherapy at the annual meeting of the association of Friends of the Sorbonne, and brought a cured dog with him to strengthen his argument. A member of the Municipal Council of Paris, Ambroise Rendu, present at that talk, was strongly impressed by Richet's claim that he had developed an efficient cure of tuberculosis. With Rendu's assistance, Richet was appointed in 1905 as the president of the administrative council of the Jouve-Rouves-Taniers dispensary for the treatment of tuberculosis. This dispensary had been founded in a working-class neighbourhood of Paris supported by a joint gift of 150,000 francs of Mrs Jouve-Rouves and Mrs. Taniers.[16] Richet transformed the dispensary into a major site of experimentation with zomotherapy. The patients treated at Jouve-Rouves-Taniers received daily a fresh meat extract, but also a nutritive ration of approximately 1,500 calories. The treatment lasted usually three months, and was supervised by Jules Héricourt.[17] Concluding results obtained during the first year of functioning at the dispensary, Richet claimed, showed that zomotherapy 'cured' about half of the 200 treated patients. He added, however, that the treatment did not eliminate the infection with Koch's bacillus. Zomotherapy's main effect was the restoration of the patients' strength and their work capacity. Richet conceded that it was probably more accurate under these circumstances to consider therapeutic results as an 'economic cure' rather than a medical one. This was nevertheless an important achievement, stated Richet, since instead of workers 'being a burden to their families, they are able to support them. Perhaps one should define this capacity as a true cure?'[18]

The restoration of the patient's ability to earn his living, Richet argued, was cost-effective for society as a whole. Although the price of zomine treatment was quite considerable, approximately 400 francs per patient, he declared it was nevertheless decidedly less onerous than an invalidity pension for a sick worker and his family. The dispensary, he added, fulfilled in parallel an important educative task: patients learned that tuberculosis was an infectious disease and were taught how to protect others, and to take care of themselves. Richet was proud of the results of zomotherapy at the Jouve-Rouves-Taniers dispensary but he also acknowledged that the development of tuberculosis in dispensary patients depended on both their general economic and nutritional condition. In the absence of untreated control groups it was difficult to distinguish between the therapeutic virtues of meat juice, and the effects of more general elements of treatment such as rest and adequate nutrition.[19]

This difficulty in identifying the therapeutic virtues of meat may account for the absence of scientific publications on zomotherapy at the Jouve-Rouves-Taniers dispensary. Another problem might have been economic. Zomine preparation and treatment were expensive and the dispensary lacked funds to maintain a treatment with high doses of raw meat juice for a great number of individuals over a long time. In the following years, Jules Héricourt, who replaced Richet as the head of the Jouve-Rouves-Taniers dispensary, treated tuberculous patients with only 125 grams of uncooked meat per day, in spite of the fact that Richet recommended a dose nearly ten times higher. Richet claimed that even this low dose had beneficent effects.[20] However, this claim contradicted his argument that other doctors failed to demonstrate therapeutic virtues of zomotherapy because their patients did not receive adequate quantities of raw meat juice.[21] Despite Richet's personal convictions and his scientific arguments zomotherapy remained controversial before World War II.

From a Homemade Remedy to a Commercial Preparation: Zomine

While Richet was persuaded that zomotherapy was an efficient treatment of tuberculosis, he realized that its diffusion was seriously hampered by the practical difficulty of manually extracting meat juice with a domestic press. The preparation of extract of two kilograms of meat could take up to five hours of intensive labour.22 Another problem was the fragility of the preparation. In order to be efficient, raw meat juice had to be prepared daily, using very fresh meat kept on ice during the whole extraction process. Even a short delay between the death of an animal and the extraction of meat juice, Richet explained, reduced the therapeutic virtues of raw meat. He argued that meat underwent chemical alterations following death, which could be slowed down through chilling, though not entirely eliminated:

> If one wishes to apply rigorously the principle of zomotherapy and to use live muscle tissue as an aliment, the patient should be fed the flesh of an animal killed only few minutes earlier. I tried this method once, with great success. I ordered a preparation of minced meat from freshly killed large chicken. The meat, still warm, was eaten immediately. By consequence, it reached the stomach before the development of post-mortem alterations.[23]

The obvious solution was to develop industrial methods of preparing a stable form of meat juice that could be put on the market. Faithful to the Pasteurian spirit which he energetically promoted, Richet was interested in industrial applications of medical inventions. In a poem written in 1913 to celebrate the centenary of Louis Pasteur's birth, Richet glorified the Pasteur Institute as a true 'temple of science'.[24] As Harry Paul has noted, this temple had a double identity: 'it was clear from the beginning that the institute with its laboratories and department for medical biology and rabies, and vaccine production and sales, was to be an empire of medical science and commerce. Apollo and Hermes in tandem: the double-edged alliance pushing medical research and care – no wonder their staffs are often confused in medical iconology'.[25] Richet, like other Pasteurians, viewed this alliance of health and industry as self-evident. He noted in his memoirs that Behring not only had the good luck to find the 'general principle' of serotherapy, but was also able to promptly commercialize his invention 'by the admirable factories of the chemical industry in Germany'.[26] He hoped to be able to repeat this feat with his meat extract.

The first step towards a commercialization of meat extract was its stabilization. This step was achieved by the chemists Grigaut and Guilbaud who developed a method to lyophilize raw meat juice. The lyophilized preparation, named 'zomine', could be stored for several months in a dry place.[27] It could therefore be produced industrially and sold in a pharmacy. Richet recommended the uptake of forty to sixty grams of zomine powder per day, a quantity that was equivalent to the consumption of 400 to 600ml of meat juice and one-and-a-half to two kilos of raw meat. The lyophilized extract, a red-brownish powder, was rich in salt, soluble in water, and smelled and tasted like roasted meat and blood. Some people, Richet reported, were able to eat powdered zomine, but the majority elected to mix it with other aliments. Richet experimented with zomine recipes himself. One of the best, he had found, was to dissolve the lyophilized meat juice in a vegetable broth, concentrated and well spiced but unsalted. The majority of the patients tolerated this preparation well. Zomine could also be mixed with a thick soup, mashed potatoes or other mashed vegetables and in a fruit pudding. The latter method helped to persuade children to accept zomotherapy.[28]

In 1913, Richet started negotiations with the representatives of the Antwerp branch of Lemco, the Liebig Extract Meat Company. The inclusion of zomine among items produced by Lemco was a logical extension of their already important activity which involved transforming South American-produced meat into industrial products sold in Europe. The plan was to open a Lemco-sponsored zomine production plant in Argentina which would be directed by Richet's son, Albert Richet. An agreement to open such a plant was signed in Antwerp in July 1914. Richet was interested in collaboration with Lemco, but he repeatedly stressed that his product was very different from Liebig's meat extract. While the latter was merely a nutritive supplement, zomine, he claimed, was a true medication that modulated physiological mechanisms.[29]

Zomotherapy During World War I

The summer of 1914 was not a good time to start an international commercial venture: The plan to produce zomine in Argentina ended with the outbreak of World War I. Richet found a new commercial partner, an industrialist from the French city of LeHavre, Charles Latham.[30] The war opened new possibilities for testing zomine's therapeutic properties. A personal friend of the French Minister of Health, Justin Godart, Richet obtained from the latter permission to test the commercial preparation of zomine produced by Latham at the military hospital of Côte Saint André (Val d'Isère). Richet and his young collaborators, Paul Brodin and François de Saint Girons, treated more than two hundred soldiers at the hospital diagnosed with tuberculosis, in fact experimenting on a large, though unstable population. The soldiers usually stayed a few weeks in the hospital, then were either declared unfit for service, or sent to the Front. It was impossible therefore to observe long term effects of raw meat juice. Worse, the treated soldiers did not wish to get well. Those with a relatively mild disease generally wanted to be permanently exempt from military service, and the prospect of being fed twice daily with – despite Richet's attempts to make zomine more palatable – a foul-tasting preparation in order to get better and be sent back to trenches, was not a very alluring one. Those with more advanced illness generally wanted to be cured, but, alas, zomine was effective only in relatively mild cases. Richet experimented on soldiers who agreed to undergo a cure (or perhaps were afraid to refuse it), but he was obliged to put forward a complex system of supervision to ensure that the soldiers did not cheat and ingested the prescribed dose of zomine (usually, in a soup). In addition, the treated soldiers needed to be supervised to prevent drinking (a contra-indication for zomine therapy, according to Richet): a problem exacerbated by the fact that the hospital was surrounded with taverns and bars, and consumption of alcoholic beverages, while strictly forbidden, was an 'irresistible temptation'. Richet and his colleagues stopped the treatment of soldiers found drunk or caught in a tavern, but they were aware that, in all probability, many of their patients devised ways to drink without being caught.[31]

Despite the problem of unruly patients, Côte de Saint André provided Richet with access to a captive population for the first time. There, he and his collaborators were able to conduct detailed studies of changes induced by the ingestion of zomine. The treated soldiers were weighed every day with a precision balance, underwent regular urine and blood tests, and their muscular strength was tested with a dynamometer and ergograph. These tests indicated that soldiers who received zomine gained weight, especially during the first three weeks of treatment, their muscular strength increased, and chemical analyses (secretion of urea, fixation of nitrogen) indicated that in all probability the uptake of zomine favoured an increase in muscular mass.[32] However, it was difficult to show that these positive changes resulted in improvements in patients' health. Richet noted in his diary:

> we tried many approaches, but after some time, the results became uncertain. This became rather monotonous. A rapid and intensive increase in weight, then a stationary state, and finally, in some cases an improvement, and in other a degradation of health. Moreover, it was difficult to make accurate observations, because the soldiers were anxious to be declared unfit for service, and did not want to get better. Finally, Paul Brodin and François de Saint Girons had the simple and bright idea to leave la Côte de Saint André, because there was not much we could do there.[33]

Following these problems, Richet had the new idea of using zomine to treat soldiers that suffered from a shock produced by a massive loss of blood. Thanks to Godard's mediation, Richet was appointed head of a special medical mission to study the treatment of traumatic shock. Richet, Brodin, and Saint Girons at first attempted to experiment with zomine at the teaching centre for military doctors at La Bouleuse directed by his colleague Claudius Regaud from Lyon.[34] Later, dissatisfied with the conditions at La Bouleuse, they moved to the military hospital of Vaux Varennes, where they tried zomine treatment on wounded soldiers. They had found, however, that soldiers who suffered a significant loss of blood were unable to digest the preparation, even when it was mixed with champagne. Richet also noted in his diary that his colleagues at the Vaux Varennes hospital did not believe in the curative virtues of raw meat juice. He decided therefore to abandon the zomine study and to investigate instead the possibility of treating shock by transfusion of horse plasma to wounded soldiers.[35]

In 1924, when Richet published the details of his studies conducted at the Côte Saint André Hospital in his book *La Nouvelle Zomothérapie*, he proposed a more positive view of this episode than the one he had earlier given in his diary. He admitted that the conditions for testing zomine at Côte Saint André were far from ideal: the patients were not always cooperative, and it was not possible to record the long-term effects of zomotherapy because the majority of the treated soldiers were declared unfit for service and lost from sight. Nevertheless, Richet believed that the studies conducted at Côte Saint André Hospital provided a scientific proof of the efficacy of zomine in the treatment of tuberculosis. Gain of weight and of muscular strength he now argued, contradicting his earlier comments, were always correlated with a general improvement of the patient's health. In tuberculosis, a chronic disease with an uncertain trajectory, he claimed that such objective and quantifiable measures often provided more reliable information on the patient's health status than clinical signs. Gain of weight, if evaluated frequently and with great precision, was an especially reliable indicator of positive evolution of the patient's disease.[36]

In 1917, Richet's son, Charles Richet Jr, conducted experiments on a small group of Russian soldiers with tuberculosis treated in a hospital in Cannes. These soldiers were treated with zomine for three or four months. In Cannes, as in Côte Saint André, the main indicator of modifications induced by zomine was a change in weight measured as precisely as possible in standardized conditions. In addition, Charles Richet Jr. assessed the patients' arterial pressure, level of haemoglobin in the blood, quantity of tuberculosis bacteria in the sputum, nitrogen in urine, and muscular power, and attempted to correlate these data with a detailed clinical history. His main conclusion was similar to that of his father: zomine treatment led to an increase in weight and in muscular force of the treated soldiers and it seemed to be especially beneficial in those with a less advanced disease. Moreover, Richet Jr was able to collect data on long term outcomes in some of his patients. After the war he was able to trace fourteen of the Russian soldiers treated by zomine: seven of them were declared cured or in long term remission, three improved slightly, and four were not affected by zomotherapy. The patients who did improve were in early stages of tuberculosis.[37]

Richet Sr maintained his faith in efficacy of zomine during the war. In 1917, he outlined a plan for the large-scale testing of zomotherapy in tuberculosis patients, including the use of high doses.[38] He noted in his diary: 'I have a firm hope that after the war ... zomine will have a brilliant future. It will save the lives of thousands of people, and will bring us material prosperity, well justified by its beneficial effects.'[39] However, the death of his son Albert, a pilot killed by a 'friendly fire' shortly before the end of the war, dampened Richet's enthusiasm for the industrial production of lyophilized meat juice, as it dampened his enthusiasm for many other projects. In the 1920s zomine was produced on a relatively modest scale by a small Parisian firm, Laboratoire Longuet. Publicity leaflets for this product explained that zomine was 'a plasma prepared from raw meat, dried in a vacuum and at low temperature,' and stressed the spectacular effects of zomine in dogs infected with tuberculosis. The leaflet reproduced pictures of cured dogs, but also graphs that showed rapid increases in weight and muscular force of tuberculous soldiers treated by zomine at the Côte de Saint André hospital. It was illustrated with images of a modern production chain, reinforcing the impression of a science-based cure.[40] Richet did not provide information on the commercial success of this preparation. In an autobiographic notice at the end of the last volume of his memoirs, he hints, however, that it did not sell well. He affirmed again that zomine was an efficient treatment of tuberculosis, but added that, 'unfortunately, the price of this preparation was too high to allow a regular uptake of a sufficient quantity for several months'.[41]

La Nouvelle Zomothérapie (1924) updated Richet's views on therapeutic effects of raw meat juice. The book opened with a praise of uncooked food, the natural aliment par excellence. It then compared the effects of zomotherapy with those of vitamins and hormones.[42] Richet described zomotherapy as a 'muscular opotherapy' – using a term usually employed to describe treatment with glandular extracts, such as insulin, thyroid extract or ovarian extract.[43] Richet did not present zomine as a specific therapy of tuberculosis anymore. Instead, he presented it as a candidate 'proto-vitamin' endowed with a unique ability to reconstruct muscles and blood. The parallel with vitamins was probably intended to prevent the classification of zomine as a mere fortifying tonic, a variant of Liebig's meat extract or Oxo broth. Richet's discussion of the effects of raw meat extracts oscillated between several levels of explanation: physiological, bacteriological, evolutionary and social. His general conclusion – that zomine was an especially efficient 'repairing aliment' – relied on the polysemy of the term 'repairing': the fixation of a well-identified defect (as one repairs a broken machine) and a global process of restoration of physical or spiritual wellbeing.[44]

Zomine's Networks of Meaning

Richet the clinician wanted to devise a preparation which would 'save the lives of thousands of people.' Richet the physiologist wanted to unravel the biological mechanism which gave raw meat juice its unique therapeutic virtues. His view of anaphylaxis (remember that Richet received a Nobel prize for his studies of this phenomenon) sheds light on his understanding of therapeutic action of raw meat juice. Richet first observed a violent reaction to a second contact with a sensitizing substance when, together with Pierre Portier, they injected dogs with toxins of the Portuguese Man o'War jellyfish (*Physalia physalis*). They noticed then that some dogs injected for a second time with a small, non-lethal dose of toxin died rapidly, exhibiting respiratory symptoms, very different from those of intoxication by the studied substance. The reaction was highly specific. It was induced only by a second injection of an identical substance. It was also highly individualized – the same stimulus provoked very different reactions in different dogs.[45] Richet named this phenomenon 'anaphylaxis' to stress its proximity with 'phylaxis' – a protective immunization. Anaphylaxis, he proposed, was a mirror-image immunity: second contact with a substance led to a specific harm, not a specific protection.

Other researchers had shown that anaphylactic reactions were not related to toxicity of sensitizing substances. They could be induced by any foreign protein. 'Serum sickness' and 'serum shock' – pathological manifestations induced by a second injection of therapeutic serum – was redefined as an anaphylaxis produced through sensitization by blood proteins.[46] In parallel, Richet linked anaphylaxis with a more familiar phenomenon: 'food idiosyncrasy' (today, food allergy): Some persons reacted violently to strawberries, others could not eat mussels or crab meat, and other still reacted badly to common drugs. All these reactions, Richet proposed, should be viewed as forms of anaphylaxis.[47] To Richet, sensitization by food indicated that some proteins were not destroyed in the intestine and could pass intact (or, at least, partially intact) from the digestive tract into the bloodstream.[48] He argued that food idiosyncrasy illuminated the evolutionary role of anaphylaxis. A violent reaction against foreign proteins allowed the organism to protect itself against the danger of a haphazard integration of such proteins – above all, those adsorbed through a digestive tract – into the tissues. A chaotic incorporation of elements of other living organisms could create strange 'alimentary chimeras' – bodies composed from bits of other bodies. It could therefore threaten the stability of hereditary traits acquired by each species through natural selection. Anaphylaxis might be disastrous to the individual, but it protected the integrity of the species.[49]

Richet attributed the unique therapeutic virtues of raw meat juice to the same physiological mechanism which led to the development of food idiosyncrasies and legitimated the evolutionary role of anaphylaxis: the capacity of ingested proteins to cross the intestine barrier and to become part of the body. When eating uncooked meat, 'the polypeptides specific for each foodstuff are not dislocated by cooking, and do not need to be transformed then reconstituted anew in order to become a living tissue. It is a fully formed tissue that is ingested and rapidly becomes a living tissue'.[50] One could assume that only a small fraction of 'albuminoids' from raw meat extract escaped destruction in the intestine and penetrated the bloodstream, but this was not an obstacle for efficacy of zomotherapy. Richet believed that while the lifeless world was governed by the laws of Lavoisier's chemistry, the body was ruled by a 'chemistry of imponderables', that is, chemical reactions mediated by minuscule quantities of active substances. Such substances, be they secretions of ductless glands, indispensable nutrients such as vitamins, or 'sensitizing proteins' that induced immunity and anaphylaxis, attached themselves to cells and were able to change them permanently. They governed all the major physiological reactions and biological and mental reflexes. They were also responsible for the body's capacity to remember past events: the neural and the immunological memory.[51]

Proteins from raw meat juice which entered the bloodstream were described by Richet in terms akin to those he employed to define his 'chemistry of imponderables'. They were first integrated into muscles, and later affected the central nervous system, and through it, all the cells of the body: 'the muscle and the nerve cells have a very close relationship. Every change in the nerve system affects the muscle system, and, inversely, alternations in the muscle system affect the nervous system ... By consequence, when we repair the muscle, we repair the nervous system'.[52] For Richet, raw meat juice was 'the most easily assimilated aliment' because it was extracted from living cells, and because its structure was very close to the chemical structure of the body.[53] This structural proximity also made possible a direct integration of elements contained in this preparation into the tissues. Raw meat extract was thus at the same time a foodstuff and a drug, or, to be more precise, it was a *sui generis* entity that cannot be fully translated into present-day terms.

To say that the meaning of words and concepts change over time is to state the obvious. The starting point of Thomas Kuhn's reflection on change in the sciences was the insight that terms such as 'heat' and 'velocity' have an entirely different meaning in Aristotelian and Newtonian physics.[54] Ludwik Fleck similarly argued that the significance of terms such as 'heavy' or 'warm' in the early modern period was very different to their meaning at the time he was writing because they were attached to a radically dissimilar universe of images, metaphors and symbols.[55] The display of networks of meaning linked with scientific terms and technological devices, Fleck added, undermines an overly simplistic, linear view of scientific progress. A Tom-Tom drum is undoubtedly a less efficient means of transmission of information over a long distance than a telegraph, but the experience of a person who receives a telegraphic message is not an exact equivalent of the experience (aesthetical, emotional or both) of someone who listens to information conveyed by a rhythmic sound of a drum.[56]

Historians are aware of the need to pay attention to changes in meanings of terms and concepts. They may, however, occasionally forget this principle, especially when they study a recent period and use terms borrowed from everyday language. In the early twenty-first century, just as a hundred years earlier, meat is above all a widely consumed (if not cheap) nutritious and reconstructive aliment. However, for Richet and his colleagues, raw meat juice was not merely a rich foodstuff, but a substance entangled in a complex web of meaning. In a conceptual universe in which extracts of living tissues were endowed with quasi-mystic properties, where bodies were ruled by a 'chemistry of imponderables', where the digestive, muscular and neural systems were interconnected and interdependent, and where organisms had porous boundaries and were able to incorporate proteins from other species into their structure, 'meat' meant something very different from the meanings of the word meat today.[57]

2 TREAT WITH MEAT: PROTEIN, PALATABILITY AND PERNICIOUS ANAEMIA IN THE 1920s–30s

Susan E. Lederer

In the early 1920s patients diagnosed with pernicious anaemia faced a difficult future. The symptoms of the disease included weakness, pallor and yellowness of the skin and fatigue; patients experienced palpitations of the heart and breathlessness when they attempted physical effort, troubling disturbances of the digestive system, including sore mouth, sore tongue, vomiting and diarrhoea, and numbness of the lower extremities. Even worse, most patients died within one to two years after learning about their disease. As science writer Paul de Kruif memorably remarked 'in 1925 being told you had pernicious anaemia meant the undertaker for you more surely than if the governor had signed your death warrant for first degree murder.'[1]

By the end of the decade, however, the picture of pernicious anaemia had drastically changed. In 1930 life insurance statisticians reported that mortality from the disease among white persons between the ages of fifty-five and seventy-four had been reduced by 50 per cent.[2] This dramatic change did not result from 'some extremely complicated deep science out of a white-tile-and-glass-door-knob laboratory and cooked by some abstruse highbrow investigator.'[3] Instead the solution to the problem was feeding patients a food category that most Americans had regarded with scant enthusiasm, the so-called organ meats or 'edible viscera' – heart, kidney and especially liver of animals. As physician William Murphy recalled, liver was regarded as 'cat food', barely palatable and 'hardly digestible for a human being, particularly a sick one.'[4] Once dismissed by many as merely a 'loathsome waste product', liver by 1931 and by virtue of its role in vanquishing pernicious anaemia had become 'a dignified and valued food for human beings.'[5]

This paper examines the creation of the 'liver life belt', and the implications of medicalizing a common foodstuff. The prescription for 'taking one's liver' – nearly three-quarters of a pound a liver a day – required major accommodation on the part of patients and their families. It not only compelled doctors, nurses and dieticians to seek ways to enhance the palatability of liver; it provided a boon to meatpackers, processors and butchers, who saw the price of this food article skyrocket during the heyday of liver therapy and amid the Great Depression. Like diabetes, which was transformed by the isolation and introduction of insulin, pernicious anaemia became a chronic disease requiring lifelong (or liverlong) management. Unlike diabetes, however, the liver diet could be more readily managed domestically.[6] The discovery of the material effects of liver treatment on anaemia prompted many Americans, anaemic or not, to embrace the consumption of organ meats, which in turn raised the costs of these 'special cuts' making them less affordable to those in dire need.[7] Liver's popularity with nutritionists, mothers and other American consumers endured even as the spectre of pernicious anaemia evaporated.

Before Liver Therapy

'For a long period,' noted Thomas Addison in 1855, 'I had from time to time met with a very remarkable form of general anaemia, occurring without any discoverable cause whatever'. Addison labelled this form of anaemia 'idiopathic' to differentiate it from anemias of known aetiology. The English clinician offered a vivid description of the disease, which 'with scarcely a single exception', resulted in the death of the patient. 'The countenance gets pale, the whites of the eyes become pearly, the general frame flabby rather than wasted; the pulse perhaps large, but remarkably soft and compressible, and occasionally with a slight jerk, especially under the lightest excitement'.[8] Resisting all treatment, the disease caused breathlessness, debility and finally, death. In 1872, when the Zurich physician Anton Biermer described similar symptoms and disease course, he designated the condition as 'progressive pernicious anemia', and found, like Addison, few effective treatments for the patients identified with the disease.[9] Despite a flurry of papers outlining the diffuse symptomatology of the disorder, most clinicians agreed with William Osler's dismal assessment in 1881 of available therapies for pernicious anaemia. Although he recommended iron, arsenic, blood transfusion and transfusion with milk, he sadly reported that 'all our Montreal cases have died'. Only a few of Osler's patients survived more than a year with their diagnosis.[10] More than forty years later, the outcome for patients with pernicious anaemia remained bleak. In the tenth edition of Osler's *Principles and Practice of Medicine* (published in 1925), the authors characterized the 'recurring and usually fatal anemia' as both widespread and apparently on the increase, even as they recorded the conventional therapies for the disease including arsenic (Fowler's solution), splenectomy and transfusion.[11] The same year, Boston internist Richard Clarke Cabot published a review of some 1,200 cases of pernicious anaemia just before the announcement of liver therapy; he reported that only ten of the patients in his series had lived longer than seven years once the diagnosis was made.[12]

The popular press noted the disease's toll. One of the earliest American newspaper references to pernicious anaemia occurred in 1890, reporting the death of Harriet Horne, the wife of Morristown physician William Horne.[13] But the disease also claimed the lives of better-known Americans, including assistant Army paymaster general George Glenn, Methodist Episcopalian clergyman Reverend Doctor James A. McCauley, newspaper magnate George Scripps, millionaire plough manufacturer Charles Deere, financier Edward H. Harriman, Senator Charles James Hughes (Colorado), New Mexican Governor E. C. Da Baca, Rear Admiral and arctic explorer Robert Peary, actress (and ex-wife of impresario Florenz Ziegfeld) Anna Held all succumbed to pernicious anaemia.[14] Sharpshooter Annie Oakley, actors Lon Chaney and George Siegmann (who played slave driver Simon Legree in *Uncle Toms' Cabin*), and Army generals George Bell and Robert 'Vinegar Bob' McCoy also lost their lives to the disease.[15] In the popular press, reports of deaths often followed accounts of futile, if numerous, transfusions to stave off death from the disease, but to little avail.

From Anaemic Dogs to 'Cat Food'

Diet had long played a role in thinking about anaemia, pernicious or secondary. Even William Shakespeare, noted physicians George Minot and William Murphy, had recorded that 'improper food might impair the state of the blood'.[16] The liver of animals had appeared, along with 'other unsavory viscera and excreta of animals' in the pharmacopoeia for centuries.[17] Given the conventional wisdom that 'good food makes good blood', some physicians believed that 'insufficient and unsuitable feeding' prompted poor blood, and poor blood could seemingly be altered with changes in dietary practices. The medical literature was littered with reports of dietetic treatment for the disease. In 1894 T. R. Fraser, an Edinburgh physician, ordered daily feeding of beef bone marrow to a patient with pernicious anaemia. Two decades later, clinicians Lewellys Barker and Thomas Sprunt dosed pernicious anaemia patients at the Johns Hopkins Hospital with milk administered every two hours (2.5 ounces between the hours of 7 a.m. and 9 p.m., until by the sixth day, the patient received some three litres of milk per day.)[18]

Research findings from the 'anemic dog colony' maintained by physician George Hoyt Whipple provided new impetus for adopting dietary changes in pernicious anaemia. Whipple's focus on liver and anaemia developed from interest in the production of red blood cells and diet. At the University of California at San Francisco, he created a population of research dogs by breeding Boston terriers, bulldogs, and a mixture of Dalmatian coach hounds to obtain a more or less standard-sized 'bull mongrel'. Whipple made these dogs anaemic after drawing down their blood supply, and then attempted to regenerate the animals' blood with various diets – table scraps, lean scrap meats, carbohydrates, carbohydrates and fats – to see which foodstuffs would regenerate blood most efficiently. In an effort to allay potential concern about severe bloodletting in these animals, George W. Corner, Whipple's biographer, explained

> The dogs remained well and lively even while their hemoglobin stayed as low as 40 per cent; when the investigators visited them in their outdoor runs the dogs would often come happily bounding toward them, and some of the dogs got so accustomed to the frequent collection of blood samples that they would leap on the table, lie down and stretch out their necks for the needle. The experiments were in fact scarcely harder upon the dogs than upon the investigators and technicians who had to carry on the interminable counts and estimations.

Whipple and his colleague Frieda Robscheit-Robbins argued that whereas a diet of bread and milk or cracker meal, butter and lard required weeks to regenerate the dog's blood cells, a diet of beef heart or liver produced rapid regeneration. In 1920 the investigators reported that a diet of cooked liver was more efficient than a diet of meat (muscle) in promoting blood regeneration after anaemia. In 1922 when Whipple moved to Rochester, New York to become dean of the newly created medical school, his dog colony – twenty-two adult dogs and eighteen puppies – travelled by special railroad car to their new quarters. In 1925 Whipple and Robscheit-Robbins reported that liver feeding remained 'the most potent factor for the sustained production of haemoglobin and red cells. This favourable and remarkable reaction is invariable in our dog experiments no matter how long continued the anaemia level, no matter how unfavourable the preceding diet periods may be, and regardless of the substances given with the liver feeding'.[19] Supported in part by funds from the National Live Stock and Meat Board, Whipple and Robscheit-Robbins found liver feeding superior to the feeding of animal brains and pancreases, and to the feeding of spleen and bone marrow. They reported that liver taken from chicken, pigs and cattle was far superior to fish liver.[20]

In Boston, a young internist, George R. Minot, familiar with the results from the Rochester dog colony, adapted the information to patients suffering from pernicious anaemia. Beginning with advice to private patients to increase their daily consumption of liver, by 1925 Minot had arranged for patients with pernicious anaemia at the Peter Bent Brigham Hospital to receive large amounts of raw liver. In the hospital setting, Minot and his colleague William P. Murphy were able to monitor both liver intake and to measure the haematological response to the therapy.[21] In May 1926 at the Atlantic City meeting of the Association of American Physicians, Minot described how the forty-five patients with pernicious anaemia who consumed nearly a half-pound of raw liver each day experienced a rapid rise in their red blood cell (reticulocyte) counts demonstrating the effective reversal of the symptoms of pernicious anaemia. In 1926 Murphy and Minot published a brief, now classic, account of their work in the *Journal of the American Medical Association*, describing the administration of a daily diet 'made as palatable as possible' featuring from 120 to 240 grams of cooked calves' or beef liver, 120 grams of beef or mutton muscle meat, 300 grams of vegetables – lettuce and spinach, 250 to 500 grams of fruit – especially peaches, apricots, strawberries, pineapple, oranges and grapefruit, 40 grams of fat from butter or cream, and if desired, an egg and 240 grams of milk. Perhaps not surprisingly, one of the problems that the doctors encountered was getting patients to consume a total intake of between 2,000 and 3,000 calories of these foods. Initially patients consumed as little as 1,000 calories of liver and fruits; as their condition improved, some patients became 'ravenously hungry' and even 'often anxious to eat more than the customary allowance of liver and meat'.[22]

The doctors recorded the rapid improvement of their entire series of forty-five patients on the special diet. One sign of their improved condition was the change the doctors noted in the frequency of the bowel movements (from diarrhoea to one formed stool a day) and the 'laxative effect' of the diet. A clinical index of patient's improvement came from red blood counts, which demonstrated the rapidity of red blood corpuscle increase from an average of 1.47 RBC counts in millions before the diet to an average of 3.40 RBC counts in millions one month after the diet to an average of 4.5 RBC count in millions four to six months after the diet therapy began.

By 1939, William Murphy presented evidence from some 484 of the 578 pernicious anaemia patients he had observed since he and Minot published their initial paper on the liver therapy. He reported that 378 of the 484 patients he was able to trace were alive, including a small cohort of patients who had lived more than ten years since they had received their diagnosis. Murphy acknowledged that longer life was not the most important criterion. 'What of the social and economic status of these patients whose lives are being lengthened? Are they merely existing as invalids and consequently a burden to their families and to society or do they continue as economically efficient members of society?'[23] The answer was certainly not as straightforward as Murphy may have wished. Some 61 per cent of his patients presented with neural disturbance (and in 34 per cent there was evidence of 'locomotor disturbance'). He concluded that only 10 per cent of his patients had serious problems with locomotion, whereas a few experienced several difficulties in using their hands and fingers. In spite of these problems, he claimed that the patient could be returned to and maintained in 'a state of economic efficiency' so long as the diagnosis was made early and prompt, vigorous therapy with whole liver or liver substitute was undertaken.

Many of Murphy and Minot's patients seemingly had little or no difficulty complying with the liver diet. Even after the introduction of liver extract (by 1928 there were several of these extracts on the market, which could be taken orally, intramuscularly or parenterally), some patients reportedly preferred to stick to the whole liver therapy. One of Murphy's patients, for example, who consumed approximately a half-pound of calf's liver per day for twelve years – a total of more than 2,000 pounds of liver – remained in excellent health.[24]

'As Palatable as Possible'

The results from Minot and Murphy's series fostered an enormous enthusiasm among physicians confronted with patients with pernicious anaemia. Their patients were not always so enthusiastic. The case of J. H., a forty-one-year-old carpenter, first admitted to the Johns Hopkins Hospital in 1919, illustrates the changing treatment picture for patients with the disease, as well as the difficulty of maintaining the demanding liver regimen. When attacks of nausea and vomiting and inability to work prompted J. H. to enter the hospital, his doctors found that he was weak, very pale, and possessed of a smooth tongue. He was extremely anaemic, with only 38 per cent of the normal haemoglobin expected for a man of his size. He experienced several remissions and relapses. He was in turn force fed, then placed on a restricted diet with Fowler's solution (fluid containing 1 per cent potassium arsenite) and hydrochloric acid; during his third and fourth relapses he received transfusions, producing the longest remission from symptoms that he had ever enjoyed. In July 1926 when he re-entered the hospital, he was sent home with the prescription to eat between three-quarters to one pound of liver (raw weight) every day. This 'ambulatory form of livery therapy' produced astounding results. His anaemia receded, his blood returned to normal, and he 'felt better than he had ever felt since the onset of his illness'. That is, until he stopped 'taking liver' in the summer of 1927, and his symptoms recurred. When he resumed the liver life, he quickly rebounded. As physician James Bordley explained in an extended aquatic metaphor, 'as the illness progressed the patient swam hopelessly from one wave to another being sucked farther downward in each successive trough'. Offering the liver 'life-belt' improved the patient's chances but was not a cure: 'the swimmer must forever hold fast to his preserver for he still lingers upon a treacherous sea and cannot hope to stay afloat unaided'.[25]

For some patients, it was not so much maintaining the liver diet as starting it. At the Waltham Hospital in Cambridge, Massachusetts, physicians Dwight O'Hara and J. S. Grewal reported their difficulties with a sixteen-year-old boy diagnosed two years earlier with pernicious anaemia. When the young man developed severe anaemic symptoms in the spring of 1927, physicians attempted to treat him using blood transfusions large (700 c.c.s) and small to no avail. However, the dietary management of the patient proved onerous: 'the food antipathies of a sixteen-year-old boy may be insurmountable. In vain we coaxed, teased, pleaded, reasoned, threatened, warned, menaced, and swore. For two months he would have none of us with our liver'. Fortunately for all concerned, the hospital dietician Marian Haywood offered a novel solution, liver ice cream. Blending cream, sugar, cocoa, salt and forty-five grams of ground liver and freezing the mixture, the 'delicacy' was sufficiently palatable to persuade the young man to consume some liver.[26]

Nurses joined dieticians and doctors in advocating the careful preparation of liver and the development of strategies to cajole recalcitrant patients into taking the prescribed dose. The liver, noted nurse Bertha Wood, 'must be made palatable and attractive when served'. In addition, getting patients to consume liver required ingenuity: 'the power of persuasion may be called into play to administer it to the patient'.[27] Lulu Hunt Peters, a nationally syndicated medical columnist in the popular press, advocated reasoning with patients who showed reluctance in adopting the liver diet. Eating raw liver, she conceded, 'seems repellent to us, but we eat raw oysters and raw clams without making any faces so there is no doubt that the taste for raw liver can be cultivated'.[28] Capitalizing on the seafood analogy, she recommended taking a 'liver cocktail' in small doses until the patient acquired a taste for it. Preparation of the liver for the cocktail entailed careful removal of the veins and 'tough parts', grinding the liver into a paste, and preparing a sauce from tomato ketchup, lemon juice, Worcestershire sauce, and chives. Once the sauce and liver product were combined, she suggested that the mixture be chilled before serving in a cocktail glass with crackers or wafers. (And indeed, the so-called shrimp cocktail was relatively new. The earliest reference to shrimp cocktail in the *New York Times*, for example, appeared in an advertisement for 'Pride of the Farm Tomato Catsup' recommended for preparing a cocktail sauce for oysters, clams, or shrimp cocktail for Christmas dinner. For the shrimp cocktail, the advertisement advised mixing the shrimp and ketchup together before serving in small glass dishes set at each place).[29]

If it was clear that patients required some persuasion to adopt the liver therapy, it is not clear from the historical record what physicians and nurses told patients to ensure their compliance. In 1929, for example, one of Murphy and Minot's colleagues at Harvard Medical School became interested in the relationship between some stomach secretions, especially hydrochloric acid, and pernicious anaemia.[30] To test his hypothesis about an 'intrinsic factor' in the stomach, William B. Castle fed healthy fasting subjects some 300 grams of raw finely ground beef muscle (what he called hamburg meat), and asked them to regurgitate it after one hour. Once vomited, the mixture was mixed with hydrochloric acid, sieved, and introduced into the stomach of a patient with pernicious anaemia. 'Care was exercised', Castle explained, that 'all subjects, who were healthy medical students or physicians, were free from upper respiratory infections.'[31] Presumably Castle exercised care in explaining to his pernicious anaemia patients the source of the 'meat material' they received after a fast of some six hours and a meatless diet.

Even as the liver treatment became well established the problem of palatability remained. As Harvard physician William Castle explained, patients did not always successfully maintain the liver diet for their pernicious anaemia because of the monotony and the expense of either the half-pound of fresh liver a day or the more expensive liver extracts that had quickly become commercially available. Like the diabetic patient compelled to face the necessity of lifelong treatment and expense with insulin, the patient with pernicious anaemia confronted ongoing expenses. 'The dilemma', wrote Castle in 1929, 'often assumes the proportions of a moral issue in the life of the impecunious patient who has become tired of liver.'[32]

What were the patient's options? To maintain red blood cells, the patient with pernicious anaemia generally required about 200 grams of liver per day or the extract prepared from 300 grams of liver. In 1929 most commercially available extracts cost roughly 85 cents per day. For patients who could not afford this expense, the recourse was to purchase calf's liver (the most palatable and the most expensive organ meat at 75 cents per pound). Given these alternatives, Castle proposed a method to prepare an effective liver extract at home using not calf but beef liver (roughly 15 to 30 cents per pound). By 1934, the domestic solution became less attractive when the cost of calves' liver declined to 55 cents per pound, and the daily expense of liver extract declined to 60 cents per day.[33]

At Johns Hopkins, physicians recommended liver in the form of a 'liver pulp', the result of the raw meat run several times through a meat grinder. When cold water was added to the ground liver, it was pressed through a coarse sieve or potato ricer and then served in chilled orange juice or ginger ale. Dieticians at Hopkins encouraged the preparation of liver in myriad ways, including

> Broiled liver, liver soup, liver sandwich, creamed liver, breaded liver, tomatoes and peppers and eggs stuffed with liver, liver and bacon, liver rolls, liver loaf, liver dumplings, liver with mushrooms, curried liver, liver en casserole, jellied liver, liver croquettes, Swedish baked liver, liver soufflé, liver hash, Mexican liver, liver salad, liver pudding, et cetera et cetera.[34]

References to ethnic cuisine (Swedish liver, Mexican liver) illustrated the versatility of the organ meats. It apparently did not map readily onto the understanding of the 'racial distribution' of pernicious anaemia. Whereas diabetes in the 1920s and 1930s was often identified as 'the Jewish disease', pernicious anaemia was linked to those 'races with blue eyes and light hair and complexions' rather than those races with dark eyes and dark complexions.[35] Evidence from case records at the Peter Bent Brigham Hospital in Boston, for example, suggested that those of Northern European ancestry developed pernicious anaemia more readily than Russian Jews, people from Asia, and people from Africa. 'Negroes', wrote William Murphy, 'seem to be relatively immune from the disease'. Case records from Johns Hopkins Hospital and the Cook County Hospital in Chicago, institutions in which 'approximately one-third of the admissions are colored persons' identified many fewer cases of pernicious anaemia among Negroes. (At Johns Hopkins eight of 111 pernicious anaemia patients were identified as Negro; at Cook County, eight of 256 patients were identified as Negro.) Murphy further emphasized the racial dimension when he noted that all of the patients were 'mulattoes'. Murphy's findings were shared by physicians at the US Veteran's Hospital in Tuskegee, Alabama, where only two cases of pernicious anaemia were reported among some 4,940 'colored patients'. Pernicious anaemia, echoed the physician Longcope, 'seldom, if ever, occurs in the full-blooded Negro'.[36]

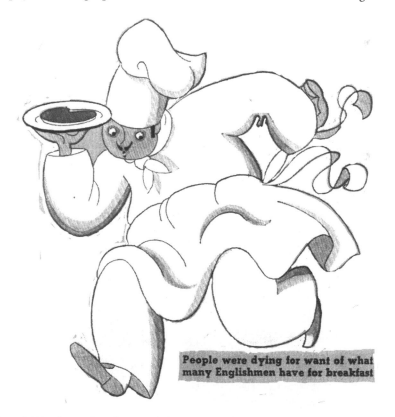

People were dying for want of what many Englishmen have for breakfast

Figure 2.1: People were dying for want of what many Englishmen have for breakfast. Source: Hannah Lees, 'Living on Liver', *Colliers*, 21 October 1939, p. 29.

In spite of a seemingly endless array of liver preparations, the problem of palatability and compliance with the dietary regimen for pernicious anaemia remained an issue. In his 1931 book *Living the Liver Diet*, Kansas physician Elmer Miner similarly emphasized the versatility of this variety of meat. He offered recipes for liver appetizer, liver loaf, calf's liver on toast, liver dolmans, liver and macaroni, liver soufflé, and liver pudding. Conceding that consuming large quantities of liver on a daily basis for a period of several years could become a 'serious and irksome affair', Miner advocated what he called 'Liver Appetizer Supreme'. This was prepared from one pound of calf's liver placed in a double boiler and then steamed in its own juices for about forty minutes. The steamed liver was then ground in a coarse sieve. The resulting pulp and waste juices were then ground in a medium sieve until it produced a liver paste, which was then mixed with warm or cold water in a drinking glass and consumed immediately. This 'palatable drink' was one that Miner used with 'complete personal satisfaction'. Consumed in this way, Miner noted, 'liver is thus taken as a medicine, and not necessarily as part of a meal'.[37]

If liver could be taken as a medicine, it was nevertheless not to be regarded as a panacea. Physicians, Miner warned, were too prone to prescribe liver for a variety of illnesses and complaints. This had the effect of placing inordinate demands on the liver supply. 'The market price has been doubled and then trebled in some instances. We therefore ask that liver as a food be spared for those who really need it'.[38] Other commentators echoed Miner's call for responsible liver consumption, as thousands who had formerly avoided liver or thought it best suited to feline consumption raced to adopt the liver life. 'The raid on liver', warned one editorial writer, 'has sent the price soaring to figures difficult for sufferers from pernicious anemia who have both poor blood and poor purses'. This writer encouraged readers to forego liver unless it was necessary for health.[39]

That the liver treatment of pernicious anaemia had driven up the price of 'edible viscera' was a truism for many observers. 'Honestly, I hate to mention liver at all in this column', wrote medical columnist Doctor William Brady in 1928, 'lest some butcher boost the price, which is already soaring almost beyond reach of plain people'. Brady acknowledged that physicians bore considerable responsibility for the increased prices of edible offal:

> we doctors are, in a way, to blame for the tremendous inflation in liver prices, too, for the choicest liver was still far below other choice meat in cost when the doctors announced the discovery that this heretofore rather despised and unappreciated article of diet would cure severe anaemia, pernicious anaemia, a disease for which no other effective remedy had been found.[40]

Medical columnist W.A. Evans echoed these sentiments in his newspaper column. The physician described numerous letters he received from readers complaining about the increased cost of liver and its disappearance from the menus of many restaurants. 'The price has gone up markedly in packing establishments, in whole meat markets, and at retail markets in large cities', noted Evans. 'The butchers justify the advance in price. They say the demand is in far excess of the supply and they know of no way to practically limit the demand to the level of supply except by raising the price'. Evans's solution to the liver shortage was to encourage readers to move beyond the conventional calf's liver to the 'healthy liver of any edible animal', and to consider the consumption of animal brains, hearts, kidneys and sweetbreads.[41]

One such animal was the hog. When H. Milton Conner selected raw swine stomach as a potential source, he obtained the stomachs from packing houses, which were instructed to remove the stomach after they tied off the pylorus 'so as to prevent regurgitation of intestinal material into the stomach'. He exercised some care to ensure that no parasitic disease (trichinosis or porcine undulant fever) would be transmitted from the animal to the human. The Mayo Clinic physician did encounter 'some opposition' from patients who balked at eating the raw swine stomach (ground in a coarse grinder before being mixed with cold cereal, salads, or sandwiches). His efforts proved more successful when he adopted a 'seprasieve' which allowed him to discard the fibrous stomach material and use only the remaining liquid in tomato, orange, cranberry or other fruit juices.[42] Of the ten patients who received raw swine stomach, six seemingly enjoyed some benefit. At the University of Michigan, professors Cyrus Sturgis and Raphael Isaacs developed a different method in preparing hog stomach as a specific in the treatment of pernicious anaemia.

In 1929 Sturgis and Isaacs obtained fresh swine stomach, removed the fat and surrounding mesentery from the organ and finely chopped the material. After drying the stomach bits at low temperatures, they repeatedly washed the stomach with petroleum benzene. The removal of the fat and the benzene washes reportedly eliminated much of the stomach odour. The product, 'which had very little taste', was administered to patients as a 'thick puree in tomato juice, being eaten as one would a thick cereal'.[43] (Elsewhere the material was described as 'like sawdust and practically tasteless'.)[44] Sturgis and Isaacs found that this desiccated, defatted hog stomach was effective in bringing about a haemopoietic remission in patients with pernicious anaemia, and that it proved even more effective to include the mucosa of the stomach rather than the muscle. The advantage of hog stomach, Sturgis and Isaacs readily conceded, was an economic one. 'As desiccated stomach is prepared from tissue which is ordinarily regarded as waste material, and the process of manufacture requires only a few simple steps, the cost of the final product should be less than liver extract'.[45] Given that liver or liver extract would be required for the lifetime of the pernicious anaemia patient, the economic factor was important, they argued, for patient well-being. Hog stomach did produce some problems, however. When Cyrus Sturgis appeared on a radio programme to discuss this new substance, effective for the treatment of pernicious anaemia, he made reference to the material as 'ground hog stomach', which some of his listeners apparently interpreted as 'groundhog stomach'. To the professor's dismay, he reported that he had received 'hundreds of inquiries asking where in the world I get all the groundhogs, whether there is any chance of hiring out as a groundhog catcher, and so on'.[46] It may not have been so strange to hear that the stomach from groundhogs would be useful, for William Murphy reported how liver from both deer and moose was used effectively by some patients because of its availability during the winter months.[47]

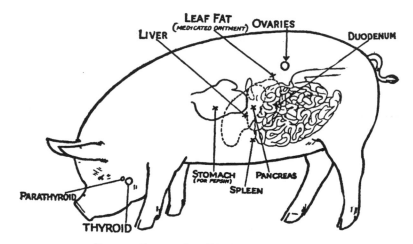

FIG. 35.—Sources of medicinal products from hogs

Figure 2.2: Sources of Medicinal Products from Hogs. Source: R. A. Clemen, *By-Products in the Packing Industry* (Chicago, IL: University of Chicago Press, 1927), p. 214.

Economic factors in the fact of increasing costs of beef liver and the organ meats of other mammals encouraged some physicians to look at edible viscera beyond mammals. In the fishing town of Aberdeen, Scotland, physician L. S. P. Davidson responded to the 'financial strain' borne by the pernicious anaemia patient by attempting to feed patients with raw fish liver. In so doing, Davidson went against conventional wisdom, for the feeding experiments conducted by George H. Whipple and Frieda Robbins suggested that fish liver was not as effective in blood regeneration as liver from mammals. Davidson's initial efforts to create a therapeutic dose of fish liver met with failure. When he placed a preparation not unlike a 'thick anchovy sauce' between layers of bread and butter and fed it to two patients with pernicious anaemia, the experiment was stopped 'because of the nausea and disgust which the material produced, and partly because it had rapidly undergone putrefaction, even when kept in the icebox'.[48] A second effort to apply the fish liver met with similar failure. After treating the fish liver with acetone to prevent putrefaction and to reduce the bulk, the fish liver product induced nausea and vomiting in a patient fed the new preparation. Despite these adverse outcomes, Davidson persevered. He developed a process in which the twenty pounds of fresh fish liver was minced, heated, and desiccated to produce a powder. This powder could then be administered to patients in orange juice, tomato juice, ginger beer or Bovril. The patients reported that the type of fish liver used influenced the palatability of the product; they preferred whiting to that of cod, monkfish, or haddock. (Among cod liver oil purveyors, some made claims that some cod were more palatable than others; see the advertisement for Nason's Palatable-Norwegian Cod Liver Oil, touted as the 'the better tasting kind now in the Antarctic with Commander Byrd'.)[49]

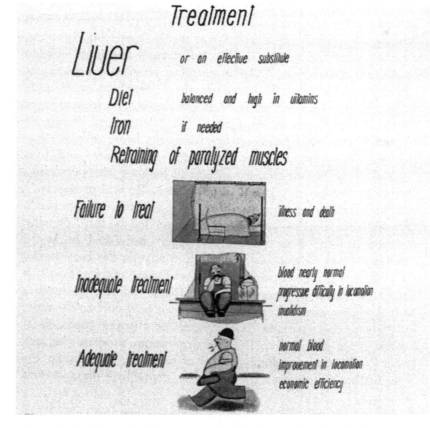

Figure 2.3: Invalidism or death in the absence of, social and economic efficiency in the presence of adequate, controlled therapy. Source: William P. Murphy, *Anemia in Practice: Pernicious Anemia* (Philadelphia, PA: W. B. Saunders, 1939), p. 118.

During the Great Depression and for several years after, physicians continued to discuss the economic dimensions of liver therapy for pernicious anaemia. One of the chief architects of the liver therapy, William Murphy devoted considerable attention to the financial aspects of treating pernicious anaemia with liver.

As this image from his 1939 textbook on pernicious anaemia makes clear, Murphy claimed that adequately controlled pernicious anaemia produced not only normal blood, but improved locomotion and enhanced social and economic efficiency. In the same text, Murphy devoted pages to the costs of the treatment, noting 'Are we not as physicians, to some extent at least, conservators of our patients' money? Should we not utilize those available means of treatment which will best serve the needs of the patient and which will accomplish the desired result with a minimum of expense and inconvenience to the patient?'[50] In some cases, this meant that establishing the cost of liver treatment included not just the substances (liver or liver extract) but also the means of its delivery. In the case of Miss B. S., a fifty-two-year-old woman who earned her livelihood as a cook, the effective treatment for her pernicious anaemia cost 62.5 cents per day (a 5 c.c. injection of liver extract). But because she paid, in addition to the cost of the drug, 50 cents per day to the district nurse who administered the injection, her annual costs for the treatment rose to some $410. Murphy encouraged her to obtain the new highly concentrated form of liver extract which required injections every six weeks, decreasing her yearly treatment expense to $10.83.[51] She might have saved even more as a cook, knowing how to prepare liver in an appetizing fashion, but finding a cure at the butcher shop was not the kind of advice that Nobel laureates dispensed to their patients.[52]

The Liver Life-Belt

In 1934 the Nobel Foundation awarded the prize in medicine or physiology to George Minot and William Murphy, jointly with George H. Whipple (Frieda Robscheit-Robbins, his long-time collaborator, did not receive any credit). By this time, the liver life-belt for pernicious anaemia had become well entrenched in American medical practice and in American kitchens. Even before the formal recognition of liver therapy for pernicious anaemia, physician William Brady recalled in 1932 the changing fortunes of liver. In 'barefoot days', the medical columnist recalled, 'we developed a furtive air from trying to get by the butcher shop to patronize the town pump without being halted with a "Hi, buddy, take this along home to your mother" – the butcher's way of disposing of a surplus of liver'.[53] From a surplus, waste product, liver was transformed into a commodity valued for its blood-regenerating, life-restoring properties.

'If you have been watching the booms and slumps in the liver market in the last five years', noted Mary Meade, the food columnist for the *Chicago Tribune*, 'you've discovered that it doesn't take bears and bulls to upset prices and send them rocketing. The job can be done just as effectively by a few words from the family doctor'. Meade explained how the link between pernicious anaemia and liver raised the price of calves' liver as high as $1.25 per pound, before it gradually returned to a more affordable price.

Not all families welcomed the liver diet, but Meade insisted that it would be 'no real sport to practice intrigue and camouflage' and inject more liver into the family meals. In addition to recipes for liver goulash, creamed liver and liver custard, she instructed readers in the art of making casserole of liver, stuffed baked liver, and beef liver loaf.

Enthusiasm for organ meats continued into the 1940s, especially when meat rationing for the war effort went into effect. As much of the domestically produced meat was being sent overseas to feed soldiers and Allies, the meat ration in the United States was set at 2.5 pounds per person per week. Poultry and fish were not restricted, nor were such organ meats as liver, tongue, heart, kidney and sweetbreads restricted (pig's feet, knuckles, scrapple, and joints also remained unrestricted). To ensure that Americans received sufficient protein during the war years, the Department of Defense recruited Margaret Mead, Kurt Lewin and other social scientists to spur the dietary changes needed. 'The homemaker controls the food consumption of the people', noted former president Herbert Hoover in 1943. 'Meats and fats are just as much munitions in this war as are tanks and aeroplanes...'[54] Many homemakers had already enlisted the organ meats in the battle against iron-deficient or weak blood. Armed with recipes for liver soufflé and liver loaf, many American women were ready to do their part by preparing liver, kidney, hearts and other viscera for their husbands and children.

3 HOW ABATTOIR 'BIOTRASH' CONNECTED THE SOCIAL WORLDS OF THE UNIVERSITY LABORATORY AND THE DISASSEMBLY LINE

Naomi Pfeffer

It is generally accepted that both the American meatpacking industry and modern endocrinology originated in the latter half of the nineteenth century. However, generally their development has not been linked. A typical history of the meatpacking industry begins shortly after the Civil War (1861–5) with the meat barons, as its pioneers came to be known, taking advantage of the widening rail network, and transporting livestock from farms and ranches, mostly in the west, to the railway hub in Chicago where feedlots, slaughterhouses and factories had been set up. The introduction of chill rooms allowed livestock to be slaughtered during the summer heat and extended the shelf life of fresh table meat which was dispatched by rail in refrigerator cars to the gathering crowds of urban consumers, mostly in the east, whose appetite for it was apparently insatiable.[1] The disassembly line, introduced in the late 1880s, was the innovation that came to define modern meatpacking. In traditional slaughterhouses one or two men performed all the tasks involved in killing, dressing and cutting up an animal. The disassembly line combined engineering and scientific management: a continuous conveyer took the carcass of a freshly slaughtered animal hanging from a chain around its legs past a series of workstations where a man stood and, in a matter of seconds, performed the same task over and over again. Rapid killing and cutting dramatically increased throughput of animals and lowered costs. Henry Ford, impressed by the speed and efficiency of the disassembly line, famously adapted it to create a revolutionary system for assembling and mass-producing cars which was named after him.

The typical history of endocrinology tends to ignore its relations to the meat industry. For example, Victor Cornelius Medvei, in his exhaustive survey of the field, claims 1855 as a significant watershed because it was the year during which Claude Bernard (1813–78), the French physiologist, launched his radical idea that certain body parts secrete substances into the bloodstream.[2] These body parts were called 'ductless glands' because they lack an exit on the body's surface, and their secretions were envisaged as chemical messengers that deliver instructions to other body parts telling them to perform specific physiological functions. The secretions are now known as hormones – the English physiologist E. H. Starling is said to have coined the term in 1905.[3] In 1936 the American endocrinologist and Nobel laureate Edward A. Doisy (1893–1986) described the process through which internal secretions had been, and were being, transformed into medicines. It had four stages: in the first a body part is recognized as a secreting organ or gland; in the second the secretion it produces is isolated and its function identified; the third results in a crude preparation, a sort of soup, of the secretion which can be used in experiments on laboratory animals or in humans; in the final stage a pure product is produced, its chemical structure is determined and it is synthesized or somehow produced on an industrial scale.[4] However, as historian Diana Long Hall pointed out, endocrinology is a field, not a scientific discipline.[5] Completion of the various stages required a contribution from one or several distinct scientific disciplines: in the field's early history these were the morphological sciences (anatomy and histology), physiology and domestic science. In Doisy's day biochemistry became increasingly important.

These stories of meat and hormones might have been told separately but are in fact closely linked. As this chapter shows, the debt of endocrinology to the meatpacking industry was particularly large during a period known as the endocrinological goldrush which began in the 1920s and lasted around four decades. Alan Parkes, a scientist who played a leading role in the British field, gave the period this name in order to convey the feverish excitement surrounding research on hormones, and how rules of scientific probity were sometimes bent in order to secure an international reputation.[6] However, the term is apposite for another reason: meatpackers, like all prospectors of gold, were enticed into the laboratory in search of profit. In effect, during the endocrinological goldrush the social world of the laboratory came face to face with that of the disassembly line. The encounter took place at the boundary separating science and business, and contributed to its realignment.

You Either Sell it or Smell It

The social worlds of scientific endocrinologists and meatpackers converged on a shared interest in extracting value out of what might be called 'biotrash', a shorthand term for organic waste characterized by the threat of rapid decomposition. Biotrash is a large fluid and subjective category. That which falls into it is simultaneously redundant, even disgusting, and potentially productive. Biotrash includes material of human and animal origin such as faeces and urine and matter 'left over' from diagnostic and surgical procedures. However the biotrash discussed in this chapter is 'abattoir waste', that is, parts of animals killed for meat that are excluded from the typical western diet.

Butchers' meat accounts for less than half of an animal. Where few animals are slaughtered, transforming the residue – bones, fat, hair, blood and offal – into by-products is labour intensive and unprofitable. Animals were often killed near to a stream or river into which biotrash could be thrown. However, where large numbers of animals are slaughtered, further processing could be profitable. Finding novel ways of making money out of biotrash was central to the economic logic and phenomenal success of American meatpackers. As historian William Cronon explains, by-products allowed the meatpackers to sell table meat at prices which undercut and drove out of business small-scale butchers.[7] Put another way, meatpackers earned their profits on the margin largely by selling things made out of stuff that traditional butchers threw away.

The meat barons famously declared war on abattoir waste. One of their favourite maxims was 'you either sell it or smell it'.[8] In their operations, a single creature was transformed into hundreds of commodities: gut was transformed into tennis racket strings, bristles became hairbrushes, hooves were boiled up into glue, scent was added to fat which was made into soap, bones were ground into fertilizer or made into knife handles, heads and offal were rendered into animal feedstuffs, and scraps of flesh were stripped off bone and other body parts and incorporated into foods such as sausage meat, tinned pork and beans and edible fats.

A novel use of biotrash was identified by the French physiologist C.-E. Brown-Sequard (1817–94), a contemporary and sometime colleague of Claude Bernard. In 1889, Brown-Sequard announced that his seventy-two-year-old body had been rejuvenated by injections of watery extracts of the testicles of young animals. Two years later he proposed that all animal organs and tissues can deliver something special to the blood, and advised physicians to administer preparations of them to patients suffering from an intractable disease.[9] The system of medicine he inspired is known as organotherapy. It enjoyed considerable publicity in the popular press. Meatpackers began producing proprietary lines of organotherapies, either cocktails of different tissues or preparations of desiccated single glands. Armour & Co., the largest of the Chicago meatpackers, produced its own range under the 'Glanoid' brand. Organotherapies were marketed through the same wholesale and retail channels that had been established for other by-products such as margarine, brushes and glue.

By the first decade of the twentieth century, a meat trust, a secret corporate alliance that fixed prices and carved up markets, had enabled the five largest Chicago meatpackers – Armour, Swift, Morrisey, Wilson and Cudahy – to capture more than half of the American meat market from their competitors. By the end of World War I meatpackers were contributing one-tenth of the USA's gross national product, and the industry was larger than any other food or consumer durable good industry including automobiles.[10] The Federal Trade Commission accused the meat barons of obstructing competition through their control of the chain of supply from ranch and farm gate to kitchen table. In 1920 the federal government used the Sherman Antitrust Act 1890 and the Clayton Antitrust Act 1914 to 'bust' the trust. It forced the sale of moneymaking subsidiaries such as butchers' shops, cold-storage warehouses, and market newspapers and journals, a punishment which pushed some meatpackers towards bankruptcy.[11] Meatpackers were allowed to keep their disassembly lines.[12] Faced with limited opportunities for developing their interests in related industries, they looked favourably on any novel method of exploiting biotrash. They had vast amounts at their disposal: by the 1920s, some disassembly lines were capable of processing 2,500 animals each day, the annual product of several farms or a whole ranch. By the 1940s, meatpackers were producing around seventy-five non-food 'by-products' and had acquired considerable stakes in several new and expanding industries divorced from food, which, as we shall see, included modern pharmaceuticals.[13]

Physiologists following in the footsteps of Claude Bernard viewed organotherapies as quack remedies, and as nothing more than meat extracts, and claimed any physiological potential would be destroyed by stomach acid. However, their attempts to discredit organotherapies mostly fell on deaf ears. Indeed, the market in organotherapies thrived, and they were either sold over the counter or prescribed enthusiastically by some American physicians,[14] referred to as 'endocriminologists' by their critics.[15]

Scientists were only convinced a substance had therapeutic value if it demonstrated physiological activity as a result of an experiment, usually involving vivisection (mostly of dogs), or on living people. Put another way, research subjects were found in the dog pound, amongst patients and family and friends. For instance, in 1893, George Oliver, an English physician, whose hobby was carrying out physiological experiments on family and friends, injected into his son an extract of adrenal glands which he had obtained from his local butcher's shop. The unfortunate boy's blood pressure rose and his heart began to beat more rapidly. Oliver took his extract to Schafer, Professor of Physiology at University College London, where, together, they examined its effect on dogs. At a meeting of the Physiological Society held in London the following year, they announced their discovery of a remarkable substance which was capable of dilating the pupils of the eye, opening the air passages to the lungs, causing the hair to stand on end, and stimulating blood circulation. This substance is now known as adrenalin.

Other hormones with therapeutic promise were identified. For instance, thyroxin was isolated two years after the identification of adrenalin. However, the discovery of insulin, an internal secretion of the pancreas, in 1921, the year after the meat trust had been busted, was responsible for initiating the endocrinological goldrush. Mass production of insulin was achieved through a novel collaboration between the University of Toronto, Eli Lilly & Co. – a pharmaceutical company – and Chicago meatpackers who agreed to rearrange the disassembly line so that pancreases could be cut out at an early stage.[16] Hormones held out to scientists the possibility of gaining an international reputation. Frederick Banting and John Macleod who, together with Charles Best, collaborated on the isolation of insulin, received the Nobel Prize in 1923. It is public knowledge that Eli Lilly's profits soared in 1923, with about half deriving from insulin even though its commercial distribution had not begun until October of that year.[17] There is no record of how much money meatpackers made out of the deal.

Difficulties Unravelling the Role of 'the Leader of the Endocrine Orchestra'

During the endocrinological goldrush biotrash was the chief source of research material. However, despite being produced in vast quantities, it was a scarce resource for scientists because meatpackers, for a range of different reasons discussed below, were reluctant to part with it. Fortunately for scientists working on sex hormones – oestrogen, progesterone and testosterone – their dependence on meatpackers was of relatively short duration. It took six years for what is now known as progesterone to pass through all four stages of Doisy's scheme presented in the introduction above, seven years for a testicular hormone, and fifteen years for the production of a synthetic oestrogen.[18] However, none enjoyed the level of esteem in which the anterior lobe of the pituitary gland was held, perhaps because, as sociologist Adele Clarke suggests, they are associated with sex and reproduction, topics then deemed illegitimate and which 'respectable' scientists steered clear of.[19] The pituitary gland began to be referred to as the 'master' gland, as the leader of the endocrine orchestra, as the general headquarters of the endocrine system where the status of virtually every bodily function is decided. And, mixing metaphors again, it was revered as a veritable storehouse of valuable therapeutic substances.[20] As one investigator put it in 1935 'That this small gland, which in man averages less than 0.5 gm in weight, secretes this number of hormones as separate entities throughout the entire secretory processes taxes the imagination.'[21]

Unfortunately the anterior lobe of the pituitary gland was loath to give up its secrets. It took five decades for its hormones to complete all four of Doisy's stages. Hindsight makes it easy to understand why. In the first place, the anterior lobe produces (at least) six distinctive hormones responsible for promoting activity in various body parts: growth hormone (GH); adrenocorticotrophic hormone (ACTH – the hormone that stimulates the adrenal glands); follicle stimulating hormone (FSH – responsible for stimulating specific activities in ovaries and testes); luteinizing hormone (LH – responsible for stimulating specific activities in ovaries and testes); thyroid-stimulating hormone (TSH); and prolactin which is responsible for lactation. Progress in isolating and characterizing the protein hormones was further frustrated by the rudimentary techniques then available: crystallography, chromatography, radioactive tracers and the ultracentrifuge were in their infancy during the endocrinological goldrush. Every success in the laboratory disclosed a new set of theoretical and technical problems. Researchers also failed to agree on which experimental animal was appropriate, with some championing rats and others preferring mice, rabbits or dogs. And because the stakes were high, competition rather than collaboration often ruled.

In the second place, science and technology were not the only impediments to progress in the laboratory. Unravelling the structure and function of the anterior lobe of the pituitary gland demanded cooperation and a considerable commitment on the part of meatpackers. A rearrangement of the disassembly line was all that was required for pancreases in a condition sufficiently fresh for the manufacture of insulin to be salvaged from the viscera of slaughtered animals. Recovery of a pituitary gland from its inaccessible and heavily fortified position within an animal's skull incurred additional labour costs and required investment in machinery. Heads were usually cut off animals at the fifth station of the disassembly line, following knock, shackle, stick and bleed.[22] They were thrown down a chute to the floor below where biotrash was separated for the manufacture of by products: fat was sent for refining into lard or oleomargarine; hearts for adding to sausage filler; intestines for transformation into sausage casings.[23] Sorting, cleaning and routing of biotrash were women's work and they were paid less than men on the killing floor.[24] However, cattle have thick skulls and cracking them open takes considerable physical force. Only the larger slaughterhouses of the American meatpackers could justify the expense of a 'splitting wheel' which crushes skull bones. And only a man, whose wages were higher than those of a woman, would have had the strength to operate it – he was often the only one working on that floor. Dissecting out each pituitary gland from the crushed skull took up to ten minutes. At most, one woman could collect around fifty to sixty per day.[25] As endocrinologist George Corner (1889–1981) succinctly put it, 'these small objects buried in the floor of the brain cavity are damnably hard to reach and dig out of the surrounding bone'.[26]

A business case justifying the trouble and expense of removing pituitary glands had been made prior to the endocrinological goldrush. In 1895 Schafer and Oliver had identified in the posterior lobe of the pituitary gland a substance which has a powerful oxytocic substance, that is, it makes the uterus contract. It was called pituitrin, and a watery soup of it began to be administered as an alternative to ergot, the traditional method of accelerating or inducing labour.[27] Some meatpackers produced and marketed their own brand of pituitrin; others sold pituitary glands to pharmaceutical concerns such as Parke, Davis & Co. and Eli Lilly & Co. Only minute quantities of pituitrin are present in the posterior lobe: 12,000 head of young cattle together yield just one pound.[28] Anterior lobes were not wasted but were incorporated into organotherapies.

Slow progress in the laboratory made a convincing business case in support of research into the pituitary gland's anterior lobe difficult to sustain and its terms had to be renegotiated repeatedly to accommodate changes in the meatpackers' fortunes. Evidence in support of this claim is drawn from the papers of Herbert Evans (1882–1971), anatomist and embryologist, whose laboratory at the University of California was a leader in the hunt for the hormones of the anterior lobe.[29] How American meatpackers viewed their relationship with the social world of the laboratory can only be inferred. For as Adele Clarke observed, primary sources of the meatpacking industry's history are absent, due in some part to companies protecting their proprietary interests, but also because of the turbulent labour relations that characterize it.[30]

Herbert Evans and the Identification of Growth Hormone

Evans's name is immortalized in 'Evans's Blue', a diazo dye, sometimes called T1824, which he formulated following a trip to Germany in 1911, and which is still used in the measurement of blood volume of humans and animals. However, he claimed his greatest achievement was the identification and isolation of Vitamin E, an achievement he shared with his long-time colleague Katherine Scott Bishop. He also pioneered the rat as an experimental laboratory animal and, together with Joseph Long (1879–1953), developed the Long–Evans strain of rat, one of the leading strains of laboratory rat. His interest in the pituitary gland had begun whilst a medical student and remained until his retirement in 1952. While he was studying at Johns Hopkins Hospital the neurosurgeon Harvey Cushing (1869–1939) was pioneering hypophysectomy, that is, extirpation (surgical removal) of the pituitary gland.[31] Cushing developed the technique in response to the late nineteenth-century observation in the mortuary that people suffering from acromegaly, a form of gigantism, had a tumour of the pituitary gland. This observation suggested that the pituitary gland somehow is involved in both normal and disordered growth.[32] Acromegaly affects older people whose long-bones are incapable of growth; a tumour of the pituitary gland in a young person whose long-bones are capable of growth may result in excessive height. Other syndromes associated with over- or under-production of hormones produced by the anterior lobe of the pituitary gland were subsequently identified, such as short stature in children and Fröhlich's syndrome, a childhood metabolic disease. Whenever another disease was attributed by scientific medicine to a malfunctioning or diseased pituitary gland it was added to the list of conditions which manufacturers of organotherapies claimed might be resolved by their products.

Evans's entrance into the world of pituitary hormones was dramatic. In 1921, he announced to the world that he had created gigantic rats by daily injections of a soup of beef cattle pituitary glands.[33] The rats were three times heavier than their untreated littermates, but they were not fat: large bones accounted for most of their extra weight. Culinary practices and terminology abounded in the social world of pituitary hormones. Evans called his cattle soup 'pea soup' because the pituitary gland is about the size of a pea. His recipe took under an hour to prepare.[34] In the laboratory, the gland's anterior lobe was separated out from the posterior lobe which consists of biologically different tissue, soaked in alcohol, pounded in a mortar for fifteen minutes, and the resulting sludge centrifuged for half of an hour. In 1923, he was awarded the gold medal of the American Medical Association in recognition of his demonstration of the growth-promoting capacity of the secretions of the anterior lobe.

The 1920s were difficult times for meatpackers. Both the livestock and meatpacking industries had enjoyed unequalled prosperity during the First World War thanks to a highly acquisitive public sector. Following the outbreak of peace, the military stopped buying meat, and cattlemen, swineherds and sheep men suffered the consequences of overproduction: prices plummeted a full decade before the stock market crash of 1929 signalled the onset of the Great Depression.[35] Then in 1920 the meat trust was busted. In this economic climate meatpackers were unlikely to feel benevolent towards science. A local slaughterhouse agreed to supply Evans with pituitary glands but only if he covered additional labour costs. In 1923, these amounted to $804. On top of that Evans paid $887 to hire a car and driver who collected and delivered around 400 glands daily, a yearly total of around 100,000 glands (for just under 1.7 cents per gland).[36] The University of California awarded him a grant of $1,700 which covered his costs, but the following year the slaughterhouse demanded half as much again, thereby raising the price of each gland to around 2.1 cents.

The appetite for cattle pituitary glands of scientists working in Evans's laboratory began outstripping local supply and reached a scale which only a Chicago meatpacker could meet. Armour agreed to help out, perhaps in the hope that Evans might reward the company with a discovery as profitable as insulin. For his part, Evans had a strong card to play: scientists in his laboratory had a rare skill, that of performing hypophysectomy, a procedure which renders the experimental animal into a blank canvas, a precondition to experimentation elucidating the role of pituitary hormones. Hypophysectomy involves drilling a hole in the skull close to the eye, exposing the pituitary gland, and sucking it out through a pipette. For many years, no one had managed to perform it without damaging the delicate neurological structures that surround the gland and thereby either killing the experimental animal or plunging it into a coma. This discouraging record had ended in 1916 when Philip E. Smith (1884–1970) and his wife Irene, who worked as a team in Evans's laboratory between 1912 and 1926, succeeded in performing a hypophysectomy without killing the tadpoles on which they were practising. The secret of their success was steady hands and tiny instruments which Smith painstakingly fashioned for the operation.[37] Few scientists outside of Evans's laboratory were capable of performing a hypophysectomy. Those who could were said to have golden hands because it enhanced their employability, an important consideration during the interwar years when there were few openings.[38] American endocrinologist Roy Greep (1905–97) cited it as a turning point in his career, and treated the first rat that survived his attempt at the procedure as a celebratory: the rat was named Adolph, and treated to a bed of cotton batting, and fed choice morsels.[39]

Supplying Evans with biotrash for use in research was a gamble. Armour continued to engage in the established market for organotherapies. As a result, for some years, Evans's laboratory was both supplicant and potential competitor. The risk of conflict emerged in 1930 following the announcement of the first test on a patient of a growth hormone soup prepared in Evans's laboratory out of cattle pituitary glands that had been supplied by Armour. The research subject was Miss J. M., aged nine-and-a-half, who stood just thirty-six inches tall, sixteen inches less than the average height of children of her age. A course of daily injections of a soup of growth hormone prepared in Evan's laboratory was administered by William Engelbach, a New York doctor. Engelbach declared Evans's soup superior to the expensive organotherapies marketed by meatpackers.[40] However, Miss J. M. was the first and only person to receive it. Evans claimed scientists in his laboratory were so completely occupied with basic research that they had no time to prepare growth hormone for the clinic.[41] Any threat to his relationship with Armour was diplomatically avoided.

Wartime Gland Famine

In 1938, Evans hired Choh Hao Li (1913–87), a biochemist, to investigate how the various hormones in the pea soup might be identified and purified. Born in Canton, China, Li was one of eleven children fathered by a well-to-do industrialist. In 1935, Li had enrolled as a graduate student at the University of California, Berkeley, where one of his brothers worked as a professor of business administration. Although the job was not one he would have chosen, Li accepted it because of the difficulties he was encountering in finding an employer prepared to hire a Chinese chemist (for the same reason, he had been unable to find a landlord prepared to rent a room to him and his wife).[42] Evans proved an excellent judge of scientific potential: Li was an outstanding scientist who went on to win prestigious awards.

In January 1941, leading endocrinologists and physiologists were invited to a secret conference held at Yale University. There was only one item on the agenda: how to respond to the rumour picked up by military agents that the Nazis were buying vast quantities of adrenal glands in Argentina, where the meatpacking industry was vast and largely foreign-owned, taking them by U-boat to Germany where they were made into a soup which was injected into fighter pilots who were then able to withstand the cold and disorientation experienced at high altitudes.[43] The rumour sounded plausible: research undertaken before the war had found injections of an adrenal gland soup helped laboratory rats to withstand the stress of oxygen deprivation.

Just as the development of the atomic bomb was stimulated by a rumour that the Nazis were about to produce one – both rumours turned out to be false – both encouraged federal government sponsorship of science. The Committee on Medical Research, the US armed forces' wartime agency responsible for sponsoring biomedical research deemed of strategic importance, contracted leading investigators in the field to find out how to transform adrenal gland soup into a cheap pharmaceutical.[44] Evans's laboratory was allocated the task of isolating and purifying pituitary ACTH stimulating the adrenal cortex.

Li now needed sufficient pituitary glands for investigations on both growth hormone and ACTH. However paradoxically the war effort had both stimulated pituitary gland research and created a gland famine. In 1942 meat rationing was imposed. The number of animals reaching slaughterhouses was limited by edict, the price of meat was held down, and civilians were issued coupons. Americans who before the war were eating 400 million pounds of red meat each week had to suffer the ignominy of a diet of fowl and herrings. It was relatively easy for the authorities to monitor the activities of the large meatpackers, and the throughput of their disassembly lines fell. But a thriving under-the-counter trade developed that was reputed to be shifting as many animals as the law-abiding meatpackers. Illegal meat traders treated scientists seeking glands with suspicion, as if they were agents of the Federal Government in disguise, and refused to help.[45]

Making matters worse, able-bodied men were being called up into the armed forces, and the meatpackers lacked the muscle to operate the splitting machine. As a favour to the University of California, a slaughterhouse in Oakland agreed to collect some pituitary glands but the most it could provide met just under one tenth of Li's monthly requirement of seventy pounds. By dint of begging, cajoling and calling in favours, Evans managed to obtain sufficient glands to keep Li occupied. His reward came in January 1944 when the journal *Science* announced their success in isolating a comparatively pure preparation of growth hormone.[46] The popular press heralded their achievement as an important contribution to the war effort: a substance capable of making short people taller might resolve the inferiority complex and aggression of undersized people like the Japanese. A journalist provided Evans with the first indication of the size of the home market for it: 'The world is waiting, especially we here in the East who are tired of wearing elevator shoes and submitting to other forms of artificial height.'[47] However, Evans said social engineering on this scale would be far too expensive. Two pounds of anterior lobes yielded just one-thousandth of an ounce of growth hormone.[48]

Furthermore Evans faced enormous difficulties in accumulating sufficient glands for the experiment: the meat industry was experiencing yet another crisis. In the autumn of 1946, slaughtering of cattle fell to 80 per cent of 1945 levels, and, in Chicago, 5,000 packing house workers were laid off. Armour had no glands to spare; it was hundreds of pounds behind in the production of its own pituitary hormones, including proprietary pituitrin and organotherapeutic preparations of growth hormone and needed at least twelve months to meet outstanding orders.[49] Evans was compelled to import glands from New Zealand and South America at an exorbitant price. Between 1947 and 1948 he spent more than $16,000 on glands compared to $5,000 in the previous year.[50]

Preparations for a test on a patient were made nevertheless. These included sending some growth-hormone soup to the state Virus Laboratory where it was passed through a filter which excluded bacterial-sized particles. Investigators also tested the safety of the substance by pricking their skin and smearing some on the punctures, and then when nothing untoward occurred, injecting small amounts into a muscle. It was then considered safe to administer the hormone to a child. The first 'guinea pig' was 'F.H.', a young woman aged sixteen years and eight months, who stood at just less than fifty inches tall. In the previous year, she had had the pituitary glands of two freshly slaughtered calves grafted into her stomach. In the spring of 1947, in a tiny private room in the hospital of the University of California Medical School, San Francisco, she embarked on an exacting regime of daily injections of beef growth hormone. The only food F.H. was allowed was a fortified milkshake. At the end of three months she had grown $3/_8$". Released from the hospital, she submitted to the injections for several more months. But her growth rate remained the same as before treatment. The last her doctors heard of her was when she wrote to them from Paris, France, asking permission to get married.[51] Beef growth hormone may have made rats grow into giants, but it didn't work in humans. In 1949, Armour stopped selling it.

Meatpackers become Meat-and-Medicine Businesses

Ironically, disappointment with beef growth hormone coincided with the decision of the National Institutes of Health (NIH) to shield investigators from the vicissitudes of the meat market. In 1948, its Metabolism and Endocrinology Study Section had struck a deal with Armour. For its part, Armour would collect under specific and controlled conditions 500 pounds of pituitary glands from different species and distribute them to investigators approved by the NIH. Armour, in return, would be paid the current market price of the glands, and the NIH awarded the Study Section a grant of $30,000 to reimburse the company. As additional compensation for inconvenience and any extra costs incurred, Armour would be the first company to learn of any exciting findings.[52]

The NIH's decision was a response to the first clinical trial of a substance called Compound E which famously allowed patients long crippled with arthritis to walk and even dance. Made out of the adrenal cortex, Compound E – renamed cortisone – joined penicillin and streptomycin, archetypal postwar magic bullets.[53] But forty head of cattle were needed to treat one person for one day. As there were 7 million people with arthritis in the USA, around 3,000 million head of cattle – many more than the nation's entire herd – would have to be slaughtered every year. A search for an alternative method of production began. The following year, the first clinical trial of ACTH – now sometimes called corticotrophin because it is the hormone that stimulates natural cortisone production in the body – took place and proved as miraculous as cortisone: patients racked with rheumatic fever were completely changed within 48 hours, and victims of crippling rheumatoid arthritis were able to dance a jig.

ACTH also provided Li with the means of escaping Evans's clutches. Despite his achievements, he was poorly paid and endured terrible working conditions: Evans had relegated him to a closet-sized, overheated basement laboratory through which the university's main steam lines sizzled and rats ran, and he was often obliged to leave his bed in the middle of the night to open the windows of the laboratory to prevent the excess heat from spoiling a delicate experiment.[54] While studying chromatography in Sweden in the laboratory of Arne Tiselius, winner of the Nobel Prize in 1948, Li had received offers of jobs from other American universities. As he was about to accept one of them, a cablegram arrived from the University of California: 'Come back and you can have almost anything you want'. On his return to Berkeley, Li was appointed Professor of Biochemistry and made director of The Hormone Research Laboratory which had been established specifically for him.

Li entered the race to map the structure of the ACTH molecule. But Armour refused to part with pituitary glands. The company, at this stage, no longer needed his expertise. It had established its own laboratory, and scientists in the company's employ were undertaking basic and applied research which – ironically – was building on Li's work, and resulted in the isolation in hog pituitaries of a relatively pure preparation of ACTH.[55] It was Armour's ACTH that had first demonstrated that the hormone was capable of eliciting in the clinic dramatic results similar to that of Compound E. In July the company announced it was beginning production of ACTHAR, its brand of ACTH, at the rate of sixty pounds a year. But it took 400,000 hogs to produce one pound of the hormone which was valued at $10,000.[56] Armour needed every single pituitary gland produced in its thirty-four packing plants.

The demand for hog pituitaries had leapt up in response to news of the dramatic effects of ACTH, and the price per pound rose from $8 to $25.[57] Li was saved by his friend, K. K. Chen of the Animal Products Purchasing Department of Eli Lilly, who agreed to use his connections in the meat industry and secure a large quantity of sheep pituitary glands. Unfortunately for Li, in 1953, Armour and American Cyanamid beat him to the finishing line. Li claimed he would have won if confirmation of his results had not been delayed by a fire in the warehouse where his stock of frozen glands was held.[58] Furthermore his method proved to be too involved and expensive for commercial application: 360,000 sheep pituitary glands yielded only two grams of ACTH at a cost of $28,000.[59] That same year Armour opened a $12 million laboratory and manufacturing centre for its pharmaceuticals.[60]

Conclusion

Success achieved during the endocrinological goldrush was dependent not simply on intellectual and technological supremacy so much as the capacity to lay claim to abattoir waste in much the same way as success in the 'real' goldrush depended on the capacity to lay claim to valuable real property. Medical historians Jean-Paul Gaudillière and Ilana Löwy identify in scholars and science policymakers a tendency of rarely admitting in public the importance of industry for fundamental research.[61] Hiding industry's often crucial role, they argue, creates an unrealistic division between the production of knowledge and the market, and allows biomedical research to be idealized as a noble disinterested pursuit free of the corrupting influence of the market. However Gaudillière and Löwy envisage scientists as consumers, perusing manufacturers' catalogues for the best state-of-the-art instruments and the purest reagents. It is undoubtedly the case that industrialists are admitted into the university laboratory via the cash nexus. But much biomedical research requires biotrash for which no market exists.

Another characteristic of waste is its capacity to transform. By the time the endocrinological gold research came to an end, the boundary separating disassembly line and university laboratory had been realigned. Some meatpackers had become meat-and-medicine businesses, but the social world of the university laboratory had also been altered in a variety of ways. Evans is reputed to have been a difficult man who irritated almost everyone who came into contact with him, a tendency which goes some way to explain why he was never awarded the high honours some claim he deserved.[62] The technical expertise in and growing reputation of Evans's laboratory had initially strengthened his bargaining power. But the logic of the meat market, its strategic importance in the United States during the Second World War and Armour's decision to invest in its own laboratory liberated the company from any dependence it had on academic investigators. However, Evans attempted to maintain the illusion that the social worlds of the university laboratory and disassembly line were distinct, perhaps in an attempt to protect the high-minded values of science from contamination by the reputation of the disreputable and powerful Chicago meatpackers. Other scientists working in the field found ways of profiting through their engagement with the meat market. For instance, Ernst Laqueur (1880–1947), a German biochemist working at the University of Amsterdam on sex hormones, in 1923, reached an arrangement with Saal van Zwanenberg, the director of a Dutch slaughterhouse, which resulted in the creation of a new company, the Organon Limited Company for the Manufacture of Organ Preparations on a Scientific Basis, with Laquer serving as its scientific director.[63]

4 WHAT'S MEATPACKING GOT TO DO WITH WORKER AND COMMUNITY HEALTH?

Donald D. Stull and Michael J. Broadway

and thou shalt say, I will eat flesh, because thy soul longeth to eat flesh...then thou shalt kill of thy herd and of thy flock, which the Lord hath given thee... Ye shall not eat of any thing that dieth of itself...

Deuteronomy 12:20, 21; 14:21

Most Americans come to know meat only through the grocery store and the restaurant. But meat must be made, and it can only be made by the slaughter of animals. In fact, the Judeo-Christian tradition forbids the eating of animals that die by other than human hands. The slaughter and dismemberment that transform 'animal to edible', to borrow Noëlie Vialles's[1] telling phrase, may be essential in the making of animals into meat, but most of us prefer to remain ignorant of where our meat comes from.

The Jungle,[2] Upton Sinclair's damning expose of the packing-houses of Chicago, is now more than a century old. But for all the years and all the progress touted by industry spokesmen, knockers still start the killing. And, today's stickers and gutters, tail rippers and head droppers, chuckboners and short ribbers, still use steels to hone the edges of their knives as they turn hundreds of cattle or hogs by the hour into meat.

Packing-houses remain, as they were a century ago, massive factories, employing thousands of workers. But instead of the Serbian and Polish workers of Sinclair's day, today's meatpacking plants are crowded with immigrants and refugees from Mexico and Guatemala, Somalia and Sudan. Immigrants remain attracted to packing-house jobs because command of English is unnecessary, and because the wages they earn on the 'disassembly' lines are better than they can expect elsewhere.

In Sinclair's day, cattle were raised on the plains and prairies of North America and shipped by rail for slaughter in packing-houses in the stockyard districts of Chicago, St. Louis, Denver and other major Midwestern cities. But the Kansas

City stockyards have been razed; the pens and barns of the Fort Worth stock-yards now hold honkytonks and boutiques instead of cattle and hogs; and the stock pens of Toronto's meatpacking district have been replaced with the largest Home Depot in Canada.

Urban stockyards and packing-houses are gone, but demand for the meat they once provided is not. In their place, giant modern meat processing plants have sprung up across rural North America, from beef plants on the plains of Kansas and Alberta to pork plants in Oklahoma and Manitoba to chicken plants in Maryland and Kentucky.

Packing-houses at the beginning of the twenty-first century are a far cry from those at the beginning of the twentieth. But for all their computerization and laser technology, their robotics and ergonomics, the knife, the meathook and the steel are still the basic tools of the trade. And today's plants remain, like the ones they replaced, rigidly organized, labour-intensive factories that slaughter animals and turn them into meat.

We begin with a brief historical overview of meatpacking's transformation from an urban, relatively high-wage industry with a unionized workforce into a rural industry characterized by low wages and dramatically diminished union influence. Next, we review the industry's recent health and safety record, and then analyse the effects of meatpacking on worker and community health.

Our introduction to the meat and poultry industry began in 1987, when we collaborated on a study of relations between new immigrants and established residents in Garden City, Kansas. Refugees from Southeast Asia and migrants from Mexico and elsewhere in Latin America were flocking to Garden City to work in its two beef plants, one the world's largest. We soon realized that to understand the socioeconomic forces at play in Garden City, we needed to understand the beef industry itself. Our study of ethnic relations in Garden City concluded in 1990, but our research on meatpacking's consequences for its workers and host communities had only just begun. It has taken us to farms and ranches from Oklahoma to Alberta and from Maryland to Manitoba. We have listened to packing-house workers describe their work over beers and stood alongside them as they wielded knives and saws on the killfloor. We have listened to them describe dismal working conditions and disabling injuries in court-rooms and living rooms. And we have worked with educators, clergy, healthcare providers, police and concerned citizens first in Garden City, and later in Lexing-ton, Nebraska; Guymon, Oklahoma; Webster County, Kentucky; and Brooks, Alberta, Canada, as they grapple with the massive changes and daunting chal-lenges packing-houses bring to the communities where our meat is made. The two decades we have spent studying the meat and poultry industry have taught us the human cost of our meat for those who make it and for the communities in which they live and work.[3]

Cutting Costs and Workers

Meatpacking has always been marginally profitable and dependent upon immigrant labour. In the early 1900s meatpackers attempted to increase productivity by lowering wages and increasing output. They did this by replacing skilled butchers with unskilled workers. They replaced German and Irish workers, who had dominated the industry since the early 1880s, with recent immigrants from Eastern Europe. The founder of one of America's largest meatpacking firms at the turn of the twentieth century, Philip Armour, admitted that his company deliberately tried to deter unionism by replacing experienced workers, who might be disillusioned, with newly arrived immigrants. But rather than target a specific nationality, the company preferred hiring immigrants from many different countries, hoping to hamper communication between workers. When strikes did occur, African Americans were recruited as replacement workers.[4]

Sixty years later, the same capitalist imperatives of cutting costs and boosting productivity underpinned the so-called IBP revolution. In 1960, Iowa Beef Packers (IBP) built its first plant in Denison, Iowa, two hours northwest of Des Moines. By locating the plant in a cattle-producing region, rather than adjacent to urban stockyards, IBP lowered its transport costs and reduced the bruising and shrinkage associated with shipping cattle long distances. At the same time, it eliminated stockyard middlemen by purchasing cattle directly from farmers and ranchers.[5]

The Denison plant, unlike its urban counterparts, was a one-story structure that allowed 'on the line dressing'. The animal is first stunned; then suspended by a hind leg before moving continuously along an overhead rail past stationary workers who each perform a single task necessary to dismantle the carcass.[6] The company's founder acknowledged the goal behind the 'disassembly' line was 'to take the skill out of every step of butchering'.[7] IBP used this 'deskilling' to justify paying lower wages and benefits and avoid the terms of the existing industry-wide union master contract. This strategy was enhanced by locating plants in right-to-work states, such as Iowa, Nebraska, Kansas and Texas, where it is harder for labour unions to organize. The company also lowered costs by using economies of scale to construct large-capacity plants close to supplies of fed cattle on the High Plains. These plants have low unit costs per animal slaughtered and are able to spread fixed costs (electricity, water) over two shifts, making them more profitable to operate than smaller plants.[8]

Union efforts during and after World War II produced a master contract establishing industry-wide work standards and wages that were 15 per cent *above* the average manufacturing wage in 1960. Faced with a lower-cost producer, IBP's competitors broke union contracts, sought pay cuts through collective bargaining, or went bankrupt. The net effect was a steep decline in meatpacking wages, and by 2002 they had fallen to 25 per cent *below* the average manufacturing wage.[9]

Declining wages are only part of the story. Demand for beef is seasonal, and workers' hours are increased or decreased with fluctuations in cattle supplies and consumer demand. It is true that packers offer health and life insurance, paid vacations, and yearly bonuses, but workers are not eligible for such benefits for several months. Many do not last that long.

Low wages and disagreeable working conditions contribute to high employee turnover. For its first twenty-one months of operation, *monthly* turnover among line workers at IBP's Lexington, Nebraska, beef plant averaged 12 per cent.[10] When IBP opened the world's largest beef plant in Finney County, Kansas, in 1980, turnover reached as high as 60 per cent a month.[11] Turnover is lower for established plants, but, even so, it far exceeds that of most other industries. Worker turnover for established beef plants in Kansas and Nebraska averages 6–8 per cent a month, and a 10 per cent monthly turnover has been reported for an established pork plant in Iowa.[12]

The industry's insatiable appetite for workers means local labour pools are quickly exhausted, and plants recruit from far and wide. Employees are often paid bonuses of $150–200 for recruiting new workers if they remain on the job past the probationary period of 90–120 days. This practice fosters chain migration and the emergence of immigrant enclaves, usually from specific sending communities, in packing towns.[13] The sudden population growth accompanying the establishment of meatpacking plants in rural areas exacerbates problems of healthcare provision, since these areas are traditionally medically underserved.[14]

Disassembling Cattle; Disabling Workers

Carlos was in his late twenties; he did not speak English. He started work at IBP on June 20, 1988, and was injured on October 15, 1989. He made $7.25 an hour 'pulling ribs', which involved grabbing a piece of meat in one hand and pulling the rib out of it with the other – which hands he used depended on whether he was pulling right ribs or left ribs. He made the same motion – a hard jerk – twelve times a minute. As he was doing this on October 15, he heard a pop and felt a sharp pain on the end of his fourth rib. He told his foreman – Walter – that he couldn't go on. Walter sent him to the nurse, who just rubbed it. For the next three–four weeks he'd go in to work and the nurse would rub it down, and he would continue to work. Finally IBP sent him to Dr. X, the company doctor. Dr. X saw him for three weeks and said he couldn't do anything for him, then sent him to Dr. Y, who diagnosed Carlos as having a stress fracture and recommended he return to work on 'light duty'. He was returned to light duty on January 23, 1989, and assigned to pick small pieces of meat off the bone and inspect boxes as they went by on the line. After about four hours the supervisor – Mike – told him to go home; they didn't have a job for him till he could do full work. They have not recalled him or paid him.

Carlos's attorney asked the judge to grant him temporary partial disability, since he could do light duty but IBP would not allow him to come back to work. IBP's attorney argued that Carlos's injury was not work related, since you couldn't break a rib doing that job. Carlos's attorney countered that a stress fracture was well within the line of possibility for this type of work. IBP's attorney questioned Carlos about riding and training horses, suggesting this as a plausible explanation of his injury. Carlos maintained that although he had trained horses on a ranch in Mexico, he had not ridden since he came to the United States ... The judge denied temporary total and temporary partial disability and ordered an exam by Dr. Y.[15]

Work in a meatpacking plant has always been dangerous. In 1917, eleven years after *The Jungle* was published, and long before the federal government required companies to report worker injuries or illnesses, the welfare director of Chicago's Armour plant reported that 50 per cent of the company's 22,381 workers became ill at work or were injured over the course of the year. Barrett[16] attributes the high injury rate to using sharp knives and working in a damp and cold environment, as well as the speed at which work was accomplished.

By the time we began studying meatpacking in the 1980s, workers were required to wear hardhats, safety glasses, earplugs, steel-toed and rubber-soled boots, and an amazing array of additional gear intended to protect them from injury. Even so, meatpacking had the highest injury and illness rate of any industry in America throughout much of the last quarter of the twentieth century.[17]

Meatpacking's reported occupational injury and illness rate hovered between 30.4 and 36.9 per 100 full-time workers from 1975 to 1985 – around three times the average for manufacturing overall. From there meatpacking's rates sharply increased till they peaked in 1992 at 44.4/100.[18] Skyrocketing injury and illness rates made meatpacking the target of congressional committee hearings and the Department of Labor's Occupational Safety and Health Administration (OSHA). In the late 1980s and early 90s, OSHA successfully secured record fines against several meatpacking companies for underreporting injuries and unsafe practices. The unwanted publicity, coupled with declines in the packers' labour pool and rising workers' compensation costs, forced companies to pay more attention to safety.[19]

In 1993 OSHA published its *Ergonomics Programs Management Guidelines for Meatpacking Plants*.[20] The guidelines were designed to help employers identify and correct worksite ergonomic-related problems. Government researchers working with union and management representatives recommended the establishment of packing-house ergonomic teams consisting of production workers, supervisors and maintenance/engineering staff.[21] Ergonomists try to improve equipment and tool design, while new workers receive training and conditioning to protect them from injury, supervisors are held accountable for accidents on their crews, and incentives are offered for reducing accidents.

The most significant illnesses and injuries in meatpacking are associated with musculoskeletal disorders, arising from repetitive motions, most notably, carpal tunnel syndrome: 'a condition in which the nerve passing through the wrist to the hand is pinched and compressed because of fast repeated forceful motions'.[22] It 'can frequently lead to severe nerve damage, and the crippling of the hand or wrist, making it impossible for workers to grip or pick up everyday objects'.[23]

Between 1979 and 1986 the incidence of repeated trauma disorder among meatpacking workers increased by nearly 300 per cent, reaching a rate of 479/10,000 full-time workers, while the comparable rate for manufacturing workers was just 22/10,000.[24] In response, Secretary of Labor Elizabeth Dole initiated a study of repetitive motion injuries in 1990. Ten years later, President Bill Clinton concluded this process by issuing a set of ergonomic standards designed to reduce on-the-job repetitive motion injuries. According to OSHA, the standard would prevent more than 4.6 million injuries over 10 years.[25]

Within days of taking office in 2001, President George W. Bush signed a repeal of the ergonomic standard, stating that his administration would pursue a 'comprehensive approach' to ergonomic injuries. This approach consisted of issuing voluntary guidelines to specific industries and changing injury reporting requirements. In 2002, a new work accident report form was introduced that lacked a column for musculoskeletal disorders. A year later OSHA decided employers do not have to record when workers report ergonomic injuries.[26] The effect has been dramatic.

Between 2000 and 2004 meatpacking's occupational injury and illness rate dropped from 24.7/100 full-time workers to 13.3, while the comparable figures for repeated trauma went from 812/10,000 workers in 2000 to who knows what in 2004,[27] when the government no longer collected the data! Whether this most recent decline is real, due to underreporting or changes in reporting procedures, or aided by Bureau of Labor Statistics (BLS) sleight of hand that fails to classify plant cleanup crews as meatpacking workers because they work on contract – or, more likely, a combination of all four – the fact remains that rates have declined since the early 1990s. Even so, the reported injury and illness rate for meatpacking is still twice the manufacturing rate.

Responding to charges by Human Rights Watch[28] that the meat and poultry industry blatantly disregards its workers' safety, J. Patrick Doyle,[29] president and chief executive officer of the American Meat Institute, pointed proudly to the fact that 'injury and illness rates in the meatpacking industry have been declining steadily over the past 15 years ... If [Human Rights Watch] can't accept the idea that we do the right thing just because it's right and we have a strong collective conscience, maybe they can believe that we do it because it's also financially beneficial and required by federal regulations.' As proof of packer commitment to safety in the workplace, the American Meat Institute points to the *Ergonom-*

ics Program Management Guidelines for Meat Packing Plants it developed jointly
with OSHA and to the cooperative alliance it entered into with OSHA in 2002
to 'foster a culture of illness and injury prevention in meat plants'.[30]

'Safety First' at Running Iron Beef[31]

Running Iron Beef (a pseudonym) is owned by one of North America's biggest
food processing companies. The plant we studied in 1994 slaughtered about
5,000 head of cattle a day, six days a week, and employed over 2,000 workers.
Two-thirds of the workforce was Hispanic, one-fourth white, one-tenth Asian.
But overall figures are misleading: three-quarters of the plant's officials and managers were white males, and 7 per cent were white females; 11 per cent were
Hispanic men and 2 per cent Hispanic women. The majority of workers classi-
fied as unskilled were Hispanic men (61 per cent), followed by Hispanic women
(13 per cent) and white men (12 per cent).

Its employee handbook said that Running Iron Beef 'is dedicated to quality
and safety . . . to 'doing it right the first time', and 'doing it safely at all times'.
'Safety first' appeared on bulletin boards and walls throughout the plant. Safety
was highlighted and reinforced in celebrations and rituals. It was prominent in
corporate and plant competitions, awards, training meetings and paperwork.
Supervisors who failed to turn in their safety-meeting records were rebuked on
bulletin boards and in company memoranda. Injured employees could be called
into upper management's morning meeting to explain how they were hurt and
suggest what the plant might do to prevent such occurrences.

'Safety' was always written first on maintenance supervisors' 'to-do' lists. But
as they went to and from their office and the plant floors, they discussed work
priorities, allocation of time and effort and strategies to solve pressing problems.
They didn't talk about safety, except to laugh and say 'Safety second!'

'Nothing gets fixed until someone gets hurt', was the most prevalent and bitter complaint heard from line workers. Part of the problem was that many in
positions of authority 'pass the buck' to avoid being held accountable. That 'they
only fix it after someone gets hurt' was born out by management's regular discussion of problems after, rather than before, they resulted in physical harm to an
employee. This pattern repeated itself at all levels in the plant.

When we carried out our research in 1994, Running Iron Beef's full-time
safety coordinator had been in place for three years. His job was to identify
potential problems and ensure they were rectified. The safety coordinator had
responsibility but no authority. Every month he recommended improvements
in equipment and crewing. Invariably, many were repeats from previous months
because safety recommendations were often in direct conflict with the needs of
line supervisors and floor managers to keep production rates up. Superintendents

and supervisors 'don't want to see the chain shut down'. The safety coordinator told us he had even been told he would be put back on the chuckboning line if he shut down the line for any reason.

Safety regulations require workers on certain lines to wear safety glasses, but a foreman of one such line didn't believe they were necessary, so he didn't enforce the rule or write his people up for not wearing them. If one of his crew didn't wear glasses or lost them, and was called on it by the safety coordinator, the foreman just got the worker another pair. Eventually the problem was resolved in the safety coordinator's favour, but it took a reprimand of the foreman by the assistant plant manager. Still, the safety coordinator had to complain over and over. 'It takes an injury to get anything done', he told us. 'It takes people to buy into an issue to get them to enforce the regulations. Safety is not the priority; production is.'

Getting Hurt and Workers' Compensation

It was common opinion among line workers that, as a workers' compensation workshop leader aptly put it, 'If you get injured at Running Iron, you're gonna get fired'. Workers on light duty 'get disrespected just because they are injured, even though they may have put in ten or twelve good years here – that's not right', according to a utility leadman, the second in command on a line crew.

> 'In the first 45 days they can fire you for any reason, and the union can't do anything', according to one union steward. 'Trainers are not supposed to be in the line, but they get put in the line if they're short crewed. Put them in the line and injuries go up because foremans [*sic*] push new hires like everybody else. The company tells us to tell them if things are wrong. You tell them and you tell them and you tell them, and nothing happens. Pretty soon, you just don't give a shit. And if you report something to the USDA [inspector], the company gets mad'.

Injured workers are often viewed as malingerers who want to work the system to their advantage. In the morning meeting, for example, the case of Eusebio (a pseudonym), who had a shoulder strain, was brought up. He got a lawyer to help him get a job change. According to the manager reporting on this case, 'It doesn't matter what he does, he hurts. When he drives to work it hurts. He has the perfect lawyer answers to everything. 'Yes, I'll do whatever you want, but it hurts'. Senior managers commonly believed malingerers get a lawyer, who encourages them to 'milk the company' so the lawyer can get his cut of the settlement. While this may have been true on occasion, managers avoided facing the reality that injury in the service of the company wrecks the health of many workers. Managers did, of course, recognize that injury and illness are very much a part of their industry and that loyal employees may be left debilitated at the end of long years of company service. They shrugged, laughed ironically and attributed such injuries to 'just plain old packing-house wear and tear'.

Line workers said the 'workers' comp problem' is not people faking it, as management contended, but 'it's people getting hurt'. If you were injured, the company gave you a hard time and tried its best to avoid its legal obligations. For example, some workers said the company tried to get around the law on things like paying mileage for trips to the doctor. Company doctors had a reputation for putting Running Iron's interests over those of injured workers. Once injured employees were returned to work, critics charged that they were often ill-informed of their restrictions or supervisors just ignored them.

Managers commonly contended that the rise in workers' compensation claims was due to fraud, attorney greed, and the 'Mexican dream': getting a good settlement from workers' comp, moving back to Mexico and buying a *ranchito* (little ranch). This attitude was especially prevalent among managers who remembered the 'old days' when you 'worked through' pain and injury. Old-timers swapped war stories and showed each other their scars. They reminisced of days when supervisors patched up injured workers with Super Glue and electric tape, then sent them back to the line. 'Workers were sore back then but they worked through their soreness. People are not as hard working now and don't want to put up with it'. Such stories were a matter of pride, and though the tellers made the point of how things had changed, they seemed almost nostalgic for the days when it was a rough and ready industry. Nostalgia for the old days was no doubt influenced by supervisors' responsibility for daily production quotas.

Chain speed and crewing are important factors in maintaining a safe work environment. Sufficient crewing is essential to productivity. According to several plant managers, 'Corporate' just counts bodies, but it is the ratio of qualified to unqualified bodies that really matters. And even though people go off probation after forty-five days, they can't be expected to qualify till ninety days have passed. One week in July 1994, for example, one in five workers on first-shift Fabrication (where the carcass is broken down) had been on the job less than ninety days.

Safety Meetings

Supervisors were required to hold monthly safety and quality meetings. These meetings were supposed to last thirty minutes but supervisors invariably tried to finish in fifteen because of the cost. Workers often pointed out problems, but supervisors usually brushed these points aside, saying, 'Yeah, yeah, we'll look into it'. Supervisors didn't want to let meetings turn into 'bitch sessions', and they didn't want to let them run on because workers were 'on the clock' but weren't 'getting product out the door'. So, these meetings were often held on days when the shift was ending early, or supervisors stopped the shift early to avoid paying overtime.

Clear communication and demonstrated effectiveness were missing from safety meetings, despite the regular, ritualized attention these meetings received. Meeting effectiveness was compromised by: 1) language barriers between many supervisors and their crews; 2) the eagerness of first-shift workers to leave work and the second-shift supervisors to get their crews out on the floor; and 3) what workers perceived as supervisors' lack of sincerity regarding quality and safety, which reflected a plant-wide mismatch between the ideal of safety and the daily reality of keeping the line running.

A safety meeting following first shift one afternoon was a case in point. The line supervisor was an Anglo who later claimed to speak Spanish 'well enough to get by'. But during the meeting he spoke only in English to his 'safety rep', a slight Latina. When he finished each phrase, she spoke to the crew – about thirty mostly Mexican men – in Spanish. When he spoke, he looked at her, never at his crew. He was very stern, lecturing his crew to keep their knives in their scabbards when they weren't in use, or they would be fired. The men listened in silence, some smiled slightly when they heard the translation. The supervisor then dismissed them with a perfunctory '*hasta manana*' ('until tomorrow'), and they bolted for the door.

Nursing should play a key role in plant safety, but the morning meeting pattern of dealing with problems rather than preventing them extended to the company nurses. When 'Corporate' suggested to nursing staff that they do more prevention and check-up activities, they reacted fearfully that such measures would actually result in more injuries to report and, therefore, more problems for them to deal with.

Safety messages suffered from the same troubles that plagued much of Running Iron's communication. But these problems went beyond inadequate and often incorrect translation and interpretation, which presented serious problems in and of themselves. More fundamentally, they related to the intrinsic conflict of talking 'safety first', but placing prevention second after today's injury, lost time or broken machinery. Written slogans about safety were poorly translated into Spanish, absent in Lao and Vietnamese, which were also spoken by a number of workers, and did not reflect reality on the floor. Written curricula and orientation about safety actually reinforced employee unwillingness to report safety problems because responsibility for safety was placed on individual workers. Training was so general and 'canned' that it was not responsive to new training needs. When employees did report safety issues, they could not always expect a response. This led them to conclude that reporting was not worthwhile. Of course, if potential safety problems were not reported they were not discussed at safety meetings, which resulted in more injuries and less trust.

All I hear is safety this and safety that. It's all I hear 90 per cent of the time. We got into it, well, that meeting we had last week, we had one employee who came here and was complaining about where he was working. He was having trouble with it. When he went back, I went over to talk to the foreman. He said 'Okay.' That was it. This was on a Monday. On Thursday morning the employee went back in and told him, 'Hey, I'm still having the same problem. They haven't fixed it.' And the foreman just shook his head and shrugged. A couple of hours later the employee cut his finger off.[32]

'They Don't Just Kill Cows, They Kill People. They Kill Them Inside'

Work on a meatpacking line is 'manly' work: workers must be tough, hard and, at times, mean. 'We don't change their diapers for 'em', is the attitude of management, from 'the suits' in corporate board rooms through plant managers down to line supervisors. Line workers must 'pull their count'. Those who can't are quickly shown the door.

Out on the floor, the pressure is constant: 'get the product out the door' as quickly and as cheaply as possible. Despite protestations to the contrary, formal training for line workers is minimal and of poor quality. 'Watch a film and hit the floor' is how one former IBP worker described his orientation. It was no different when Stull went through Running Iron's new-hire training in the summer of 1994.

Hourly workers are constantly pushed to go faster, and competition between shifts is encouraged. Supervisors relentlessly push crews, armed with stopwatches and the ever-present threat to 'show the slow ones the door'. Lines designed to run at 280 head an hour may put out 430 head an hour. Workers constantly complain they cannot do their jobs right because chains run too fast and lines are 'short crewed'.

Meatpacking wears its hourly workers out and then wears them down – physically, mentally, and emotionally. As a former meatpacking worker and union representative put it: 'They don't just kill cows, they kill people. They kill them inside'.

Poor training, dismal and dangerous working conditions and constant pressure to pull count are a sure formula for high turnover, especially in the dangerous knife and saw jobs. Plant managers dream of annual turnover rates of 36–50 per cent. In fact, they don't even talk in terms of annual rates or turnover. They speak, instead, of monthly rates: 7 per cent turnover sounds so much better than 84 per cent, after all. Besides, monthly rates more accurately reflect the constant movement of workers in and out of the plants.

Meatpacking plants must have a steady supply of new workers. Workers are recruited through a combination of techniques: print and electronic advertisements run constantly in meatpacking towns and areas of high unemployment; bonuses are paid to employees who recruit new workers who make it past the probationary period; travel loans and promises of transitional housing (at shelters in host communities) are used to entice applicants in distant towns. What is waiting for those who travel long distances for these jobs is often misrepresented, and the resources of local communities are exploited without permission or compensation.

Turnover is tacitly encouraged because it helps keep wages and workers' compensation costs down. It also mitigates against union organizing. As in the days of *The Jungle*, today's meat and poultry companies rely heavily on vulnerable classes of labourers to work on their lines – minorities, women and especially immigrants. They can be paid less. Industry executives also believe they will work harder, put up with worse working conditions and be less likely to organize or assert their rights (even if they know them). And the very presence of immigrants on the line serves as a warning to native-born workers that they can always be replaced.

What all this means is that turnover is the dominant demographic process at work in communities that host meatpacking plants. Population mobility is felt in every aspect of the community – housing, traffic, healthcare, social services, crime, schools and more. For example, in 1997, the year Seaboard Corporation opened its pork plant in Guymon, Oklahoma, there were over 2,000 new residential utility connections in town, but by the following April (1998) only one-third were still active. Garden City, Kansas, a community we have studied since 1987, was home to two major beef processing plants during the 1980s and 90s. Among the many problems it faces as a result of recurrent population mobility is an elevated rate of pupil turnover in its public schools: 35–45 per cent of students are not enrolled for the entire year, and in some elementary schools annual turnover exceeds 100 per cent.[33]

Packers initially recruit young men, the demographic group with the highest mobility levels, but over time the newcomer profile changes to include young families. The community health implications of this change are illustrated in Brooks, Alberta, a town of 13,000, 120 miles east of Calgary. In the late 1990s when Lakeside Packers was hiring about 2,000 workers to staff a newly expanded beef plant two miles outside of town, Brooks experienced an explosion in alcohol-related incidents. The number of persons detained by the Royal Canadian Mounted Police (RCMP) because they were a danger to themselves tripled – from 128 in 1996 to 398 a year later. Persons detained for other provincial liquor-act violations doubled – from 165 to 308 – during the same period.[34] Several highly publicized fights broke out between newcomers and established residents outside of local bars. In September 1997 over 100 people were involved in a brawl, and when the RCMP appeared on the scene they were attacked by the mob.[35] Alcohol-related problems also affected the packing plant – between fifty and seventy-five workers routinely failed to report to work the day after payday because they were incapacitated from drinking the night before.[36]

Lakeside's recruitment practices contributed to these problems by targeting young men in areas of high unemployment in Newfoundland, Nova Scotia and British Columbia. Men between the ages of eighteen and twenty-four have the highest frequency of heavy drinking, while single persons are three times more likely to have alcohol-related problems than married persons, and Atlantic Canada has the highest proportion of persons reporting alcohol-related problems.[37]

The population spike that accompanied the plant's expansion exacerbated the shortage of healthcare professionals. Difficulties in finding a local doctor and taking time off work to schedule a visit with a family practitioner forced many newcomers to use the local hospital's emergency room (ER) for routine medical care. Between 1996 and 1997 visits to the ER jumped 20 per cent, while Brooks's population increased by just 10 per cent.[38]

New Immigrants, Packing-Houses and Community Health

Domestic labour sources are quickly exhausted, and packers turn to immigrants and refugees to staff their lines. At Lakeside, immigrants and refugees account for about 60 per cent of the labour force and an even higher percentage of line workers. Following on an expansion in its slaughter capacity, a protracted labour dispute in 2005 and increased competition for workers from a booming oil and gas industry, Lakeside is working hand in hand with Alberta's provincial government to recruit workers directly from China, El Salvador, the Philippines and the Ukraine.[39] Thus far, Lakeside's recruitment bonuses, and sponsorship of immigrants and refugees by family members, have drawn about 3,500 refugees to Brooks from the Sudan, Ethiopia, Somalia and the Democratic Republic of the Congo, as well as Pakistan and Afghanistan. In just seven years – from 1998 to 2005 – Brooks was transformed from a typical western Canadian small town with a smattering of minorities into a multicultural and multilingual community where 100 different languages and dialects can be heard.

Accompanying population growth from in-migration was a spike in the town's birth rate – from 17/1,000 in 1996 to an estimated 19/1,000 in 2005. This was in marked contrast to what happened in the rest of the province, as Alberta's birth rate dropped from 14/1,000 to 12/1000. In absolute terms, the number of babies born to women with a Brooks home address went from 165 in 1996 to 247 in 2005 – a 50 per cent increase. The multiplicity of newcomer languages and cultures creates serious challenges for healthcare providers. In pre-natal care, for example, Muslim women prefer to be seen by a woman and are reluctant to discuss their health concerns with men. The idea of couples attending Lamaze classes is also alien to them.

The local hospital has attempted to address the language issue by subscribing to US-based Language Line, which advertises itself 'as providing fast, accurate, confidential language interpretation in 150 languages'. But this service, which requires the patient and staff member to each wear a headset, is not really suitable for emergency situations where decisive intervention may be needed. An ER nurse noted that patients sometimes resort to miming their symptoms, leaving nurses and doctors to guess the ailment.[40]

The emergency room continues to be the area where many newcomers access the healthcare system. A nurse explained the problem this way:

> A Lakeside employee who works the B shift will come home late at night and take a look in on their children and if one doesn't look quite right they will take them to the ER at 3.00 a.m. This makes little sense from our perspective, since follow-up visits are usually called for and the patient ends up seeing another doctor who then has to become acquainted with the original diagnosis. And it, of course, overloads the ER.[41]

Refugees may also suffer from post-traumatic stress syndrome. A Brooks High School English as a Second Language teacher noted that some refugee students commonly deal with a variety of stressors, including:

> a new environment, imagine going from a hot desert environment to Brooks in the winter. They may be adjusting to a new family situation, perhaps the trauma of seeing friends or relatives killed, plus they have the added pressure of wanting to fit in with students here. Many have to work to help pay the rent, or have a little spending money of their own, or some may be required to send money back to relatives. That's a lot of stuff to deal with and they do remarkably well.[42]

Adults are subject to similar pressures, but as one person who works closely with the refugee population put it, there is 'nobody in Brooks with the type of expertise to diagnose post-traumatic stress syndrome'.[43] The academic literature is rife with studies documenting the greater risk for refugee children of developing mental health problems, such as alcohol abuse, drug addiction, delinquency, depression and post-traumatic stress.[44] The challenge for communities like Brooks is to equip newcomer children with the life skills necessary to become fully productive members of the host community.

Newcomers to meatpacking towns place demands on healthcare services by virtue of their low socioeconomic status. In Canada's 1996 National Population Health Survey only 19 per cent of persons with less than a high school education rated their health as excellent, compared to almost 30 per cent for those with a university education; while 73 per cent of those in the highest income level reported excellent or good health, compared with just 47 per cent in the lowest income group.[45] Most jobs in a packing-house and a good many of the spin-off jobs they create in the service sector are relatively low-paying and require minimal education. Thus, most newcomers to packing-house towns are likely to need more medical services than middle-class residents.

The number of Brooks residents who failed to graduate from high school *increased* by 745 between 1996 and 2001, and this group's share of the population increased from 41 to 43 per cent. By contrast, the equivalent population declined from 48 to 40 per cent in the nearby town of Taber (2001 pop. 7,671), which is in line with provincial trends. As Brooks experienced an influx of less-educated adults, average earnings fell relative to the rest of the province – from 104 per cent in 1996 to 93 per cent in 2000.[46]

The creation of thousands of low-paying jobs, combined with housing shortages, sent rents soaring, and some newcomers found themselves unable to afford to feed themselves or their families. Food is a basic prerequisite for good health. Poor nutrition during pregnancy is linked to low-birth weight and preterm delivery, which add to healthcare costs, while infants and children who fail to eat a balanced diet may suffer from growth and developmental problems, attention deficits and weakened resistance to disease. Packing-house communities often recognize this problem and establish community food banks. The Brooks Food Bank opened on 1 October 1998, and has grown ever since. In 2002 it served 1,746 adults and 1,638 children, by 2005 the equivalent figures were 2,412 adults and 1,595 children. Nearly three-quarters of the food bank's clients work at Lakeside. There is even a special sack full of groceries for single workers who live in company-provided trailers on site because there are only six microwave ovens to serve some 300 workers.[47]

Mental Health and the Uninsured

South of the border, Garden City, and surrounding Finney County, Kansas, have confronted a different set of healthcare challenges. In 1980, soon after IBP opened the world's largest beef processing plant in Holcomb, ten miles west of Garden City, people began moving to the area. Within two years, admissions from Finney County residents to the area mental health centre jumped 65 per cent, suggesting that some newcomers had difficulty in adjusting to life in southwest Kansas.[48] But admissions declined after 1982, which counsellors attributed to linguistic and cultural barriers faced by the growing number of Southeast Asian refugees who came to work in the plants. A Vietnamese doctor who settled in Garden City explained that: 'The traditional way of dealing with personal problems is within the family, to seek help from a total stranger, like a counsellor, would be alien for most Vietnamese.'[49]

Throughout the 1990s, Finney County placed in the bottom 10 per cent of Kansas counties for children lacking immunization, teen pregnancies and lack of prenatal care. The county's poor performance was attributed to the lack of 'access and availability of health resources for low-income minority households',[50] since only 2.96 full-time equivalent primary-care physicians out of 15.8 in Garden City would accept Medicaid patients. To fill this vacuum, United Methodist Western Kansas Mexican-American Ministries Care Centers and Clinics (better known as Mexican-American Ministries or MAM) provides basic healthcare for persons without medical insurance for Garden City and surrounding southwest Kansas. Services are provided in English, Spanish and Low German. Founded in 1987, MAM's Care Centers and Clinics recorded 6,000 primary care visits in 1990; by 1995 this number increased to 17,652; in 2000 it reached 22,207. For 2004 it was just over 23,000, of which about 19,000 were in Garden City. Although the demand for services slowed between 2000 and 2004, MAM's executive director cautioned: 'It does not mean there was no more need – it simply means that we do not have the capacity to meet that need'.[51]

A Christmas Day 2000 fire at one of the two main engines of Garden City's economy, the ConAgra beef plant on the town's east end, put nearly 2,300 employees out of work. Three years later, the discovery of a single case of bovine spongiform encephalopathy (also known as BSE or mad cow disease) in Washington State led to the loss of export markets for US beef. Finney County's remaining beef plant, now owned by Tyson Foods, reduced weekly hours for employees to thirty-two and then twenty-four by the fall of 2004. The resulting drop in take-home pay put many families, already struggling to make ends meet, well below the federal poverty line. Together, these two events added to the community's healthcare woes. The loss of the community's second largest employer led many people to leave, and the county's population dropped by an estimated 3.3 per cent between 2000 and 2004. But some former ConAgra workers and their families have stayed, and during this five-year period, the number of individuals receiving public assistance for medical care rose 35 per cent, while total expenditures jumped from $14.2 million to nearly $20 million.[52]

Meatpacking Worker and Community Health

What's meatpacking got to do with worker and community health? The answer is, in fact, a great deal! Meatpacking is labour intensive and dependent upon unskilled labour. It is one of North America's few remaining manufacturing industries where a high school diploma, previous work experience, and the ability to speak English are *not* necessary for employment. Working on the line in a packing-house is unpleasant and physically demanding. Workers remain on their feet most of the day and perform the same repetitive motions hundreds or thousands of times during their shift, whether it's 'dropping heads' or artfully cutting meat into retail portions which will be vacuum-packed and sent directly to a supermarket's meat counter.

The packers' relocation from urban to rural areas to be near cattle supplies and save transport costs means that companies quickly exhaust locally available labour supplies and recruit workers from farther and farther afield. This translates into dramatic population increases due to the rapid influx of immigrants and refugees – and continuous population mobility – in packing-house towns throughout North America. Newcomers put a greater demand on healthcare services by virtue of their low socioeconomic status, since less-educated individuals report more health problems than those with higher education. But meeting everyone's healthcare needs in such communities is often compromised since rural areas generally suffer from a shortage of physicians and other healthcare professionals. Long hours, unpredictable work schedules, and heavy patient loads often translate into physicians' unwillingness to accept new patients. In Brooks – and similar communities elsewhere – low-wage workers and their families often resort to the ER for routine healthcare needs. In Garden City and other packing-house towns in southwest Kansas, the uninsured and underinsured rely on Mexican-American Ministries, which is funded primarily through grants from non-profit organizations and donations.

Language and cultural barriers add to the challenges of newcomer healthcare delivery. In Brooks, many newcomers lack English language skills, which complicate patient diagnoses. On the surface, providing translators seems a simple expedient, but some clients may refuse to share their particular symptoms with someone from the same community for fear their condition will be publicized. And programmes like Language Line have practical limitations. While this problem will eventually be solved as the second generation achieves English fluency, it remains a barrier. And no sooner has the host community begun to accommodate one immigrant population than another arrives on the scene to present new linguistic and cultural challenges, which can create practical difficulties, given the shortage of medical staff in rural areas.

Lessening injury rates and meatpacking's overall impact on community health would require the industry to lower line speeds and take other measures to reduce employee turnover. But such steps are unlikely, given the economics of North American meat production. For plants to be profitable, their slaughter capacity must be fully utilized. Several years ago we reported on a new generation of meatpacking plants in New Zealand that appeared to address many of the ills of the North American industry. These plants are smaller than their North American counterparts, processing about 500 cattle a day rather than the 5,000 a day common in major US plants. But despite a slower line speed, worker productivity is higher per animal slaughtered, and worker turnover is about 7 per cent a year compared with North America's average of about 7 per cent a month.[53] These innovations have yet to be adopted by any of the major US-based meatpacking companies – and it is doubtful they will be.

Communities and workers are virtually powerless to alter the nature of modern meatpacking, since they have no control over the production process. Packers seduce rural communities with the promise of economic development and job creation, and for many small towns with stagnant or declining economies these jobs seem too good to pass up. But, as our research has shown time and time again, these jobs come with a host of hidden costs to the health and well being of workers and host communities alike. Only when there are no more communities willing to accept this Faustian bargain, will the packers be likely to change.

Acknowledgements

This paper has been revised and updated from the one we originally presented at the workshop on 'Meat, Medicine and Human Health in the Twentieth Century', National Institutes of Health in Bethesda, Maryland, USA, 14–15 November 2006. A much abbreviated and altered version of that paper appeared earlier as: M. J. Broadway and D. D. Stull, "'I'll Do Whatever You Want, But It Hurts": Worker Safety and Community Health in Modern Meatpacking', *Labor*, 5:4 (2008), pp. 27–37.

5 IS REFRIGERATED MEAT HEALTHY? MEXICO ENCOUNTERS THE CHICAGO MEATPACKING 'JUNGLE', c. 1910

Jeffrey M. Pilcher

Attitudes about the healthfulness of foods are embedded in wider cultural beliefs. In the United States, except for a vegetarian counterculture, meat has generally been considered an essential part of a healthy diet. Economists have even attributed late nineteenth-century improvements in nutrition and public health largely to the greater availability of protein made possible by the technologies of mechanical refrigeration and industrial ranching.[1] Admittedly, the feedlots and packing-houses which broadened access to meat have also produced serious public health scares, yet these have largely concerned the incidental contamination of processed meat, not its basic nature. Today, fears focus on E. coli infection and 'mad cow' syndrome, whereas a hundred years ago, adulteration resulted from industrial preservatives such as boracic acid or from accidents caused by low safety standards – to use Upton Sinclair's unsettling example of workers who fell into vats where 'they would be overlooked for days, till all but the bones of them had gone out to the world as Durham's Pure Leaf Lard!'[2]

When North American technologies were transferred to other cultures, however, they often raised more fundamental questions. For example, meat technologies transferred to Mexico at the beginning of the twentieth century generated suspicions about the healthfulness of meat and of the ways in which it was processed. Entrepreneurs from the meatpacking capital of Chicago attempted to convince the local population of the value of refrigerated meat in the first decade of the twentieth century. Yet despite a high status accorded to meat and generally low levels of consumption, Mexicans proved reluctant to accept the new product because of a cultural preference for the taste of freshly slaughtered meat. The foreign investors therefore faced two significant challenges; the production problem of establishing a cost-effective industry in a tropical environment unlike the Great Plains of North America or the Argentine Pampas and also the marketing problem of convincing Mexican consumers that North American refrigeration produced healthier meat than traditional methods. The incipient packing industry ultimately failed both hurdles, in part because of precarious finances, the strength of local competitors, and, most significantly for this paper, consumer beliefs about the unhealthiness of refrigerated meat.

The example of Mexican meat illustrates the cultural tension between healthfulness and taste – what is supposed to be good for you and what tastes good. Studies of taste preferences often emphasize the evolutionary advantages among early humans of highly caloric foods, sugars and fats, and the aversion to bitter foods associated with poisons. Yet, beyond health considerations, the human sense of taste is extremely complex – based on smell and texture as well as flavour – and it differs widely across cultures. Many bitter toxins developed as self-defence mechanisms by plants, including the capsaic acid in chilli peppers and the caffeine of coffee and tea, have become popular tastes within particular societies. Different tastes for meat, such as 'high' or rotted game, likewise illustrate this point.

North Americans first encountered Mexican meat on a large scale in the 1980s with the Tex-Mex fad of fajitas, but this great novelty of thin strips of skirt steak seared quickly on a hot fire was simply the traditional Hispanic *carne asada*. By contrast, Anglo-Americans had long preferred thick roasts and steaks, cooked under a broiler or on a grill, which browned the exterior while leaving thick layers of juicy meat inside. Such methods worked best with the marbled flesh of fatty animals, aged to increase the tenderness still further by releasing enzymes to break down connective muscle tissue. An 1841 cookbook explained: 'Fresh beef is better for being kept three or four days in moderate, and much longer in cold weather. One reason why beef is not so good or wholesome in summer is, that it must be eaten too fresh, and while the fibre is tough, or it will spoil'.[3] Confronted with the stringy flesh of Spanish Creole cattle rather than well-marbled cuts of Aberdeen Angus or Hereford, Mexican cooking emphasized the rich taste of freshly slaughtered meat, and tenderized it through techniques such as stewing and making fajitas. A migrant worker from Guanajuato, living in Los Angeles in the 1920s, explained: 'I don't like the meat, that is to say, the meat here [in the United States], because it is not fresh'.[4] Thus, the differences between US and Mexican cultures of meat pervaded every step of the supply chain, from the feedlot to the supermarket to the kitchen to the table.[5]

However ingrained cultural attitudes may have been, transformations in taste and perceived healthfulness were an unavoidable consequence of the modernization of food production. Martin Bruegel has described the century-long struggle to teach the French to eat canned food instead of fresh, a campaign that ultimately succeeded in large part because of shortages during World War I.[6] Even shoppers in the United States reacted to refrigerated meat with much the same reluctance that Mexicans showed, and only an overwhelming cost advantage assured the transition to refrigerated supply.[7] These experiences highlight an obvious but important point: personal tastes and attitudes about health depend on the availability of food.

To explain the early failure of industrial meatpacking in Mexico, this essay begins by describing the complicated health debates surrounding meat in late nineteenth-century Mexico, including both cultural preferences inherited from the colonial era and the struggle by medical authorities to assert control over the butchering trade. The narrative then turns to domestic attempts to modernize provisioning, first under the direction of the Mexico City council and then as part of an incipient beef trust held by northern cattle barons. Both attempts failed, in part through incomplete adoption of the refrigerated technology, and also because of resistance from local livestock merchants and meat cutters, who rightly feared being reduced from independent tradesmen to an industrial proletariat like their counterparts in Chicago's meatpacking 'jungle'. Finally, the essay examines the ill-fated attempt by foreigners to create a fully refrigerated industry. This experience, in turn, serves as a basis for questioning the narrative of inevitable technological progress enunciated by the modern-day meatpacking industry.

Meat and Health in Mexico

Not only are attitudes about health culturally embedded, they also evolve over time. Nineteenth-century Mexicans began to adopt Enlightenment notions of public health, focusing on disease and the individual, in place of early modern concepts encompassing urban order, but butcher guilds fiercely contested attempts by medical authorities to regulate their business. Merchants were particularly successful in asserting their autonomy in the first half-century after independence in 1821, a period of palace revolutions and foreign invasions that made effective governance virtually impossible. Only under the dictatorship of Porfirio Díaz (1876–1910) did political stability allow officials to regain a measure of control, and by this time, population growth had overburdened provisioning systems established to feed Mexico City in the eighteenth century. Popular attitudes about meat likewise persisted from the colonial era despite the fashion for northern European foods like roast beef that swept through the elite, particularly during the Porfirian era.

For thousands of years, Mexican peasants had subsisted on a basically vegetarian diet, with maize and beans as their primary sources of protein. In pre-Hispanic times, the only domesticated animals were turkeys and small dogs, both of which were considered gourmet delights. Ecological anthropologists of the 1970s attributed the notorious practice of Aztec cannibalism to protein hunger, ignoring the fact that the nobles who reputedly ate their conquered enemies were already well fed on fish and game.[8] Even commoners shared in this bounty during annual religious festivals–a social order similar to the medieval Catholic calendar of feast and fast. The rapid spread of European livestock after the conquest coincided with the dramatic collapse of the indigenous population to assure cheap meat, at least for a few decades. Native Americans acquired new tastes for pork and beef, which they could rarely satisfy in subsequent generations. Nevertheless, this brief era of plenty continued to influence attitudes about meat in New Spain. Colonial authorities maintained European associations between meat and masculinity, believing that only a steady diet of meat allowed hard work in the silver mines, despite the ubiquity of Native American porters carrying tremendous loads while eating little more than tortillas and chillies.[9]

The Mexican belief that the wholesomeness of meat was intimately connected to its freshness was evident in both sanitary regulations and culinary culture. From the early days of the colonial period, market officials decreed that meat had to be sold on the same day that it was slaughtered, and shoppers denounced butchers who sold leftovers. Violations of these rules were common, particularly in times of meat shortages, but popular attitudes and official requirements clearly viewed freshness as the essence of healthfulness.[10] Colonial cookbooks likewise insisted that meat be cooked promptly; even when recipes called for marinades, they were applied for as little as a few hours or perhaps overnight. Exceptions can be found, for example, an eighteenth-century manuscript cookbook by Dominga de Guzmán specified an aged *carnero* for mutton stew, although with the revealing description 'bien manido' (well rotted).[11]

After independence, Mexican elites sought to demonstrate their savoir faire by hiring French chefs, yet they did not allow kitchen workers free rein in meat cookery, demanding that imported recipes be adapted to local tastes. Foreign cookbook authors made their preferences clear; Wenceslao Ayguals de Izco explained that a roast had to sit for five days before putting it over the fire, while the Catalan gourmet Narcisso Bassols, insisted that 'the preparation of a good biftek requires that the tenderloin not be from meat slaughtered the same day'.[12] By contrast, Mexican culinary guides adapted their recipes to local tastes. In 1896, Vicenta Torres de Rubio explained the necessity for aging meat for English *rosbif*, and after giving a cooking time of two and a half hours, she warned: 'This is *a la inglesa*. But as not all tastes correspond to the English point of doneness, I will indicate another procedure more adequate to our inclinations and customs'.[13] The most sophisticated realized that the French foods served in Mexico City restaurants bore little resemblance to Parisian fare, but this mainly gave them the opportunity to disparage their less-travelled countrymen. Antonio García Cubas gave the following commentary upon finding the French term *rôtis* misspelled on a Mexican menu as '*Rots*. Free translation 'ragged ones' (rotos), allusion of our street people (léperos) to the frock coat crowd, but translated by the cognoscenti (instruidos) as roast'.[14]

Cooking techniques in turn depended on the work of butchers, and in the colonial era, powerful merchant guilds had dominated both the provisioning and regulation of meat in Mexico City, although they were subject to municipal oversight. Following Iberian tradition, the city council contracted out sales of beef and mutton as a semi-private monopoly known as the *abasto de carne* (meat supply). Livestock merchants bid for the abasto contract, promising to provide abundant quantities at a fixed and fair price for one or more years. The city also maintained fixed prices for pork, based on the costs of production, which were determined annually through the ceremonial slaughter of a sample of hogs known as the *experiencia de cerdo* (pork experiment).[15] The technical skills of butcher craftsmen had assured the guilds considerable authority over production techniques, but a special tribunal called the *fiel ejecutoria* still supervised public abattoirs and meat markets. Health and pollution remained constant concerns for court deputies, who inspected livestock to ensure that it was well-fed and free of disease. Nevertheless, regular consumer complaints indicate that this ideal was not always attained. By the late eighteenth century, when abasto merchants were unable to satisfy demand during the summer, an official testified that illicit butchers smuggled two or three hundred steers into the city each month 'dead and completely rotten'.[16]

Health problems multiplied with the breakdown of government oversight in the early national period. Shortages grew so extreme during the wars of independence that in 1813 the viceroy abolished the abasto system and declared free trade to encourage greater supplies. The government also privatized the municipal abattoir at San Lucas, allowing private slaughterhouses to proliferate throughout the city. These measures may not have increased the overall availability of meat, but critics painted a fly-by-night image of individuals slaughtering cattle in every public thoroughfare and 'selling the meat by the by'.[17] The resulting surge of pollution and unwholesome meat continued to plague the city for decades. In 1839, General Ramón Rayón noted 'the unbearable foulness, the putrefaction of blood, the inadequate disposal of manure' from private corrals.[18] A municipal commission also warned of the 'grave danger to public health' posed by illicit sales of corrupt meat from clandestine slaughterhouses in the suburbs.[19] Another official later recalled that 'they slaughtered cattle in a corral on the side of the granary [recogidas], facing south, in another at the Cacahuatal [Street of the Peanut Field], in those [two] on the Garrapata [Street of the Tick, appropriately], and in all of the hidden ones of the city, without order, many without paying taxes, neither the import fees [alcabala], nor the municipal [duties], and without any policing'.[20]

The Mexico City council re-established the San Lucas slaughterhouse in 1848 following the US invasion, but health authorities struggled for decades to regulate the industry. Prominent livestock merchants conspired against the first inspector, Colonel Francisco Carbajal y Espinosa, driving him from office in 1851, and his successors made little effort to challenge the powerful meat cartel. Only in 1872 did control of the slaughterhouse pass from political appointees to medical professionals under the Board of Health (Consejo Superior de Salubridad). Veterinary medicine had made important advances during the nineteenth century, and Mexicans were at the forefront of this international movement. The diagnostic technology of the microscope allowed health professionals to screen livestock for dangerous diseases such as trichinosis, which Mexican experts discovered independently of their European colleagues.[21] But fully utilizing this scientific knowledge depended on the active collaboration of butchers, who had been accustomed to acting as the primary assurance of quality through their skills in selecting livestock and preparing meat, and conflicts between the two were inevitable, particularly when inspectors challenged the property rights of merchants.[22]

The provisional nature of medical authority was demonstrated by an episode in 1894, when a health inspector noticed a particularly bad smell emanating from the stall of a butcher. The inspector consulted with local market officials, who agreed that a rump roast and its accompanying viscera were discoloured and decomposing, and promptly impounded the meat. Nevertheless, laboratory workers analysed the roast, although apparently not the viscera, and pronounced it clean. The butcher never got his meat back and pressed charges with a local judge, who issued an arrest warrant, not for abuse of authority, but for issuing a false expert opinion. The inspector was promptly freed from jail, but word of the scandal appeared in the pages of a popular newspaper. The Health Board feared that similar incidents in the future could destroy its credibility and referred the matter to city attorneys with a note emphasizing the 'transcendence of this case' for sanitary inspection.[23]

In addition to concerns about sanitation, the need to increase supplies of meat became an important theme in the discourse of national health at the turn of the century. Intellectuals worried that shortages of meat would impede industrial development and lead to excessive consumption of *pulque*, the intoxicating and nutritious drink of the masses, with consequent threats to public order. High meat prices not only undercut living standards, they were also considered to be a genuine threat to the nation. As one editorialist observed, with meat in such short supply, one could hardly be surprised by the feebleness of national productivity. 'The truth is irrefutable: in the US, the number one country in meat consumption, the workers are robust and the output abundant'.[24] Worse still, workers unable to afford meat filled their stomachs with pulque instead, thus contributing to drunkenness, the country's greatest problem according to many leaders. The newspaper *El Imparcial* made this connection clear by calling for the Mexico City council to raise taxes on the indigenous alcoholic beverage while lowering the duties on meat, thereby encouraging the poor to drink less and eat more.[25]

Meat was viewed as an essential element of Mexican progress in the late nineteenth century. Nevertheless, assuring abundant and healthy supplies of animal protein remained a burdensome task, as it had been since the colonial era. While the elite fancied themselves dining on sophisticated Parisian cookery, albeit prepared to their own tastes, ordinary workers often could not afford this expensive commodity, and when they did buy it, it was frequently from unlicensed clandestine slaughterhouses. Transforming this antiquated provisioning system was therefore a top priority of the Porfirian government.

Modernizing the Meat Industry

President Díaz's administrative elite placed enormous faith in imported technology to solve the nation's problems. In modernizing the meat supply, however, they had to choose between two competing models, and the appropriate technology for Mexico was not at all obvious. When the city council finally constructed a new slaughterhouse in the northern suburb of Peralvillo, they attempted to create a hybrid approach adapting US technology to Mexican conditions, which satisfied neither producers nor consumers. A remodelled version of the Peralvillo slaughterhouse, even when operated more openly as a private packing-house, likewise proved inadequate for local conditions.

Meat provisioning constituted an important focus of trans-Atlantic health reform and two competing slaughterhouse designs emerged in the mid-1860s, the La Villette abattoir in Paris and the Union Stockyards of Chicago. The former, conceived by Baron Haussmann as part of his monumental reconstruction of Paris, exemplified a rational approach to urban design. The centrepiece of La Villette was a great iron and glass hall with sufficient space to house all the cattle consumed in the French metropolis, while providing each animal with an individual stall in which it was carefully tended and then slaughtered by a skilled craftsman. Meanwhile, the Union Stockyards grew haphazardly, as *Scientific American* reported, into a 'true labyrinth of sheds and enormous halls that communicate in various ways by passages, staircases, and suspension bridges'.[26] This ungainly tribute to Yankee tinkering, built in haste without an overall plan, nevertheless represented a radical new industrial approach based on private packing-houses and mass-production techniques in which each worker performed a single, repetitious cut in a veritable 'disassembly' line. La Villette, by contrast, remained an old-fashioned municipal slaughterhouse, however meticulously designed.[27]

By the 1890s, the need to modernize the San Lucas slaughterhouse had become pressing. The facility had grown haphazardly over the course of the nineteenth century from a simple colonial corral into a maze of separate departments for cattle and sheep. Generations of service without adequate water for cleaning had left it with a 'constant bad odour perceptible at a great distance, owing to the violent putrefaction of blood and other organic materials'.[28] Although originally designed for a daily slaughter of 150 cattle, a municipal report described the practice of 'conducting 250 or 300 cattle into a closed perimeter inside of which the butchers, with great danger to themselves, killed the animals in crowds, here and there, causing confusion and terror through the bloody spectacle. The butchers, with cold blood, notable valor, and at times a ferocious pleasure similar to that of the bullfighter, released from misery, in a few moments, their numerous victims'.[29] The business journal *El Economista Mexicano* also blamed San Lucas for allowing livestock merchants to perpetuate a 'closed corporation of a medieval form'. Destroying the guild would be simple, the editorial declared, if the city only possessed an adequate slaughterhouse where all were free to slaughter cattle. Better still would be a great packing-house like those in the United States, Argentina or Uruguay.[30]

Perhaps because of this attitude, the Mexico City council contracted with a St Louis firm, although the cartel of livestock merchants operated more like Parisian jobbers than like the meatpacking companies of Chicago. As a result, when the New Peralvillo Slaughterhouse finally opened in September 1897, it functioned along the lines of a private packing-house rather than a municipal abattoir, albeit without refrigerated storage and market facilities. Work proceeded in a serial fashion, intended to maximize efficiency over the course of a workday, rather than the usual pre-dawn frenzy, which ensured that retailers had their meat at the market by 10 o'clock in the morning, when Mexican women preferred to shop. The resulting delays, compounded by deficient construction and summer flooding, prevented butcher shops from receiving shipments of fresh meat until as late as 9 o'clock at night. Over the long term, the assembly line method of production threatened to upset the balance of market share within the merchant clique because the first butchers to get their meat to market would receive consistently higher profits, due to the premium for fresh meat, and could eventually drive their competitors out of business. Such an outcome was precluded, however, when a series of industrial accidents – which killed two workers and seriously injured two more – combined with production delays to force the government to close the Peralvillo abattoir and return the slaughter to the corrals of San Lucas.

Rather than rebuild a municipal abattoir, the city council eventually concluded that it would be more efficient simply to privatize the system entirely. This decision caused the merchants even greater fears about an incipient meat trust because the winning bid came from the family of Luis Terrazas, who virtually monopolized the economy of the cattle-rich northern state of Chihuahua. The Terrazas meatpacking firm, La Internacional, already operated three modern packing-houses in northern cities and hoped to use the Peralvillo contract to gain a foothold in the capital's market as a step toward building a national business comparable to Swift or Armour in the United States. Indeed, when Peralvillo reopened in 1905, the Terrazas management scheduled the slaughter so that their own cattle were butchered first and competitors were not served until after the workers had taken a leisurely brunch.[31]

Nevertheless, a complaint by the wealthiest merchants brought prompt action from the Porfirian government, which ordered La Internacional to change the schedule so that the local cartel and the Terrazas went first on alternate days. The resulting competitive struggle caused a brief fall in prices, but the two parties allegedly reached a secret agreement to divide the market, and wholesale prices soon began to rise again.[32] Smaller merchants, without privileged access to high officials, resorted instead to illegal slaughter. Residents of the working-class Colonia Santa Julia, for example, saw their butcher chasing after a mortally wounded steer that was trying to escape down Matamoros Street.[33] With the competition of leading merchants for the premium markets and clandestine slaughter on the low end, profits at Peralvillo fell far short of expectations. La Internacional was forced into bankruptcy protection during the Depression of 1907, thus concluding the first Mexican attempts to import meatpacking technology from the United States.[34]

The Rise and Fall of 'El Popo'

A common failing of these early Mexican meatpacking ventures lay in their incomplete adoption of industrial technology. Performing the slaughter in Mexico City rather than in livestock-raising areas of the country meant foregoing the cost savings from shipping dressed carcasses, about half the weight of a live animal even before losses in transit. At the same time, Mexico City producers lost the economies of scale achieved by Chicago packing plants that supplied cities throughout the eastern United States. Other unrealized profits lay in the sale of industrial by-products such as fertilizer and glue made from blood and bones.[35] The potential for modernizing the Mexican livestock industry therefore continued to attract the notice of foreign capitalists. Swift & Co. made tentative investments in the 1890s, but John W. DeKay's Mexican National Packing Company was the most significant attempt to establish a US-style packing-house. Although intended primarily as an export business, the company needed domestic profits to support its operations while breaking into the fiercely competitive London market. Having mastered the technology of meatpacking in Chicago, DeKay soon discovered that knowledge of Mexican culture was just as important for the success of his venture.

DeKay first surveyed the possibilities of building a packing-house in the cattle country of Michoacán about 1900, but construction languished until 1906, when the publication of Upton Sinclair's muckraking novel, *The Jungle*, made Mexican exports to Europe appear commercially viable. With British financing, the Mexican National Packing Company quickly completed its Uruapan packing-house, and in February 1908, it made its first shipments of chilled beef by refrigerated railroad car to Mexico City.

Local success depended on persuading Mexicans that North American consumption habits were superior to their own, and to that end DeKay formulated an elaborate marketing plan. A refrigerated branch house at Rancho del Chopo, near the Mexican National Railroad terminal, served as the hub for receiving meat from railroad cars and passing it along to local butchers. The company began its retail chain with just two outlets, but they were carefully chosen for maximum exposure. To educate the masses about US standards of hygiene, DeKay established a model market on the busy thoroughfare San Juan de Letrán, which ran just east of the Alameda Park, a popular gathering place for all levels of Mexican society. A second, more upscale shop opened on Viena Street in the exclusive Zona Rosa (Pink Zone). DeKay intended the shop to cater at first to the large colony of US expatriates living in the district, but he also counted on the Mexican elite penchant for foreign fashions to add a native clientele as well. Moreover, he advertised heavily in the prominent English-language daily, the *Mexican Herald*, touting the company's 'clean, wholesome, and properly prepared meats'. The products bore the label 'El Popo', after the lofty volcano Popocatépetl, both for nostalgic appeal to Mexican consumers and because 'DeKay Meat' made a poor brand name.[36]

The Popo marketing strategy mirrored the larger Porfirian development project aimed at inculcating the Mexican masses into modern European lifestyles. The foreign colony and the elite were supposed to demonstrate such benefits of modern technology as refrigerated meats to the local middle classes, who in turn served as an example for the working classes, indoctrinating them in bourgeois manners. Diffusing the ideals of polite society was essential not only to avoid class conflict but also to ensure the success of mass production in Mexico. DeKay's business model depended on selling large quantities of meat at low prices, and an elite clientele alone could not provide sufficient demand to utilize fully the Uruapan packing-house. To reach this mass market, he later diversified his advertisements beyond English-language newspapers to the local penny press, thus hoped to establish Popo-brand refrigerated meat as an essential element of Porfirian modernity.[37]

DeKay's success also depended on the support of the Mexican government, which was equally eager to assure foreign capitalists that they could invest their money safely. When British shareholders arrived to inaugurate the packing-house, President Díaz invited the party to Chapultepec Castle, promising to lend his personal prestige to the enterprise by escorting Madame Díaz to the company's retail meat shops when they opened in the capital. Such favourable publicity would be a vital step in convincing Mexican customers of the value of the new methods of preparing meat. Moreover, to ensure that local butchers learned the lesson, he offered to have the Board of Health issue regulations requiring the trade to be organized according to the company model.[38] Díaz's cabinet joined in facilitating the company's opening; Vice President Ramón Corral arranged for federal inspection of the Uruapan slaughterhouse to avoid marketing delays, while Treasury Secretary José Yves Limantour negotiated a contract to provision the Mexican Army and other public institutions for twenty years at prices 10 per cent below retail value.[39]

Even with this apparent official favour, El Popo still faced a significant challenge in winning domestic consumers away from their traditional butchers. In April 1908, Mexican merchants responded to the foreign competitor by placing advertisements in prominent newspapers, *El Imparcial* and the *Mexican Herald*, informing readers: 'Refrigerated meat is useful on long sea voyages or to send to distant markets, but understand it well, it is only as a matter of absolute necessity.' The ads not only implied that the Popo brand tasted inferior to freshly slaughtered beef, they also cast doubt on the company's claims of sanitary benefits from refrigerated meat. 'It loses its juice, it becomes discolored, it is insipid and acquires a rare tenderness, due, perhaps, to the beginning of decomposition. How can a government inspector answer for the good sanitary condition of meat ten or fifteen days after inspection?'[40] Nor were newspaper placements the most innovative or effective promotional work undertaken by the butchers. In May, for example, El Popo offered a $100 reward for information leading to the arrest and conviction of 'certain persons, falsely representing themselves to be Agents or inspectors of the Superior Board of Health of Mexico, [who] have visited several butcher's shops saying that refrigerated meat is unhealthy and liable to decomposition.'[41]

The question of who would win this competitive struggle, the foreign meat-packer with his slick advertising copy or the local butchers with their sharpened knives, was never properly decided, for the slaughterhouse owners were planning their own strategy for handling the foreign rival. The Terrazas had already experienced a costly price war against the Mexico City merchants in 1905, and the global depression left it even less prepared to sustain an extended competitive battle with the British-financed Popo. The powerful family therefore used government connections to force a settlement with DeKay. Treasury Secretary Limantour, ever alert to mutually profitable joint ventures between domestic and foreign capital, was receptive to such a deal. Like the New York financier J. P. Morgan, he saw mergers as an ideal way of consolidating industry to avoid destructive competition. Just how he manoeuvred DeKay to buy Peralvillo from the Terrazas remains one of the deep, dark secrets of Porfirian political economy. In negotiating the contract, DeKay tried to gain concessions that would help cement the local market. In particular, he requested a monopoly on the slaughter of meat in the city, exemption from federal taxes and, most revealingly, a government regulation requiring all meat sold in Mexico City to be refrigerated. Not only did Limantour refuse all of these privileges, but the asking price for the slaughterhouse came to $2.5 million pesos – five times the cost of construction.[42]

Paying such an exorbitant price for a Mexico City facility went against DeKay's plan for providing low cost meat from small, efficient packing-houses in the livestock raising areas of the country. But having sunk his money into building the Uruapan packing-house, he simply had no choice. Thus, he proclaimed victory, declaring that the purchase of Pelavillo demonstrated that the Mexican public preferred refrigerated meat, and set about renovating the slaughterhouse.

DeKay's claims notwithstanding, local acceptance of company products was not a foregone conclusion. In the summer of 1908, the industrialist pointed to the declining numbers of livestock slaughtered at the municipal abattoir to prove that demand was strong for Popo meat. A newspaper advertisement proclaimed already in June that the Mexican National had captured half the meat sales in the capital. In testimony given years later, DeKay had inflated Popo's share to a fantastic 85 per cent of the market, but even the smaller figure would represent a remarkable achievement after just a few months. A government bulletin indeed indicated that while more than 11,000 head of cattle were butchered in each of the first three months of 1908, the numbers began to drop rapidly in April. Slaughterhouse workers processed fewer than 7,000 in June and scarcely more than 5,000 in August, although hog supplies remained steady throughout the year. Yet DeKay's claims sound much less impressive after factoring in seasonal variations, which regularly reduced the summer slaughter to about 75 per cent of the winter high. Moreover, if competition from Popo was undercutting the local importers, one would expect prices at the Peralvillo to drop significantly. In fact, they rose throughout the spring before levelling off in the summer, a strong indication that the decline in slaughter at Peralvillo resulted from overall market scarcity rather than cutthroat competition from Popo.[43]

Even an additional 25 per cent fall in cattle at the slaughterhouse represented at best a qualified success for the company. Much of the demand for Popo came from government contracts to supply schools, prisons and the army – scarcely an indication of consumer preference. Another significant market for the company's meat lay in the so-called American colony, which numbered upwards of 10,000 people by this time. Expatriates from Canada, Britain and the United States commented frequently on the poor quality of work by Mexican butchers and were delighted to purchase familiar cuts of aged beef. Admittedly, DeKay had secured exclusive contracts with several local merchants, although these agreements had probably come with promises of heavy discounts. Nevertheless, DeKay contradicted his own claim of the superiority of refrigerated beef from Uruapan over the freshly slaughtered products at the Mexico City slaughterhouse. Despite the price advantage of shipping refrigerated meat over livestock, when he purchased the slaughterhouse from Terrazas, he immediately converted the Michoacán packing-house to the preparation of canned meat, an indication that he already understood the struggle he faced in converting local consumers to US tastes. The greatest betrayal may therefore have been not the Porfirian government forcing him to purchase Peralvillo at an inflated price but rather the Mexican public, which remained sceptical of the promises of refrigerated meat.[44]

Taking control of the Mexico City slaughterhouse was a mixed blessing in the competitive struggle with local butchers, quite aside from the heavy debt incurred. The original contract, signed by the Terrazas family, required Peralvillo to operate as an awkward hybrid of public abattoir and private packing-house. Rival merchants thus had free access to the facility, although company employees performed the actual slaughter. Moreover, DeKay's attempts to reorganize operations were subject to approval by Health Board officials. In December 1908, as the company began butchering additional cattle for export, it ran up against a statutory deadline for completing the slaughter by ten o'clock in the morning, a rule intended to ensure the availability of fresh meat to all merchants. DeKay explained that he intended to refrigerate the meat rather than sell it immediately, and the Board of Health offered to hire additional inspectors, as long as the company paid their salaries, to allow work to continue until six in the afternoon. This compromise did not satisfy DeKay, who argued that slaughtering livestock in the early morning hours did not allow sufficient light for sanitary inspection, and therefore the workday should run from six in the morning until six in the afternoon. Health officials privately agreed, having attempted a similar reform in 1890 only to reinstate the early morning slaughter when consumers complained about the lack of fresh meat in the markets. This information naturally galvanized DeKay's demand for daylight shifts, which would assist his larger goal of converting the Mexican public to refrigerated meat, but the Health Board refused to adjust the schedule.[45]

Even while pursuing exports through a marketing agreement signed in February 1909 with the British retail magnate, Thomas Lipton, DeKay continued his competitive battle against local merchants. Advertisements emphasized the purity of Popo meats and denounced traditional butchers for selling 'offal and impure meat products such as would not be disposed of for human food in any other part of the world'.[46] The packer's belief in the superiority of Anglo-American cuts blinded him to the taste of Mexican consumers for organ meats. Moreover, these newspaper placements claimed that the only safe meats for sale in the city were Popo meats, as if the livestock slaughtered on the importers' accounts at Peralvillo were not government inspected as well. Another ad juxtaposed photos of the Mexican National's modern automobile and tram delivery cars with one of the competitors' horse-drawn carts (inaccurately) labelled: 'doing the meat business *contrary to law*'.[47] What the competitors told their customers about Popo meat remains unknown, but the butchers also engaged in direct action, carrying out industrial sabotage that undermined the claims of wholesomeness. Taking advantage of sanitary regulations requiring the ventilation of meat shops, night-time vandals tossed iodine through the iron bars on company stores, making it impossible to open until the floors had been disinfected and deodorized. On another occasion, they used syringes to spray acid over the meat.[48]

Despite the heavy advertising, DeKay relied on price to build market share in the face of a strong consumer preference for fresh meat, and this campaign ultimately proved too costly. Throughout the summer and autumn of 1909, Popo retail stores practically gave their meat away, selling for as little as twenty centavos a kilo, one-fifth of their competitors' prices. By year's end the company was operating on $2 million pesos in short-term, unsecured loans from DeKay's banker and treasurer, the aptly named George Ham. The financial burden proved too great for his US Banking Co., which collapsed in a run by depositors in January 1910.[49] Ham was jailed for fraud, but DeKay skilfully tied up the packing company's finances in bankruptcy court for another four years. Nevertheless, political instability caused by the Mexican Revolution of 1910 made it impossible to regain control at Peralvillo, and in 1914, he lost everything in a failed gambit to sell the company to the short-lived military dictatorship of Victoriano Huerta.[50]

Conclusion

In retrospect, although Popo advertisements insisted on the healthfulness of refrigerated meat, DeKay's marketing strategy depended not on objective science or consumer choice but rather on monopolizing local supplies. Admittedly, if he could have achieved the economies of scale needed to provide cheap meat, the urban working classes would surely have developed a taste for it, preferring refrigerated *biftek* (beefsteak) to a bleak diet of tortillas and beans alone. Unfortunately, the global distribution of income prevented DeKay from offering affordable meat to the Mexican masses – his goal had been to supply British markets anyway. Alternately, he might have built a solid local market among the meat consuming middle classes if he could have driven the independent importers out of business. In the United States and later Britain, the packing corporations achieved such a stranglehold, transforming the supply chains from fresh to refrigerated meats and thereby pushing the local butchers and livestock raisers to the edge of the market.[51] El Popo had fewer financial reserves to engage a more difficult struggle against merchants with long experience operating on the edges of the legal trade through semi-clandestine slaughter. Moreover, the Porfirian government did not provide the dictatorship that DeKay had counted on. He particularly regretted the government's refusal to require that all meat sold in Mexico City had to be refrigerated. But the Health Board held a far more realistic view of the limits of sanitation than did DeKay, and in any event, did not share his taste for North American cuts of meat.

His personal failure notwithstanding, DeKay anticipated the future of the Mexican meat supply, both its promise and its drawbacks, but only after further advances had taken place in food technology. Although butchers continued to provide freshly slaughtered meat to Mexico City consumers until nearly the end of the twentieth century, the refrigerated packing industry revived in northern Mexico in the late 1940s when an outbreak of foot-and-mouth disease closed the border to live cattle exports. To ensure that imported meat complied with US standards, the Mexican federal inspection law of 1953 was simply a translation of USDA regulations. Once the threat of aftosa had been contained, Mexican packing-houses languished until the 1970s, when industrial processed food, particularly fast food hamburgers, took off. Grass-fed Creole cattle proved superior to marbled Aberdeen Angus in these so-called 'manufacture beef' applications, and as a result, slaughterhouses spread to the states of Tamaulipas, Veracruz, Tabasco, and Chiapas, encouraging tropical deforestation.[52]

Mexico City was finally drawn into this refrigerated industrial supply chain through administrative fiat rather than consumer choice. In 1992 the neoliberal government of President Carlos Salinas de Gortari closed the municipal slaughterhouse as part of a campaign to abolish the welfare bureaucracy that had subsidized food to the popular sectors. Needless to say, the change led not to the widespread availability of prime sirloin steaks but rather to the consumption of lean cattle that had lost its fresh taste without any corresponding gain in tenderness from the time spent under refrigeration. From a health perspective, the question remained of whether the transition to modern meatpacking would provide the urban poor greater access to animal protein. An editorial in *La Jornada* described this basic trade off when the municipal slaughterhouse closed: 'The population will suffer changes in their customs and will begin to know, on a massive scale, frozen meat. It is possible that with this measure they will succeed in lowering prices and that this will redound to the benefit of hundreds of thousands of inhabitants of Mexico City, who have given up eating meat on a daily basis owing to the high prices of this product'.[53] More than a decade later, the promise of lower prices and greater popular access to meat had not been realized.[54]

Viewing the process of dietary modernization from the Mexican perspective throws new light on triumphalist industry narratives. Corporations have worked to distance consumers from the food chain, eliminating any association between living plants and animals and cellophane-wrapped products in supermarkets. Advocates of capitalism tout its success in satisfying consumer desires and ensuring the health of consumers, but the experience of meat demonstrates the industry's determination to dictate preferences and disregard risks. One legacy of the 1960s counterculture is a contrary – if still limited – cultural attitude toward health in the United States that challenges the industrial belief of more is better and follows instead the Mexican example of smaller portions of fresher food.[55] Now more than ever, wealthy consumers need to learn such lessons from the global south if we are to check the power of multinational corporations over the global food chain.

6 CONFUSED MESSAGES: MEAT, CIVILIZATION, AND CANCER EDUCATION IN THE EARLY TWENTIETH CENTURY.

David Cantor

Writing in *The Natural History of Cancer* (1908), the British medical practitioner William Roger Williams adduced what he called 'overwhelming evidence ... that the incidence of cancer is largely conditioned by nutrition'.[1] In his experience most of those affected with the disease in the early stages were 'large, robust, well-nourished, florid persons, who appear[ed] to be overflowing with vitality',[2] whereas 'the small, pale, [and] ill-nourished'[3] seldom fell victim to the disease. No factor, he claimed, was more likely to promote cancer than excessive feeding. Cancer was a rejuvenescence most likely to occur when there had been sudden or violent change in the environment, especially from poverty and want to riches and plenty. It was particularly associated with 'the gluttonous consumption of proteids – especially meat'.[4]

Williams's views capture several themes that recur in early twentieth-century discourses on diet and cancer on both sides of the Atlantic: that cancer was a disease of civilization, of excess, of nutrition and, for many, of meat. The implications for cancer control were clear. If individuals modified their diet, they might reduce their risk of cancer, and perhaps stem the growth of cancers already established in the body: dietary modification might also help them through the trauma of surgery and other treatments. But, if Williams or the many other writers on this subject hoped that cancer campaigns would encourage the public to change their meat consumption, they were to be disappointed. These campaigns did not generally include recommendations on diet and nutrition in their public education campaigns, except to suggest that moderation in diet was important to a healthy life. Focusing on the American Society for the Control of Cancer (ASCC), this paper explores why meat had such a small place in American cancer education programmes in the early part of the twentieth century, and what this tells us about such programmes – what was included in them, what was excluded, and why.

Founded in 1913, the ASCC argued that for cancer control to succeed Americans had to be persuaded to seek medical help as early in the development of the disease as possible. To promote this policy, the ASCC organized a major public education campaign that urged people to consult a 'recognized' physician as soon as they spotted one of the 'early warning signs' of the disease, to go for a regular medical check-up even if they felt well (since cancer could develop without symptoms), and to undergo treatment – generally surgery or radiotherapy – the moment a physician or pathologist diagnosed the disease or one of its precursors. But, the ASCC also worried that popular beliefs about cancer could undermine these educational efforts. Among the many threats to its message of early detection and treatment, the ASCC suggested, was the public's belief that diet and nutrition could cause, cure or prevent cancer.

In some ways, the ASCC's response to diet and nutrition was very similar to its response to heredity. In the case of heredity, I've argued elsewhere,[5] the ASCC sought to educate the public into the belief that cancer was not a hereditary disease, not because it believed there was no hereditary component to cancer, but because popular belief that cancer was a hereditary disease might prompt people to delay seeking qualified medical help. From this perspective, it was better for public education programmes to deny that cancer was a hereditary disease than to risk the possibility that such beliefs might encourage people to put off consulting a physician too long. This paper makes a similar argument for the exclusion of diet and nutrition from cancer education programmes. There were some important differences between its response to heredity and diet, as I will argue later, that illuminate the variety of strategies the ASCC used to manage public beliefs and attitudes.

Meat was central to the ASCC's concerns about diet and nutrition. As William H. Woglom, the editor of the journal *Cancer Research*, put it in 1922, it was 'the food which is most often blamed for cancer.'[6] Against the backdrop of such comments, the organization came to fear that public interest in cancer and meat – perhaps more than any other food – was a major reason why people delayed seeking medical help for the disease. Instead of turning to recognized physicians, people tended to reduce their consumption of meat in the vain hope of staving off cancer, and to disregard the warning signs of the disease in the mistaken belief that a change of diet prevented its onset. For this reason, the ASCC argued that advice on reducing meat consumption had no role in cancer education, despite the fact that some scientists and physicians believed that there was a causal relationship between meat and cancer. In ASCC's view, it was best to ignore or downplay the latter beliefs: they only confused the public.[7]

The ASCC's concerns were given added urgency by what the organization saw as the confusion of public messages about meat and cancer. In part, the problem was physicians, such as William Roger Williams, who promoted the idea that excessive consumption of meat might be cause of cancer. In the view of the Society, the messages put out by these physicians served to undermine its own educational efforts to persuade people to seek early detection and treatment, and were often indistinguishable from the messages put out by those the ASCC labelled as 'quacks'. The situation was complicated by the growing interest of the media in cancer. This interest had been deliberately cultivated by the ASCC as a means of raising public awareness of cancer. But, to its dismay, the organization also found newspapers and magazines quite willing to publish the views of physicians and 'quacks' who presented very different messages about cancer to one the ASCC wanted to promote, including the view that reducing meat consumption might help to prevent or cure cancer. At times the ASCC came to despair that it could ever control to profusion of media messages about cancer. Its response was to concentrate on its central core message of early detection and treatment, and to highlight the uncertainties involved in determining whether meat had a causative role on cancer.

The Popularity of Diet

The ASCC's anxieties about public attitudes to meat must be set against a profusion of medical and popular literature on diet and cancer. On the medical side, Indexcat identifies 161 publications on diet and cancer from 1880–1961, with 129 of these references in volume 4, 1936–55.[8] But, this does not include many books and articles on cancer or diet in which the relation between the two is one subject among many. Contemporaries believed there to be many more than 161. 'A bibliography on the subject of diet in relation to cancer would extend to many hundred titles',[9] noted an English Ministry of Health publication in 1926. And in 1937 the insurance statistician, Frederick Hoffman, reviewed the writings of over 200 'authorities' on the subject, a review that he acknowledged was partial. It only covered publications available in the library of the Biochemical Research Foundation of the Franklin Institute in Philadelphia.[10]

If medical writings on diet and cancer were prolific, they were dwarfed by the vast literature on the subject in the popular press. The ASCC routinely complained that diet and nutrition were among the most common explanations of the origins of the disease found in popular magazines, newspapers and elsewhere. Such publications, it protested, regularly promoted diets that would prevent the disease, and diets that would cure it, often accompanied by questionable scientific explanations as to why they worked. So great was the flood of popular literature that cancer agencies often felt overwhelmed, and despaired of ever being able to effectively challenge public belief in dietary explanations of cancer. The ASCC tried to build alliances with newspaper and other publishers to get their doubts before the public, but publishers continued to print such stories, and the organization worried that it could never stem the tide.[11] Despite its efforts to undermine the idea that diet and nutrition were important to cancer control, the organization's voice often seemed lost in a sea of opposing opinion.

To compound the issue, physicians complained, the stream of literature on the role of diet in cancer was only one part of a much broader flood of popular literature on the subject of cancer. In 1917, one of the founders of the ASCC, the New York surgeon William Seaman Bainbridge (1870–1947) argued that the campaign against cancer faced at least two difficulties: a confusion of media messages about cancer, and an inability on the part of physicians to agree on the facts of the disease. The result was that the public was bewildered and surgeons found themselves both attempting to correct a host of mistaken ideas, and struggling to explain a lack of medical consensus on many issues, including the role of meat in cancer causation and prevention.

> No one is more frequently importuned for what the patient, or the patient's friends and family, consider the final word concerning this or that piece of information – or misinformation – gathered from the columns of the daily press, from the 'popular medical lecture,' from the club, or from the medical meeting which the public may attend at will. Over and over the surgeon is asked: '*Is* cancer contagious?' '*Should* every little wart and mole, or every little lump and bump, be removed?' '*Will* I have cancer if I eat meat?' '*Must* I eat rice to prevent having cancer?' '*Does* persistent indigestion mean cancer of the stomach?', and so on, according to the hobby of the particular author or lecturer under whose temporary tutelage the individual has passed and according to the peculiar psychological constitution of the said individual.[12]

It was a never-ending task attempting to combat such questions, and while the surgeon might become something of an expert in answering them, they kept coming, and he [*sic*] might despair of ever stemming the flood.

Meat and Civilization

In the view of the ASCC, public confusion about the role of meat in cancer was, as Bainbridge noted, exacerbated by the lack of agreement among physicians as to the role of meat in cancer. Some said that there was no relationship, and others that there was a relationship. Even among those who agreed that there was a relationship, there was little agreement as to its nature. Some writers argued that excessive meat consumption caused cancer; others that it was caused by a lack of protein in the diet. As William P. Graves, the professor of gynaecology at Harvard Medical School, noted in 1921, 'Many unproved theories [of the cause of cancer] have been enthusiastically exploited. Among these the question of diet has played a prominent part. Some have pointed out the dangers of cancer in meat eating, others have seen a like danger in vegetarianism.'[13] The point was echoed by Frederick Hoffman in a 1937 survey of the medical literature on cancer and diet. In his view, the field comprised an amazing amount of contradictory theories and results: 'There are those who strongly advocate a vegetarian diet, while others...emphasize the urgency for a high protein diet as a measure of prevention, and possibly useful for curative purposes'.[14] On both sides of the debate, there was also little agreement as to how diet might cause cancer, or at what stage of the disease a dietary intervention was most likely to succeed. Yet, if they disagreed on many things, writers – critics of meat and its supporters – tended to agree on one thing: that cancer was a disease of urban-industrial civilization, and that civilized dietary practices were in part responsible.

Among those who argued that a diet *high* in meat caused cancer, commentators tended to share a belief that excessive meat eating was characteristic of urban-industrial civilization, and that cancer was one of the consequences of such practices. One argument was that cancer mortality had risen at the same time as meat consumption rose in Western Europe and North America, and even more so in New Zealand, Australia and Argentina and, in their view, there was a causal relationship between the two trends, from rising meat consumption to rising cancer mortality.[15] Cancer was less prevalent, if not unknown, they claimed, in countries and among peoples who did not consume such quantities of meat. The evidence for this was partly historical: it was commonly noted that people in pre-industrial Western societies consumed far less meat than people in later urban-industrial societies and that the incidence of cancer in the former was lower. The evidence was also partly anthropological: Tales from travellers, missionaries, imperial administrators, physicians and anthropologists suggested that cancer was much rarer in so-called 'primitive' races across the globe whose diet was primarily vegetarian.[16] There was also evidence from the influx of foreigners into Chicago, where their willingness to eat meat (especially inferior grades of meat) denied them in Europe was associated with increased rates of cancer mortality.[17]

All this suggested that meat was a problem of civilization. The vast quantities consumed in urban-industrial civilization led to all manner of ills, including cancer. In the view of many of these writers, a return to a more primitive, natural diet might begin to solve the problem. This is not to say that these writers necessarily rejected everything about urban-industrial food production: few, if any, wanted to do away with all the changes in agriculture, transportation, food preservation or storage that made possible the feeding of huge urban populations. Instead, they tended to argue for a leavening of such developments with the health beliefs and practices of 'primitive' and pre-industrial peoples, uncorrupted by civilization's progress – a return that often involved a reduction in meat consumption, if not its rejection entirely.[18]

For these writers, cancer control would come about by reforming eating practices. For some, reform focused on the individual: cancer, from such a perspective, was the result of personal dietary choices that people made in their day-to-day lives that could be overcome by individuals choosing to reduce or eliminate eating meat. For others, reform involved broader social interventions: cancer, the argument went, was the result of changes in farming practices, the production and distribution of meat, the poor quality and variety of food available in the rapidly expanding cities, modern methods of food preservation, the sheer quantity of meat available, or the availability of new and exotic meat products made possible by the growth of international trade and transportation. Cancer control, from such a perspective, might rely on encouraging people to change their habits and consume less meat. But it also meant changing the social, economic and cultural conditions that shaped peoples' choices.

Those who argued that a diet *low* in meat caused cancer are more difficult to characterize. They seem to be in a minority compared those who criticized meat, and their publications are more difficult to identify. So let me rely on the Idaho physician, Edwin E. Zeigler, as an example. In 1935, Zeigler argued that cancer was a disease of civilization, rare among primitive races.[19] But whereas others pointed to the increase in meat consumption as a cause of rising cancer mortality, Zeigler argued that in fact the civilized diet contained relatively little meat. The essential difference between civilized and 'primitive' diets was in the type of carbohydrate food consumed: some diets comprised predominantly acid-forming grains; others comprised base-forming foods, such as the potato and beans. In his view, the incidence of cancer was in proportion to the consumption of alkaline foods: The disease represented a failure of the body's defences against alkalosis, and he recommended a heavy protein diet as a countermeasure including all kinds of meat, seafood and fish, but also grains and nuts. He also recommended avoiding fruit and vegetables, and alkaline drugs. Ziegler's assumption that heavy protein diets were acid-forming was attacked in one review of his book. 'In his eagerness and enthusiasm to prove his thesis', the anonymous reviewer sniped,[20] 'he has selected the data that support his theory and omitted all evidence to the contrary'. But the broader argument was not dismissed by all. Hoffman, for example, extensively surveyed this book in his 1937 work on diet and cancer, perhaps the major survey of the subject in the 1930s. Hoffman characterized Zeigler as someone who had materially expanded the pioneering work of William Roger Williams among others.[21]

To the extent that Zeigler's book can be regarded as a guide to broader medical attitudes regarding the relation of meat to cancer, it suggests that proponents of meat in fact shared much with their critics. Both sides of the debate about the role of meat in cancer control linked cancer to broader concerns about civilization. In their view, civilized diets were essentially carcinogenic, and only a return to a more natural, primitive diet – be it one that included meat, or one that did not – would help to counter cancer. At a time when the ASCC argued that cancer was not taken seriously as a national concern, such arguments promised to raise the public visibility of this group of diseases by tying their emergence to broader cultural anxieties about civilization and decline. It also promised to link cancer to growing interest in holistic and Hippocratic approaches to clinical medicine, and to broader concerns about food and food reform.[22]

Dismissing Meat

Such promises might have raised the public visibility of the cancer, but they formed no part of the ASCC's programme of cancer control. Created in 1913, by a small number of physicians and lay supporters, the organization was dominated by physicians who saw early detection and treatment as the key to cancer control.[23] Their assumption was that cancer was a local disease in its early stages which later spread throughout the body. Treatment was most likely to be successful when the disease could be isolated and removed or destroyed in its local, circumscribed condition. Once the disease had spread to other parts of the body, they argued, it became more difficult, if not impossible, to treat. The core tasks of cancer control were, therefore, to identify the disease or the risk of the disease at the earliest possible stage, to get patients to their physicians as soon as the disease or the possibility of disease was identified, and to ensure their early treatment by experts using a recognized means of treatment, generally surgery, x-rays and radium.

For the physicians who ran the ASCC, popular interest in meat and other foods as causes of cancer threatened to undermine such an approach to cancer control. In the first place, the ASCC worried that a focus on diet might encourage people to delay seeking early help. In its view, delay was often the result of an excessive fear of the disease and its treatments, which encouraged people to look for any excuse not to go to their physician. Dietary beliefs provided just such an excuse. On the one hand, if people believed that their diet was healthy and unlikely to cause cancer, they could easily use this as a reason to avoid their physician if they spotted any of the early warning signs of cancer. On the other hand, if they believed that their diet was unhealthy and might be the cause of cancer they could easily succumb to a paralysing fear that nothing was to be done, or change their diet in the mistaken belief that this might cure the disease. Either way, the result was likely to be that people waited too long to see their physician. The problem was particularly difficult in the early stages of the disease, which was often unaccompanied by pain, so there was little to drive the patient to the physician, and much to allow delay. From this perspective, the ASCC believed, it was better to question any role for diet as a cause of cancer than to risk giving people an excuse not to seek early treatment.[24]

The problem was particularly acute, the ASCC believed, because – as we have seen – diet and nutrition were widely promoted as solutions to cancer in the popular literature. Magazines and newspapers routinely discussed dietary causes of the disease and nutritional interventions against it, as did the new medium of radio. Meat producers and their advertisers lauded the value of meat and meat products as building strength, preventing cancer and aiding recovery, and vigorously questioned any suggestion that it might cause cancer as the work of 'faddists'.[25] Vegetarian publications picked up on the medical literature that suggested that cancer was a product of meat consumption, as did a range of other publications concerned with health reform. For example, the health reformer, John Harvey Kellogg, argued that cancer was on the rise in flesh-eating countries, and was rare among those he labelled 'flesh-abstainers'.[26] Such comments made it difficult for the ASCC to persuade the public that diet had little or no role in cancer. It was a tiny organization until the 1940s, and – as noted above – often felt overwhelmed by the quantity of advice literature on this subject.

The problem was further compounded by the fact that many popular writers who saw a role for meat or its absence in cancer control were themselves physicians.[27] In the view of the ASCC, these physicians were mistaken. Yet – worryingly – they served to confuse the public which, it believed, was unable to distinguish between scientifically-recognized approaches to cancer control and those of dubious provenance. Nor did the public get much help from their family physicians, who, the ASCC claimed, often misunderstood the disease, failed to understand the importance of acting early, and were ignorant of the latest developments in cancer therapy – alternatively overly optimistic or overly pessimistic about the disease and its possibility of treatment.[28] They also promoted erroneous views, including that diet caused cancer and might be used to prevent or cure the disease. For Bainbridge, once a patient had reached a physician, 'the condition and not a theory is the paramount issue'.[29] It was not necessary at this stage, he claimed, 'to bring forward figures, mostly of ancient origin, to convince the patient that he must beware absolutely of a meat diet if he would escape cancer'.[30] The necessity was to treat the disease.

Such anxieties on the part of the ASCC seem to have worsened during the 1920s, and the organization began a vigorous campaign to turn physicians away from dietary interventions. 'Attempts to cure cancer, or to influence its growth, by diet have been widely advocated but with no success', it noted in a 1927 pamphlet *Essential Facts about Cancer* aimed at physicians,[31] 'When we realize the widespread occurrence of cancer in the animal kingdom, affecting herbivorous as well as carnivorous animals, of the most varied diet, we see how futile is the attempt to prevent or to cure cancer by any modification of diet in man'. It is a measure of the growing importance of this issue that such comments were not present in earlier editions of this pamphlet published in 1919 and 1924, a reflection perhaps of mounting concerns about food faddism.[32] By the end of the 1920s the AMA also weighed in with a number of radio reports asking 'Does Meat Cause Cancer?' The answer was generally no.[33]

To add to its difficulties the ASCC also became increasingly concerned about the willingness of quacks and food faddists to promote diet as a means of preventing and sometimes treating cancer. In its view, these practitioners tempted patients away from programmes of early detection and treatment, so contributing to delay, and ultimately to the death of the patient. According to the organization, such preventive measures were of little value, and the therapeutic use of diet was worse than useless. Yet it was often a difficult thing to distinguish between the alternative and orthodox. Some popular critics of meat such as John Harvey Kellogg were themselves physicians, others such as the Englishmen Rollo Russell and J. Ellis Barker drew extensively on medical writers to justify their claims.[34] The ASCC thus began a vigorous campaign to discredit those who provided such advice literature. As the surgeon James Ewing put it in 1926 'The semi-medical literature of the day abounds in advice for the avoidance of cancer by dietary and hygienic measures. One of the largest sellers among recent books laid the whole blame for cancer upon constipation. [Possibly authored by the British medical practitioner, William Arbuthnot Lane] The public should be informed that there are no panaceas of this sort'.[35]

Credibility and Cause

The ASCC's efforts to downplay claims that meat (or its absence) caused cancer were thus incorporated into broader attacks on 'quacks' and food faddists, and into attempts to educate family and other physicians and the media about cancer. The organization also sought to educate the public about the early warning signs of the disease, to go for a regular check-up from a recognized physician, and to get competent medical attention the moment the disease or the possibility of the disease was identified. In its educational efforts it asserted that knowledge about the role of diet and nutrition in cancer was highly uncertain, and sought to undermine the credibility of those who claimed it was not.

Credibility could be attacked in many ways. Sometimes the ASCC questioned the motivations of those who promoted dietary approaches to cancer; sometimes it questioned their competence; sometimes their knowledge. Quacks and faddists were routinely portrayed as more interested in profits than patients: they were secretive and untrustworthy individuals, who could do much harm to those who sought their assistance.[36] Those who promoted diet were also portrayed as unable to do much for their patients, ignorant of cancer and modern methods of intervening against it, blinded by their own enthusiasm, and divided as to how diet or nutrition caused the disease, or what role it might have in control. For the ASCC such divisions were a godsend. The lack of consensus helped it undermine the credibility of dietary approaches to cancer by highlighting the interests behind the various approaches. The English radiologist John F. Hall-Edwards writing in 1926, echoed the point. Public interest in cancer and food was largely promoted by 'Food Faddists', people who had an 'axe to grind'.[37]

If the ASCC and its supporters attacked advocates of diet for inconsistency and self-interest, they also attacked them for failing to offer sufficient proof of their claims. The British medical practitioner, William Roger Williams, whose *Natural History of Cancer* was quoted at the start of this paper was a particular object of attack. James Ewing dismissed William's suggestion that meat might be a cause of cancer with the comment that: 'It is conceivable that overnutrition should facilitate overgrowth, but it is not so clear why overnourished tissues should tend toward neoplastic instead of normal growth'.[38] The Dutch pathologist, H. J. Deelman, speaking at the ASCC conference on cancer in 1926 urged Williams to: 'Bring proof of what you are writing!'[39] In his view Williams provided no – or inadequate – evidence to counter claims that the differences in mortality rates he attributed to diet were not due to some wholly different mode of living or due to racial peculiarities. The American epidemiologist, George Soper endorsed Deelman's paper, arguing that it implied that epidemiology needed a higher-quality of person.[40]

Soper's comments point to a further means by which critics attacked those who promoted diet and nutrition as causes of cancer: they began to question the reliability of their statistical reasoning. As has been noted, many of those who argued that meat was a cause of cancer pointed to statistical evidence that correlated a rise in cancer mortality with a rise in meat production and consumption during the nineteenth century, or that compared the prevalence of cancer or cancer mortality in so-called 'primitive' and pre-industrial peoples with their prevalence in populations in so-called 'civilized' nations. Others also highlighted evidence that showed a temporary arrest of mortality in Denmark and the UK following the First World War when meat consumption fell.[41]

In the first half of the twentieth century, however, such arguments were increasingly criticized by physicians and statisticians. Some, such as the surgeon William Seamon Bainbridge attacked the association of meat and cancer by challenging the historical interpretation of the impact of meat on rising cancer statistics. 'As regards the consumption of meat – chilled or frozen meat being especially singled out for condemnation – it may be noted that the increase in the deaths recorded from cancer in England was apparent long before chilled or frozen meat reached that country in any quantity, or toward the end of the seventies of the last century'.[42] For others, statistical arguments that suggested a causal relationship between meat consumption and cancer tended to confuse causation and correlation. As William H. Woglom argued in 1922, 'It would seem that the youngest student of logic could point out the fallacy here. It is this: that the parallel course of two events is no proof that one of them causes another'.[43] Indeed, Woglom argued that the correlation between rising meat consumption and rising cancer incidence was a fiction. In his view, meat consumption was declining, and there was no proof of an increase in the number of cases of cancer.

There is also evidence that a new generation of medical statisticians were beginning to weigh into the argument, though perhaps more so in Britain than the United States. Evidence for such an intervention comes from a 1926 British Ministry of Health report.[44] The authors of the report – a Ministry medical official, S. Monckton Copeman, and the statistician Major Greenwood[45] – argued that the confusion of correlation and cause was common, especially in the case of diet and cancer. In fact, they claimed, the statistical case for a causal relation between the increase in cancer mortality and the growth of meat consumption was actually no stronger than the statistical case for the assertion of a causal relation between the increase in cancer mortality and the growth of the Socialist Party.[46] The last association was absurd, the authors noted: no rational person could imagine any direct relation of cause and effect between the two, but statistically it had the same meaning as the other association. The only difference was that intelligent people could imagine ways in which increased consumption of animal protein might prejudice normal cellular metabolism and lead to cancer.

So how were people to decide whether an association was causal? Copeman and Greenwood argued that it could only be decided by performing what they called an 'experiment'. In this case, an experiment involved studying the cancer mortality of populations living under conditions which, except for diet, were comparable with those experienced by populations in which cancer was a large and measurable factor of mortality. The advocate of vegetarianism, Rollo Russell, had already conducted such an experiment, in which he had explored cancer incidence and mortality in Cistercian and Benedictine monasteries where meat comprised respectively no part or a small part of the diet. Russell had found a lower rate of cancer mortality among the monks compared to the general population, confirming his arguments for a vegetarian diet.[47] Monckton Copeman and Greenwood, however, criticized his statistics for a lack of precision: the age distributions and exact numbers of those exposed to risk were not available, and the evidence that death from cancer had really not occurred, they claimed, was not conclusive.[48] They argued that their own study of the incidence of cancer in English religious houses lent no real support to the contention that among such populations the relative incidence of cancer was low. Fatal cancer occurred in populations abstaining from flesh food.

The report itself might not have solved the question of whether diets high in meat caused cancer, but the English Ministry saw other lessons coming from its publication. George Newman, the Chief Medical Officer noted that one of the reasons why his Ministry decided to publish the report was 'as an indication of the kind of proofs that have to be sought before the various popular dietetic theories of cancer can be accepted.'[49] And this argument would have found support across the Atlantic among those, like Soper, who hoped to increase the quality of people coming into epidemiology, and those organizations – like the ASCC – which hoped to challenge those who proposed dietary interventions against cancer. The historian Harry Marks has shown how experiments of the sort carried out by the English Ministry were increasingly employed by a group of American 'therapeutic reformers' to direct medical practice against the competing claims of groups with an interest in (over)prescribing drugs.[50] Such experiments were likely also employed to direct American medical practice against those who sought to promote dietary interventions against cancer.

Prevention

If the ASCC attempted to challenge those who promoted a role for meat (or its absence) in cancer by redefining causation, they also attempted to challenge it by redefining prevention. Those who argued that meat or its absence was a cause of cancer tended to use the term 'prevention' to mean averting the onset of cancer before it started by changing people's environment or habits. But, such a meaning of prevention was increasingly marginalized within the ASCC, which tended to employ the term in a more therapeutically-oriented way. The point can be made by the *Prevention of Cancer Series,* a series of pamphlets published by the AMA between 1915 and 1924, aimed at the public and the medical profession.[51] Despite its title, the prevention series focused primarily on early detection and treatment: preventing the further development of the disease, rather than prevention in the sense of preventing its onset. Indeed, the term 'prevention' was rarely used in any of the pamphlets, except the title. The principle point of the series was to educate physicians and the public about the nature of cancer, its detection, and the (surgical) interventions that could be deployed if a cancer was identified. Prevention – in the sense of preventing its onset – was subordinated to therapy.

But, by labelling the series 'prevention of cancer' the ASCC not only subordinated prevention in its traditional sense to cure, it also recast it in therapeutic terms.[52] Thus, authors referred to 'preventive' measures such as the encouragement of healthy wound healing, and the removal of sources of chronic irritation like moles, warts or bad teeth that might lead to cancer.[53] They also sought to portray the surgical removal of cancers already established in the body as a form of 'prevention'; preventing their further growth in the body, and preventing mortality from this group of diseases. The notion of prevention as preventing the onset of disease never entirely disappeared. Indeed, some members of the ASCC continued to see prevention in this sense as a solution to the cancer problem.[54] But, even among this last group, dietary interventions were rarely recommended, and, in practice the ASCC devoted very few resources to such approaches. The notion of prevention as early detection and treatment dominated ASCC approaches to cancer control.

Complications

The ASCC's efforts to downplay popular interest in a causal relationship between meat (or its absence) and cancer did not go smoothly. Advocates of this causal relationship challenged the ASCC's claims, urging people to ignore them, and to continue with dietary interventions. The British medical practitioner, Sir Arbuthnot Lane, for example, encouraged people to turn to a body of 'common knowledge' to counter the view of experts in the field. The public might be informed by authorities that diet played no role in the causation of cancer, he noted, but it was 'common knowledge that our health and happiness depends largely on what we eat, and that any excess in the matter of food or drink brings with it a certain retribution in the guise of some intestinal or general disturbance',[55] including cancer. Lane's voluminous popular writings contributed to such 'common knowledge', allowing him to simultaneously validate his own expertise and the expertise of the public that supported him.

A further complication in the ASCC's efforts to undermine claims that meat caused cancer was that its physician leaders saw an important role for meat in promoting meat and other nutritional interventions in maintaining health and bolstering the constitution. In the first place, while the ASCC publicly downplayed a role for diet and nutrition as causes of cancer, physicians among its leaders often portrayed meat as part of a healthy regime, something that could maintain good health if used in moderation. Patients would routinely ask them about diet and other aspects of life, and while physicians questioned their value in preventing or curing cancer, they generally argued that in moderation they were not harmful. 'A sedentary life, meat eating, and wearing corsets are not especially dangerous', noted George Soper in 1923, ' but should not be carried to excess for general health reasons'.[56] 'No particular type of diet had any known influence on the incidence of cancer,' the pathologist/physician James Ewing warned his readers in 1926, arguing that the public needed to be warned against dietary panaceas for cancer:[57] 'On the other hand one may preach without limit moderation in all things'. The problem was that in a world in which the public routinely read that diet could prevent or cure cancer, these dietary suggestions could be misconstrued, and physicians feared that by providing such advice they might inadvertently encourage the public to turn to diet and nutrition to combat cancer. It was a tricky problem. Patients' needed to be persuaded to maintain a healthy diet; but they also needed to be persuaded not to see diet and nutrition as panaceas for ills against which they were ineffective. The result was a seemingly never-ending cycle in which the ASCC's physicians urged their patients to moderate their diet to maintain health, and then, to ensure that such advice was not interpreted to mean that diet might help to combat cancer, they simultaneously sought to undermine claims that diet would cure or prevent cancer.

In the second place, the ASCC's effort to challenge public belief in a relationship between diet and cancer was also threatened by a related problem. Not only did physicians encourage their patients to maintain a healthy diet, they also used diet and nutrition to sustain patient strength through what could be a long, uncertain and painful course of treatment. Cancers and its treatments were often associated with a catchexia or wasting, which physicians sought to combat by means of dietary interventions. The result was much the same as with the advice that they dispensed on healthy-eating. Patients, physicians worried, might see such dietary interventions as cures for the disease, rather than as *supplementary* interventions that sustained patient strength so that they survived the disease and its treatment. Once again physicians found themselves having to manage their patients' beliefs about diet and cancer; ensuring that any supplementary dietary interventions were not confused with the dietary and nutritional therapies promoted by quacks, food faddists and 'ignorant' physicians.[58]

The ASCC thus constantly worried that its physicians engaged in practices that could confuse the public as to the real roles of diet and nutrition in cancer, just as they worried that their public advice – that diet and nutrition had no role in cancer control – might raise questions for patients about the nutritional advice and interventions that physicians gave. The consequence was that it continually had to monitor patients and the public for any signs that its control message was being misinterpreted. It seemed an endless task, for the public – the ASCC feared – was always misinterpreting its message, and raising questions about physician expertise. The issue was compounded by two further problems. The first was growing laboratory evidence that diet had an important role in the successful uptake of transplantable cancers in laboratory animals. (The problem was that when these animals were transported from one institute to another, tumours which had previously been easily grafted onto a particular type of animal often seem no longer so easy to transplant: changes in the animals' diet were quickly pinpointed as a possible cause.)[59] The second problem was Frederick Hoffman, the Prudential's insurance statistician and a member of ASCC. While most physicians on the ASCC questioned a role for diet in cancer causation, Hoffman took a very different position. His 1937 *Cancer and Diet*, a massive

767-page book, concluded that 'overabundant food consumption unquestionably is the underlying cause of the root condition of cancer in modern life',[60] though he tended to disagree with the theory that meat consumption was favourable to cancer, arguing instead that a high protein diet was opposed to malignant tumour formation.[61] The ASCC repeatedly told the public that diet had little or no role in cancer control: Hoffman gave a very different message.

Deny and Question

Hoffman's comments return us to the main point of this essay; the question of why in its public education programmes the ASCC undermined the idea that meat might cause cancer. I've argued that this was not because the organization necessarily rejected the idea that there might be a dietary component to cancer causation, or even that meat might contribute to the disease in some way. Instead, I suggest that it was because the ASCC feared that any mention of diet or nutrition threatened the mainstay of its anti-cancer efforts – early detection and treatment – by dissuading people from seeking expert help until after the possibility of successful intervention was gone. This concern that people might delay was given urgency by the fear that many so-call 'quacks' and food faddists encouraged the public to believe that meat could cause cancer, and so contributed to a likelihood for people to delay seeking early detection and treatment. For all these reasons the ASCC tended in its public education programmes to undermine claims that meat might promote cancer.

The situation was complicated by the media's attitude towards cancer. While the ASCC was increasingly enthusiastic about using newspapers, magazines, radio and film to promote its message of early detection and treatment, and to break down the silence and stigma around this group of diseases, it also worried that the media was as much a threat as a help. Newspapers, radio and magazines routinely promoted alternative interventions against cancer, including dietary and nutritional interventions. It often seemed impossible to control such alternative messages, and the problem was compounded by the mixed messages about cancer coming from physicians, some of whom promoted dietary interventions through the mass media. To the ASCC and other cancer agencies, a focus on one message – early detection and treatment – helped to counter such problems. It distinguished the ASCC's message from that of the mass of other messages circulating in the media, and so helped to marginalize dietary and other interventions.

At the beginning of this essay, I drew a parallel between the ASCC's response to heredity and its response to diet and meat. The ASCC tended to reject a role for heredity in cancer for much the same reasons that it sought to undermine suggestions of a role for diet and nutrition, including meat, in cancer. But the

ASCC's response to diet and meat does not seem to have been as strong as its rejection of heredity. While its public education campaigns often bluntly stated that heredity was not a cause of cancer, they were often more circumspect in their attitude towards diet and meat. In the case of the latter, the ASCC's public education efforts tended to emphasize uncertainty about the relationship between meat and cancer, and to shift attention towards the role of meat in general nutrition. From such a perspective meat was not harmful to general health if consumed in moderation and in the right circumstances, and might even help to promote health. Public faith in eating meat was thus undermined not so much by outright rejection as in the case of heredity, but by creating public uncertainty about its role in cancer.

This is not to say that ASCC public education efforts always opted for outright rejection of a role for heredity in promoting cancer, or that their discussions of meat always emphasized scientific uncertainty. On the one hand, there is ample evidence to show that some ASCC public education programmes discussed animal studies that indicated a hereditary component to cancer, while raising questions about their applicability to programmes of cancer control in humans. On the other hand, there are statements such as that in 1926 of James Ewing quoted above that bluntly state that diet had no known influence on the incidence of cancer. Instead, I emphasize tendencies in the ASCC's public education programmes, with public discussions of heredity tending towards outright rejection, and public discussions of meat and diet tending towards statements about scientific uncertainty. Against what seemed an overwhelming flood of media reporting on the role of heredity and meat in cancer, the ASCC seems to have adopted at least two strategies to focus public attention on the need for early detection and treatment: One was the blunt denial of a role in the cancer causation; the other was to use scientific disagreements to promote public doubt. The ASCC might have lamented public confusion over diet and cancer, but it also found it useful to promote confusion by raising questions, and so undermining the credibility of claims that meat or its absence might cause cancer. At the same time, confusion served to acknowledge those among its members who held a minority position that diet might be a cause of cancer. Most significant for this book, the ASCC's stand in the meat and cancer debate was less an expression of its convictions on the scientific merits of the issue than a 'communication strategy' in tune with the major focus of its cancer control programmes – early detection and treatment.

7 WHAT'S FOR DINNER? SCIENCE AND THE IDEOLOGY OF MEAT IN TWENTIETH-CENTURY US CULTURE

Rima D. Apple

Barbeque, hamburgers, bacon and eggs, fried chicken: quintessential American[1] foods – meat. They are emblematic of the ideology of meat – the belief that meat is the indispensable article of food. Statistical studies of our consumption patterns and persistent tropes in popular culture confirm these icons of the American scene, with the paradigmatic diet serving meat at two or three meals a day. Through periods of abundance and scarcity, through debates over the benefits and dangers of meat for human health, meat has remained the centrepiece of the American table and American culture in the twentieth century. Nutritionists could and did claim that so much meat was unhealthful or unnecessary and advised the families to eat less meat. Economists could and did bemoan the high cost of meat-rich diets and advised consumers to use meat substitutes such as cheese, eggs and grains. Manufacturers of potential alternatives like oatmeal elaborated on this counsel, celebrating the health benefits of their non-meat products. Yet, nutritional scientists also urged people to eat meat for their health, both physical and mental. Meat producers from farmers to packagers hyped the advantages of meat in the diet. The drive to educate Americans, primarily female consumers, about the place of meat in a healthful diet illustrates the public interplay of science and culture.

Women and the Ideology of Meat

From the colonial period, Americans had been known as meat eaters. Even so, it was two aspects of nineteenth-century culture that cemented the ideology of meat in the United States: The first was Americans' increasing fascination with and faith in science; the second, the growing insistence that women needed modern science in order to raise healthy families.[2] As nutritional sciences evolved in this period, researchers produced detailed studies of foods, categorizing them as proteids or albumens; carbohydrates; and fats. The proteid or protein element was the most crucial for human diets, indispensable for health and vital for building and repairing muscles.[3] The best form of protein came from animals, making meat the most significant factor in the diet. Reflecting contemporary science, nineteenth-century American domestic literature promoted the ideology of meat to the women of the household.[4] Catharine Beecher and Harriet Beecher Stowe published the most popular manual in this genre, *The American Woman's Home* (1869). The sisters' philosophy was simple: 'the woman who wisely adapts the food and cooking of her family to the laws of health removes one of the greatest risks which threatens the lives of those under her care'.[5] They did not expect homemakers to be scientific experts, but they did encourage women actively to seek out scientific and medical information in making decisions about family care.

Combining scientific analysis with acute observation on American diet, Beecher and Stowe despaired that:

> the Americans are proverbial for the gross and luxurious diet with which they load their tables; and there can be no doubt that the general health of the nation would be increased by a change in our customs in this respect. To take meat but once a day, and this in small quantities, compared with the common practice, is a rule, the observance of which would probably greatly reduce the amount of fevers, eruptions, headaches, bilious attacks, and the many other ailments which are produced or aggravated by too gross a diet.[6]

They were convinced that Americans ate too much meat and that the nation would be healthier with less meat. The sisters spoke largely of and to educated middle-class women but the popularity of meat was not limited to this group. Though consumption varied by region, race, class and ethnicity, nineteenth-century Americans generally consumed huge quantities of meat.[7]

Beecher and Stowe were not alone in stressing the importance of modern science, especially for the homemaker, an emphasis underscored in the twentieth century. Women had a duty to serve wholesome and nutritious food at each meal. Not infrequently, women's obligation reached beyond the home to the nation at large, as one educator asserted in 1903:

> Food is the basis upon which physical life is supported. The intellectual, and to some degree, the moral vigor is measured by the physical state ... The history in general of the individual and of a nation where properly selected and prepared foods have been habitually used, is that of moral, intellectual and physical strength.[8]

The fate of the country rested in the woman's kitchen. Over time, the rhetoric became somewhat less picturesque but the point remained. Women needed nutrition education in order to protect their families and society. If their children struggled in school, if their husbands were not productive, if their families were not successful, the fault lay in the family's diet, evidence that the woman had failed in her responsibility.

Nutritionists, doctors, teachers, home economists, food manufacturers and reformers all directed their instruction to women. In classes, books, magazines, advertisements and exhibitions, they employed the language of science – whether that science came from the laboratory, the field, or the copywriters' pen – to educate women about healthful foods. 'Do you know,' wrote one Cornell University home economist in 1949,

> that the food you [mothers and future homemakers] choose can make a difference in the growth and development of your children? That the food you select can make a difference in the number of active years you and your husband will have? That the right food may prolong the vigor of life?[9]

Women's role as wife and mother, as housekeeper and protector of her family's health and well-being, legitimated the growth of the burgeoning domestic advice literature industry of the late nineteenth and twentieth centuries, a medium that directly and indirectly documents the ideology of meat.[10]

Defining Meat and Meat Consumption

What is this crucial element in a healthful diet? To some, the word 'meat' may conjure up images of steaks and roasts, in other words, expensive cuts of beef. Yet many writers did not limit meat to food from cattle. They included lamb and even poultry; that is, warm-blooded animals, both birds and mammals. For other commentators, the category of meat comprised even more. A 1903 Cornell University pamphlet for 'farmers' wives' listed meat as beef, mutton, pork, veal, and fish.[11] More recently, studies by the US Department of Agriculture (USDA) considered beef, pork, lamb and veal as 'red meat', adding in chicken, turkey, fish and shellfish to calculate 'total meat consumption'.[12] In other words, they included pork as 'red meat', though in these decades pork producers often advertised their product as 'the other white meat'. Chicken and turkey were not red meat, but were meat, as were fish and shellfish.[13] Frequently, the word 'meat' was not defined at all. Throughout the twentieth and into the present century, the definition of meat remains problematic.[14]

Evidence of the power of the ideology of meat lies in the rates of meat consumption. Unfortunately, inconsistent definitions of meat hamper any straightforward analysis of consumption patterns. So too, does the lack of consistent statistical studies over the century. Scattered, incommensurate studies of consumption were often confounded by various, and sometimes absent, definitions of meat. For example, in 1920, Columbia University chemist H. C.

Sherman estimated that 32.7 per cent of the 'bill of fare of the average American' was expended for meat, including poultry and fish, though the sample used in this study is not clear.[15] Other research of the same period compared the foods purchased by 500 unspecified contemporary families with that bought by 400 families 'about twenty years ago' and concluded that Americans were eating 8 per cent less meat than two decades earlier.[16] What did the category 'meat' include in this study? How representative were the families? A different type of analysis, released by the National Restaurant Association in the late 1940s, disclosed that America's top dishes were, in the words of two historians of vegetarianism, 'a meat lover's dream': ham and eggs, prime ribs, chicken, lobster, New England boiled dinner, fried oysters, baked Virginia ham, breast of capon, filet of sole and devilled crab. Given the source of the study and the names of the meals, these appear to be favourite restaurant orders, but still they point to the ideology of meat.[17]

Roger Horowitz's *Putting Meat on the American Table* provides a more finely tuned set of statistics highlighting the place of meat in the United States. Focussing on 1909, 1942 and 1965, he shows how meat consumption grew over the century. The lowest third income group did not buy as much meat as those in higher income brackets in a given year but each group followed the same trend over time. Among all groups, beef consumption dropped significantly from 81.5 pounds in 1909 to 69.4 pounds in 1942 but then rose to 104.7 in 1964. Pork consumption dipped only slightly between 1909 and 1942, from 67.0 to 63.7, and continued to drop to 58.7 in 1965. Poultry saw a different trend: from 14.7 in 1909, up to 20.7 in 1942, up to 40.9 in 1965. Most significantly, the overall consumption of meat, the prominence of meat in our diet, showed only a small drop in 1942, from 169.9 to 161.0 pounds, and then a dramatic increase by 1965, 208 pounds. Horowitz also found that the differences between the rural and urban populations shrank through the century; the difference between low-income and high-income groups remained, though it was less than earlier. Meat eating differed across regions of the country, but this difference was more in kind than quantity. As Horowitz explains: 'whether cooked over open fires or gas ranges, eaten in the homes of Slavic immigrants or African American sharecroppers, more meat and better meat were measures of the good life'.[18] The ideology of meat did not mean that consumption patterns were identical across ethnic groups, geographical areas, income brackets and generations. Yet, as these studies demonstrate, over time and in general, Americans lived the ideology of meat.

Though incomplete, such statistics document the scope of meat eating in the United States. But they don't tell us why Americans ate meat so voraciously. Answers to this critical question varied over the century as scientific discoveries disclosed new aspects of human nutrition, as economic circumstances changed, as technological advances transformed the modes of meat production and transportation, and as political conditions altered the social connotations of meat. Until the end of the century, most of the arguments for and against the centrality of meat in the diet focused on its effects on the body. Many described its benefits, both nutritional and therapeutic. Others were equally adamant about the problems meat produced in people. Consistently, women were told that contemporary science provided the best guidance for healthful eating.

Scientific Arguments for Meat Eating

With the scientific evidence employed early in the century, commentators were torn between advocating and denouncing dietary meat. The ambivalence of Whitman H. Jordan, director of the New York Agricultural Experiment Station, indicated the confusion evident even among scientists studying nutrition. Jordan's 1912 *Principles of Human Nutrition*, a volume widely used in home economics courses, explained that protein wastes were eliminated through the kidneys and therefore, 'generous protein consumption' taxed this organ of the body.[19] Jordan warned that '[protein] greatly promotes the growth of bacteria in the intestinal tract'; it excites the development of uric acid and consequently 'tends to rheumatic troubles'. Moreover, evidence that 'human beings have been grown and maintained in activity on a vegetable diet' established that people did not require meat.[20] Still, all these negative attributes did not automatically condemn an animal-based diet. On the one hand, Jordan noted that most successful communities, by which he meant the United States, England and other European countries, consumed large amounts of meat. 'On the other hand', he reminded his readers, 'the inhabitants of China and Japan are, to a large extent vegetarians ... It is fair to inquire, too, whether the small stature of the Chinese and Japanese is not related in some measure to their diet'.[21] Given such confusing claims, what was the best manner of feeding the family? Jordan's response was evasive, shaped more by cultural and economic factors than physiology.

> Undoubtedly, if American people would cut down its consumption of flesh foods, it would result in an advantage to health and would lighten the cost of living. On the other hand, the ease and completeness with which meats are digested by most persons, the efficiency for constructive proof of meat proteins, and the absence of any conclusive proof that moderate meat eating is harmful, are good arguments for the reasonable use of meat in families of comfortable circumstances.[22]

Though Jordan detailed many health problems that could arise from meat eating, and some of the benefits, ultimately he determined his position by the cultural stature of flesh protein. In effect, meat is a status symbol.

Jordan could not settle on the healthfulness of meat but others had no such difficulties. Throughout the century, advocates found many reasons to celebrate the positive attributes of meat for adults as well as children. Animal protein was good because it cured anaemia, it encouraged the digestive juices and thus aided digestion, it complemented other foods and made them more attractive. Contemporary ethnographic studies confirmed the healthfulness of meat. The lives of Eskimos and of the explorers who lived with them provided evidence that all meat diets were highly successful.[23] Meat contained high-quality protein to build strong muscles and was also a good source of thiamine, iron and phosphorus.[24] The iron content of meat was especially important for women's health. By the end of the twentieth century, nutritionists particularly were concerned that women wanting to lose weight would cut back on meat in order to save calories. They insisted that women needed meat for its iron and urged them to 'eat red meat, fish, or dark-meat poultry at least once a day. These animal foods contain *heme* iron, the type that our bodies absorb and use best', they reminded dieters.[25]

By mid-century, a popular theme in promoting meat involved the value of its eight essential amino acids. In her widely read *Let's Eat Right to Keep Fit*, Adelle Davis, nutrition guru of the period, instructed readers on the importance of protein in keeping them young, and thus healthy. She explained that 'Only when protein of excellent quality is supplied can each cell function normally and keep itself in constant repair'.[26] With adequate protein the body produced sufficient energy and 'life is made easier'.[27] Davis warned her readers that all protein was not the same; its value was related to its amino acids. Humans need twenty-two amino acids, fourteen of which can be manufactured by the body. The remaining eight, the so-called essential amino acids, must be obtained from food and proteins that contain all eight are called complete or adequate. Davis informed her readers on the role of the amino acids in nutrition and on how to identify suitable sources of protein. Her guidelines:

> Protein from muscle meats, used in roasts, steaks, and chops, are complete but contain fewer of some essential amino acids that do glandular meats and are therefore less valuable. On the whole, animal proteins, such as meat, fish, eggs, milk, and cheese, contain more essential amino acids in greater abundance than do vegetable proteins; hence they have superior value.[28]

Davis's twentieth-century stature was similar to that of Beecher and Stowe in the nineteenth century, and for many of the same reasons. Davis rejected paternalistic medical authority but sought answers in the contemporary medical and scientific literature, which she then provided her readers. Her spurning physicians and their patriarchal stance, while embracing the advances of modern science and medicine, made Davis a heroine to millions of children of the counterculture and many middle-class mothers as well who appreciated her technical but caring approach to family nutrition.[29] By the early 1970s, her books sold hundreds of millions of copies. Davis's discussion of amino acids was not unique in the period, but her advocacy served to popularize the concept and sustain the ideology of meat through much of the century.

Others, however, were not convinced that meat was healthful, or at least that the prodigious quantities of meat consumed in the United States amounted to good nutrition. Before the emphasis on amino acids, commentators early in the century frequently remarked on a connection between excessive meat intake and conditions such as rheumatism, gout and the like, as well as autointoxication.[30] The arguments of these writers were similar to those of Whitman H. Jordan, but their conclusions were different. Mary Davis Swartz, leading nutritionist of the period, published a typical analysis in the popular magazine *Good Housekeeping*. She recognized that people considered meat an, if not the, essential element of American diet. After all, it was relatively simple to prepare; it was an uncomplicated central point of a meal; it contained a high percentage of protein; generally, 'it is a valuable food, supplying nutriment in a pleasing and digestible form'. Meat had many positive attributes, she acknowledged, but, when we ate too much meat, the body excreted the surplus through the kidneys in the form of urea. In addition, there were purins in meat, which cannot nourish the body. These were changed into uric acid, and when not properly eliminated through the overworked kidneys, they could give rise to gout, rheumatism and also putrefaction, leading to autointoxication.[31] Balancing all the benefits and all the difficulties, Swartz advised that Americans eat less meat.

Similar analyses led other commentators to go further, to promote vegetarianism. Dr John H. Girdner saw nothing at all positive about meat eating. He compared humans to physically stronger animals, such as horses, cows and elephants that thrived on vegetables, not meat. He compared healthy, peace-loving peoples such as those from India who eschewed meat, with the warring British who ate meat. Then, he contrasted the fighting prowess of the Japanese, non-meat eaters, with the Russians, meat eaters. (Girdner was writing in 1907, shortly after the Japanese defeated the Russians in the Russo–Japanese War.[32]) Clearly, meat eaters were not superior. In addition, meat-eaters were susceptible to 'a large number of human ills', like tuberculosis from infected cattle, and even typhoid fever from raw clams and oysters, as well as to gout, rheumatism and kidney diseases. A physician would order patients with such conditions to cut all meat from their diet. So, Girdner reasoned 'My point is this, Why wait until disease appears before quitting a flesh diet? The proteid which meat supplies to the body can be obtained from a lacto-vegetable diet, minus the poisons'.[33]

Few went as far as Girdner to advocate vegetarianism, despite assertions that meat eating was unhealthful. Following the discovery of vitamins in the first third of the twentieth century, nutritionists, researchers, and medical practitioners frequently wrote about these mysterious micronutrients in 'corn, olive oil, and green stuff'.[34] Yet, meat continued as a fundamental ingredient in American cooking. Commentators believed that consumers would find a wholly vegetable diet 'boring' and that people accustomed to eating animal protein two and three times a day would find it difficult to avoid all meat. Therefore, the more usual advice was to add a little meat to the day's nourishment, for taste, for familiarity, but not too much.[35] Nutritionist Anne Pierce accepted that 'eggs and milk and green vegetables may supplement a milk and cereal diet effectively as meats, theoretically, but meat has a savor, an appetizing value, and is tolerated and digested better in some cases than eggs.'[36] In the second half of the century, print culture denounced the saturated fat content of meat linked to concerns such as hypertension, colon cancer and diabetes. A 1984 *Newsweek* article, 'America's Nutrition Revolution', addressed our 'flourishing natural obsession' with eating for health. The piece noted medical evidence linking diet to heart disease and cancer, and conceded that nutritional experts could not agree on what the latest evidence demonstrated as a healthful diet. Nevertheless, the authors provided rules that should govern one's diet, including lowering overall fat content and 'go[ing] meatless two out of three meals'. Notice that in two out of three meals, meat was still the dietary requisite.[37]

Not surprisingly, the meat industry responded to attacks on its product, carefully pointing to contemporary understandings of nutrition and physiology to explain away claims that meat causes disease.[38] By the third decade of the century, defenders of the industry heralded scientific discussions that rheumatism is caused by an infection carried through the blood stream and that uric acid was the result, not the cause, of gout. Their crowning defence of meat was that in other parts of the world people thrive on diets that are primarily meat. Since offence is often the best defence, they also promoted the benefits of even excessive meat consumption, maintaining that 'Meat proteins have a superior nutritive value because they more closely resemble the tissues which are to be nourished than do other proteins, and can be transformed with less loss.'[39] They undercut the status of vitamin-rich fruits and vegetables with the contention that meat is therapeutic, curing pellagra, and anaemia, even scurvy and beriberi. In the last instance, 'phenomenal results were obtained in the Japanese navy in the cure of beri-beri by substituting meat for white rice in the ration.'[40] Recognizing the importance of educating the younger consumer, the American Meat Institute placed advertisements in the *Journal of Home Economics* to direct the attention of teachers to the mineral and vitamin content of meat, also noting that 'The very appearance, aroma and flavour of well-cooked meat stimulate the salivary glands and promote good appetite.'[41]

Dietary Guidelines

The most pervasive encouragement for primacy of meat in the diet was also one of the most subtle: the dietary guidelines. Despite some limited arguments about the dangers of over-consumption of animal protein or even the harmful effects of any meat eating, the ideology of meat remained strong in the recommendations proclaimed in popular nutritional advice literature and classes. Sometimes presented as lists of essential nutritional categories, sometimes in the form of pie charts, and nowadays as 'food pyramids', they were widely broadcast in newspapers, magazines and extensively-distributed pamphlets and brochures, as well as during home economics and nutrition classes, often mandatory for girls in elementary and high schools. These templates addressed the whole of the diet and therefore did not appear to privilege meat over other classes of food. Yet the very format of these graphics reinforced meat as the gold standard for protein in the human diet. For example, the United States Department of Agriculture (USDA) issued its first set of recommendations in 1917 in a pamphlet entitled *How to select foods*. With this publication, the agency established the schema of presenting foods in nutritionally essential categories. A healthful diet, the pamphlet explained, consisted of a mixture of foods from five categories: fruits and vegetables; meats and other protein-rich foods (including milk for children); cereals and other starches; sweets; and fatty foods. 'The approach', a mixture of the five groups, 'permits all food to be recommended as part of healthful diets and precludes suggestions to restrict foods in one or another group'.[42]

Over the years, different agencies produced different guidelines. By the 1930s, milk was often listed in a separate category and the number of food groups increased. A 1932 Cornell Bulletin for Homemakers organized its presentation into eight groups: milk; bread and cereals; vegetables; fruit and tomatoes; cod-liver oil; eggs; meat and meat substitutes; and butter and other fats. In recommending methods with which the mother could lower food costs, the Cornell home economists seemingly minimized the contribution of meat to the family's nutrition when they advised the woman to 'serve meat not more than once a day if you are watching every cent'. However, in several ways the prose made it clear that meat was still the standard. First, it suggested using less expensive cuts such as shank or neck to stretch the food budget. Second, it considered meat substitutes as merely substitutes: 'Fish, when low in price, may be substituted for meat ... Dried peas, beans, or lentils may take the place of meat'.[43] Meat was still the benchmark. In the 1940s, influenced by World War II concerns about the availability of food under rationing as well as nutritional considerations, the food groups were redesigned. Some recommendations listed eight groups, others seven, still others eleven. Some combined all protein foods into one group, some separated milk into its own group. All these variations served to confuse as well as instruct consumers. Such diversity provided evidence for all sorts of different diets devised by nutritionists, columnists and manufacturers. Yet, each maintained a clearly marked 'meat' group.

The situation was somewhat clarified in the 1950s when a group of nutritionists, researchers, agriculturalists and the food industry developed new guidelines for the USDA. The basic four – milk, meat, vegetables and fruits, and breads and cereals – shaped nutritional advice for decades. These labels did very specifically privilege meat. Interestingly, despite the emphasis on animal protein, the meat industry was not totally pleased with the result because for the first time the arrangement included a recommended serving size, which was a mere 2–3 ounces of cooked meat, an amount smaller than the typical contemporary portion size. (And significantly smaller than today's typical serving size as well.) American consumers were admonished to eat a more varied diet drawn from all four groups. Milk, meat, vegetables and fruits, and breads and cereals were given relatively equal weight in the graphics and in the diet. Recommendations within the meat category included beans and peas as alternative protein sources, but these appeared more as an aside. The title of the food group was meat, not protein sources. Diet lists published in widely circulated magazines such as *Parents* and *Good Housekeeping* reflected this schema, counselling mothers to allow for two or more servings of meat, poultry, fish or eggs every day, accepting 'beans, peas, and nuts as an occasional substitute'.[44] Notwithstanding these permissible alternatives, many nutrition advisors simply presented 'good quality protein foods' as 'meat, milk, poultry and fish'.[45] Regardless of whether or not the advice specified alternatives, what is most critical is that the name of the group was meat; millions of school children and millions of homemakers learned the basic four groups as milk, meat, fruits and vegetables, and bread and cereal, the foods needed for a well-balanced, healthful diet. Meat was a vital component of the family's nutrition.

An illustrative example of this type of dietary advice was the US government's 1970 pamphlet *Family Fare: A Guide to Good Nutrition*, which continued with the four basic food groups: meat, vegetable-fruit, milk, and bread-cereal, and specifically admonished mothers to provide 'some meat, poultry, fish, eggs, milk or cheese at each meal'. The continued separation of meat and milk highlighted the importance of milk for children and meat for adults. Again, the category of meat was very broad, encompassing beef, veal, lamb, pork, variety meats (such as liver, heart, kidney), poultry and eggs, and fish and shellfish. *Family Fare* did mention alternatives to animal protein such as dry beans, dry peas, lentils, nuts, peanuts, and peanut butter but these foods were not given much standing in the approved diets. The pamphlet explained the importance of different amino acids to healthful nutrition and warned:

Proteins from cereal grains, vegetables, and fruits do not provide as good an assortment of amino acids as animal proteins do, but they do supply valuable amounts of many amino acids.[46]

To be sure, 'Proteins from legumes, especially soybeans, chickpeas, and peanuts are almost as good as proteins from animal sources',[47] but almost as good was not *as* good. Consequently, the mother was reminded that 'Combining cereal and vegetable foods with a little meat or other source of animal protein will improve the protein value of the meal'.[48] Clearly, the protein standard was meat.[49]

In the 1990s, the USDA replaced the Basic Four with the Food Pyramid, a graphic to illustrate dietary advice in a form referring to nutrients such as fat, salt, and sugar rather than foods that contained them. Despite the input of numerous nutritionists and other scientists, objections from the cattle industry, the sugar industry, other nutritionists and scientists, and various politicians and government bureaucrats delayed the initial release of the pyramid. The meat partisans were particularly incensed, fearing that the proposed representation would bias readers against meat. In *Food Politics: How the Food Industry Influences Nutrition and Health*, Marion Nestle analyses the political machinations that shaped the final pyramid, released after another year of negotiations. There are now twelve different pyramids, presenting six food groups for a healthful daily diet such as 'Fats, Oils, Sweets: Use Sparingly' and 'Meat, Poultry Fish, Dry Beans, Eggs & Nuts Group: 2–3 Servings'. Intended to better represent nutritional advice and reflect specific ethnic and therapeutic diets, these pyramids are extremely confusing graphics that have not yet proven popular.[50] Most notably, the text accompanying the food pyramids continues to give precedence to meat. For example, *What's in a meal?*, a brochure issued in 1994 by the Food and Nutrition Service of the USDA, explained to day care personnel which foods were reimbursable under the Child and Adult Care Food Program. Its food pyramid had one section marked 'Meat, poultry, fish, dry beans, eggs, & nuts group', but the text used the phrase 'meat or meat alternate'; once again, meat was the standard and anything else merely an 'alternate'.[51]

Substituting Meat under Crisis Situations

The enduring emphasis on meat can obscure large-scale attempts to reconfigure the American diet. It was crises – threats to human life, the nation, and the planet – that animated concerted efforts to alter our eating patterns. These crises most clearly documented the persistence of the ideology of meat. First and foremost among these crises was war, during which a lack of readily available and affordable meat could imperil the health of the American population. Throughout World War I and World War II, American women were forcefully instructed in their patriotic duty, namely to utilize alternatives to meat. Europe could not produce the food needed to feed her population, military and civilian; the United States had to feed them.[52] This did not mean that Americans had to forego all meat. Meatless days were one option, of course.[53] Housewives were reminded over and over again that the important point in selecting food was its nutritional value, not flavour. In print and in exhibitions, mothers were urged to 'discuss diet from the standpoint of food values rather than merely from that of appetite and taste'.[54] But advisors knew that the American palate hungered for things more familiar. Soon, exotic meats such as goat, shark and seal were discussed in the popular literature and displayed in food conservation exhibitions mounted by states' councils of defence and the United States Food Administration. Women's magazines patriotically announced 'new meats' for the beleaguered housewife; they explained the nutritional value of meats such as beef kidneys, beef liver, pork ears, tripe, suggestions previously reserved for those on limited incomes, especially during periods of high meat costs.[55] Though little-known in middle-class homes before the war, they attained high status in the late 1910s as examples of one's patriotism. The continued promotion of meat, even in strange and unusual forms, demonstrates the force of this animal protein on the American psyche.

The nutrition advice during World War II was another example of the status of meat in American culture.[56] Overseas farmlands had been turned into battle fields; thus, the fields and farms of the United States needed to feed the war effort, at home and abroad. Once again, women were called upon to do their part. Advisors offered many suggestions for stretching what limited meat there was available and for proper substitutes. Home economists, in particular, touted the benefits of milk, cheese, dried beans and peas. When meat was in short supply, they recommended 'extend[ing] the meat flavour' by mixing 'meat with beans, macaroni, spaghetti, rice, vegetables, bread crumbs or cereals'.[57] Manufacturers such as Ralston Purina urged home economics teachers to promote the advantages of their products, noting that 'In these days of meat rationing, Instant Ralston and Ralston Whole Wheat Cereal serve a valuable purpose as meat-extenders'.[58] Women learned how to best utilize the ubiquitous rationing coupons found in every housewife's purse. Rationing was the 'fair way of insuring enough of America's food supply for our armed forces and lend lease, and at the same time dividing food at home so that everyone has enough to keep healthy', reminded Penny Prudence in her *Coupon Cookery*. Though her book highlighted the 'meat problem', Prudence provided little direct help to the woman looking for alternatives, beyond including more eggs and milk in the family's meals. In the recipe section, she had pages and pages of typical meat dishes, such as meatballs, breaded veal chops, and the like, though she did include other meat ingredients such as pork knuckles, oxtail, 'braised hearts with noodles', and 'brains and eggs'. She provided only seven bean recipes, of which three contained some meat.[59] Other commentators educated the public on how to better utilize the meat available. They offered tips on methods of cooking and supplied charts that described various difference cuts and their use.[60] Creative use of meat would enhance the strength of the nation.

Ironically, despite the call to sacrifice, Americans' consumption of meat jumped during the war. Increased purchasing power due to greater war-related employment that brought additional workers into the labour force ratcheted up demand for more meat and choicer cuts, like steaks and roasts.[61] In addition, the imposition of rationing minimized the differences between consumption at various income levels as poorer groups bought significantly more meat than previously, while the purchases of the well-to-do declined slightly.[62] Thus, despite the admonition to save meat and to find alternatives to meat, the ideology of meat prevailed, continuing to place meat at the centre of the meal.

Warfare was not the only crisis that generated attempts to move meat from its pivotal position. At various times in the century, especially in the 1910s, in the 1950s, and in the 1970s, meat prices rose to unprecedented heights. To aid the housewife in economic straits, magazines, classes and cookbooks all discussed the ways women could feed their family healthfully on less animal protein. Typical were recipes that employed a small amount of meat augmented with rice, vegetables, or pasta. Cheese sauces appeared frequently, as did egg dishes. Most articles mentioned the use of dry beans and peanuts. Yet, in their titles and text, the primacy of meat was taken as a given. You could use 'thrifty meat alternatives', you could 'stretch meat', you 'could make a little meat go a long way', you could 'eat high on low-cost meat cuts'.[63] The ideology of meat remained central to American culture, despite financial constraints.

In the last decades of the twentieth century, patriotism and economics faded from the discussions about American meat consumption as two new challenges confronted the ideology of meat. One arose out of a concern for the safety of the American population, the other from a concern for the health of the planet. Early in the century, arguments to moderate or eliminate meat from the American diet had centred primarily on the ill effects of excessive protein intake on the individual's well-being. In later years, the problem was the high fat content of meat that was linked to heart disease and cancer. However, the growth of factory farms in the last third of the century has altered our perceptions about meat eating. Through dramatic changes in technology and fuelled by the demand for meat, factory farms have developed as large conglomerates in which cattle are housed in close quarters and fed high-protein grains, and chickens are packed into coops and fed 'scientifically balanced' feeds. Though these modes of meat production differ radically from those employed earlier in the century, food safety practices have not significantly changed since the passage of the 1906 Meat Inspection Act. The meat industry has remained a powerful lobby in Congress which has led to media exposés about modern meat production.[64] High-profile media stories have educated the public in some of the newest bacteriological and biological discoveries, using science to alert consumers to the potential risk of eating contaminated and drugged products. Over the years, consumers have received crash courses in the action of hormones in cattle, the role of antibiotics in food production, and the consequences of ingesting E. coli 0157:H7, salmonella, listeria, campylobacter, and BSE (or mad-cow disease), and the effects of pharmaceuticals such as DES.

Despite the use of antibiotics, over the last two decades of the twentieth century the media reported on more and more cases of sickness induced by infected meat. The first microbe to receive much public attention was E. coli 0157:H7, which was estimated to cause 20,000 cases of illness and to kill 400–500 people a year. The microbe was identified in tainted ground beef in 1982 reports from Oregon and Michigan. Contamination can occur when a cow's intestinal or faecal matter comes in contact with muscle meat, usually during unsanitary slaughter. The problem is exacerbated in ground beef because the grinding spreads the contamination. Cooking at a high temperature can kill the bacteria, but this is difficult to accomplish with hamburger because of uneven temperatures throughout the patty.[65] Typical stories about the cases of E. coli opened with a heart-rending story of a dying child and the devastated parents. Bob Galler's three-year-old daughter died eighteen days after ingesting contaminated hamburger. He appealed to the meat industry and the government to alert consumers to the potential risks of such situations, but to no avail until a major outbreak of E. coli poisoning in January 1993 at a series of Jack-in-the-Box restaurants in Washington and several over western states. Approximately 600 people were sickened after eating undercooked ground beef. Other outbreaks followed in many other states from Texas to Pennsylvania, with more illness and six more deaths. Since then, there have been several large-scale withdrawals of contaminated meat from the market: one in 1997 resulted in a recall of 25 million pounds of beef; another in 2002 of nearly 19 millions pounds.[66] Problems have not been limited to contaminated beef and E. coli. By the mid-1990s, salmonella infected poultry resulted in approximately 2,000 deaths a year. A 1998 *Consumer Reports* investigation of chickens bought in supermarkets across the country revealed that 63 per cent had campylobacter, 16 per cent had salmonella, and 8 per cent had both. Only 29 per cent of the samples were free of both. Over the years, campylobacter accounted for 1.5 million illnesses, nearly half traced back to poultry. Moreover, millions of pounds of hot dogs and deli meats tainted with listeria have been recalled.[67]

The ideology of meat has been so strong that while these articles graphically described the pollution of our food supply, they rarely advised mothers to stop feeding their families meat. Instead, they offered suggestions such as thoroughly washing meat and cooking it until well done in order to ameliorate such problems. After detailing the potential horrors of the supermarket meat and fish counters, the *Ladies' Home Journal* suggested shopping at popular stores, which were more likely to have a rapid turn over of stock, inspecting the cleanliness of the store, and checking the sell-by date. The author also reminded women to 'beware of displays where fish fillets are piled high on top of each other. The ones on top will be too warm'. The article ends with: 'Do your part. When you shop, buy perishables last'.[68] Even the 1998 *Consumer Reports* exposé that disclosed extensive contamination of poultry did not tell consumers to avoid chicken. Rather the magazine recommended how to protect the family by carefully selecting, handling and cooking poultry.[69] Despite all the possible problems with the nation's meat supply, the solution was not to avoid meat, but to be careful.

By the late twentieth century, the context for the ideology of meat had changed again. During periods of war, the focus had moved from the health of the individual to the welfare of the nation. By the 1990s and the early years of the twenty-first century, it involved a renewed interest in the ethics of meat eating. Dating back to its roots in Pythagorean philosophy, vegetarians had based their rejection of meat eating on the necessity of maintaining an ethical relationship between humans and non-human animals as well as non-violent principles.[70] Conditions of factory farming revitalized the enunciation of these values. Critics deplored modern production as inhumane and unnatural.[71] Yet one quirky proposal around this ethical dilemma underscores the endurance of the ideology of meat. Recognizing our attachment to meat, PETA, People for the Ethical Treatment of Animals, one of the most active organizations promoting vegetarianism, has offered a prize of $1 million to the 'first person to come up with a method to produce commercially viable quantities of in vitro meat at competitive prices by 2012'.[72] In other words, the inhumane treatment of animals is the problem, not the eating of meat. The goal is to produce meat differently, not to replace meat with a different form of protein.[73]

Conclusion

Will our greater knowledge of contamination and adulteration of meat products change American eating habits? Will concerns such as these, coupled with worries over dietary fat and other nutritional problems linked to meat consumption, finally alter what we put on the table? So far the evidence documents that changing our dietary habits is a formidable task. Statistical data are limited but one 'natural experiment' demonstrated the resilience of the ideology of meat.

A new infective agent joined the list of potential hazards in the late 1990s.[74] Bovine Spongiform Encephalopathy (BSE), also known as 'mad cow disease', became a legally reported disease in the United States in 1986. By March 1996, the British government announced a potential connection between BSE and human Creutzfeldt–Jakob Disease (CJD). The human variant though usually fatal was rare; still, it received concerted media attention. Concern over the possible spread of CJD spurred activists such as Cele Sardo and Mayra Lichter, to form the Creuzfeldt-Jakob Disease Foundation and establish a website to raise awareness about the condition and to help other families facing the disease.[75] Calls for government regulation led to increasing inspection of cattle, particularly imported cattle, and the banning of imports from countries identified as possible reservoirs of BSE. BSE was different to previous identified microbial contaminants in other ways as well. BSE cattle were sickened when fed contaminated meat and bone meal. Whereas careful handling during production, marketing or home care could mediate some of the potential problems of E. coli, salmonella, and the like, it could do nothing for meat from cattle infected with BSE. Consequently, a March 2001 Gallup poll discovered that one quarter of those interviewed said that they 'had cut back or sworn off eating certain types of meat'.[76] Subsequently, when a cow tested positive for BSE in Washington State in 2003, many other countries stopped importing US beef.[77] In the week following, cattle prices fell, consumer surveys indicated that US beef demand could fall by as much as 15 per cent, and sales of fresh and frozen beef declined. Yet an examination of household beef purchases between 1998 and 2004 showed that this dip in consumption was only slight and temporary. As the USDA Economic Research Service statisticians noted: 'The magnitude of responses in the market was difficult to estimate precisely, but the duration was clear; within two weeks, consumers were behaving exactly as they had before the announcement'.[78] True, over a longer period, we can track some decrease in the consumption of red meat, an 11-per-cent-drop between 1970 and 1999, for example. Researchers point to various factors that influence a family's eating patterns: from geographical to racial and ethnic, and, of course, economic. But what is important to note is that in same period, poultry consumption increased 102 per cent. So our love affair with red meat may be dissipating, but not our love affair with meat per se.[7]

Time and again, the same advice is repeated in women's magazines, in newspapers, in general interest magazines, in popular health magazines, in nutrition classes:

> No food is perfect, but nuts, beans, fish, and poultry are all, on balance, more healthful sources of protein than red meat. Savor a steak now and then, but only as the occasional flourish on a diet built on fruits, vegetables, and grains.[80]

Like the food pyramids, these recommendations utilize scientific arguments to stress the importance of increasing our daily intake of fruits and vegetables and of whole grains, minimizing our intake of fats and of sugars, substituting nuts, beans, fish, and poultry for red meat. But note: steak is branded a special treat, something to be desired. Our rhetoric about food still indicates that meat is the gold standard for protein. If we are serious about promoting a more healthful diet, one that moderates our meat, especially red meat, consumption we need to invent a new rhetoric that does not implicitly reinforce the ideology of meat.

8 VEGETARIANISM, MEAT AND LIFE REFORM IN EARLY TWENTIETH-CENTURY GERMANY AND THEIR FATE IN THE 'THIRD REICH'

Ulrike Thoms

It is well known that Hitler regarded himself as a vegetarian, and described himself as such. Albert Speer, for example, reported that Hitler opposed the hunt, regarding it as a relic of the feudal world. Hitler was also known to describe meat eaters as 'corpse eaters' and meat broth as 'corpse tea', and often ordered his personal chef to prepare him separate vegetarian dishes even as his retinue dined on schnitzel and goulash.[1] Henry Picker's account of Hitler's Table Talks testifies to the fact that Hitler was not motivated purely by health concerns. Indeed, in his recorded dinnertime conversations with his followers, held at the Führer's headquarters, Hitler also was known to have reflected upon the historical development of contemporary eating and dietary habits, and to have debated whether herbivorous animals were better suited to tasks of physical endurance. He also reported on the positive personal effects he experienced as a result of his vegetarian diet, claiming that after switching to a strictly meatless diet, he no longer sweated as profusely while delivering speeches at major rallies.[2] Only later, after his health began to deteriorate, did Hitler begin to mention stomach complaints in his discussions of vegetarianism. In one instance, he is recorded to have plaintively pointed to his vegetarian and very small plate, and complained, 'How am I supposed to be able to survive on this? Just take a look!'[3]

Hitler's vegetarianism highlights one of the major themes of this paper – the multiple meanings of rejecting meat as a part of one's diet. His particular interest in vegetarianism was embedded in a broader set of values, ideas and practices which together comprised his vision of German destiny, and which, among other things, led to the Holocaust. But, his was (and is) only one of many meanings of vegetarianism. Most vegetarians today would reject the values, ideas and practices that shaped Hitler's rejection of meat. Indeed, for many the idea that Hitler could be described as a vegetarian is abhorrent. In their view, vegetarianism is associated with a set of values among which peacefulness and non-violence figure large, that is antithetical to those of the Third Reich. From this perspective, Hitler's attitude towards meat is a perversion of vegetarianism, hardly worthy of the name, a political embarrassment, and it is no small wonder that they sometimes refuse him the label of 'vegetarian'. This paper is not concerned with whether Hitler really was a vegetarian. Rather, it aims to show how German vegetarianism was part of a broader set of values and ideals that had roots in nineteenth-century Life Reform movements, and that came to occupy a somewhat problematic place within the National Socialist regime. Hitler's contradictory attitudes towards meat were only one symptom of this problematic place.

Meat, Science and Social Policy in the Nineteenth and Early Twentieth Centuries

While vegetarianism can be traced back to antiquity, its meanings in twentieth-century Germany must be understood, in part, as a response to a major increase in the meat consumption that started in the previous century. The best figures we have come from H.-J. Teuteberg, who calculated from production statistics 1986 that annual per capita meat consumption in 1855 was 19.6 kilograms, and that this figure had doubled by 1895, reaching approximately 45 kilograms annually by 1914.[4] After then the trajectory of consumption becomes more complex. Consumption fell dramatically during World War I, and improved only slowly in the immediate aftermath, until it began to stabilize between 1926 and 1928.[5] Then it dropped again with the economic turmoil of the late 1920s and early 30s. Doctors as well as national economists such as Carl von Tyszka pointed to the potential negative consequences of this decline for body and soul of the future generation of the 'Volkskörper'.[6] This was the situation in meat consumption when the Nazis seized power in 1933. Only five years later annual per capita consumption stood at 53.5 kilograms. The symbolic power of the rapid increase in consumption as an achievement of the new political regime can hardly be overestimated.

Not only did twentieth-century German vegetarianism emerge against the backdrop of a massive growth in the per capita consumption of meat, it also emerged against a growing use of science to rationalize the place of meat in the diet. As is well known, physiological issues assumed new prominence in the evaluation of meat with the emergence of nutritional science in the late eighteenth and early nineteenth centuries. François Magendie's experiments with dogs helped to promote meat and protein as crucial to an evaluation of the quality of a diet, and, in the 1830s, Justus von Liebig provided a scientific justification for the idea that that the consumption of meat was the source of all muscular strength; a belief that persisted long after it was refuted.[7] But, for my story, the key innovation was the so-called Voit standard, which, beginning in 1870, established a recommended daily per capita consumption of 120 grams of protein. Carl Voit, a protégé of Liebig, argued that a large intake of protein would boost nervous and muscle energy, which could be called upon as required by the body like electrical energy. The 120 grams of protein was the right daily intake of a man engaged in strenuous physical work, Voit claimed, and more might be needed if his work was particularly demanding. While Voit's notion of electrical and muscle energy (and Liebig's vision of some form of a storage mechanism for this energy that could be released like the spring of a clock) came to be questioned, his standard (or some variant of it) provided a basis for social policy measures to ensure that dietary levels did not fall below the recommended meat rations. For example, even before the establishment of Voit's standard in 1881, late nineteenth-century prison and workhouse reformers used Voit's research results when they claimed that the inclusion of meat in regular meals for inmates was a means of securing minimal acceptable food standards for them. As a result, in 1871, meat was introduced into the formerly vegetarian diet given to prison inmates in Prussia, and the debate on the size of the meat portion in the soldier's diet persisted throughout the nineteenth century.[8]

More broadly, the Voit standard became crucial to efforts to promote national, military and industrial fitness. Put simply, meat – or the protein within it, as set out in the Voit standard – came to be seen as a key part of efforts to maintaining the health and strength of Germany's industrial workforce and its military forces, at a time when the country was struggling to establish itself against powerful rivals such as Britain and France. Such concerns help to explain why, in the late nineteenth and early twentieth centuries, efforts to promote meat as a central part of the diet focused predominantly on men (especially male physical strength, and its preservation and enhancement), and why within physiological discourse, two masculine identities emerged. The first was the figure of the working man: he carried the responsibility of providing for wife and children, and contributed to the industrial revival of Germany. The second was the soldier: the preservation of his fighting will and capacity was an even greater societal concern given the declining rates of fitness for military service among men at the time.[9] Together these male figures were portrayed as crucial to German industrial and military strength. Apart from the figures of the worker and the soldier, the process of hunting, killing and eating animals had further specifically masculine associations for many Germans that dovetailed with actual consumption habits. Etiquette books instructed men in their task of carving the roast at the table. In order to ensure male strength and masculine labour when only small amounts of meat were available, the pater familias was entitled to consume his meat whereas wife and children could go without.[10]

Against this background, and beginning in the late nineteenth century, middle-class social reformers increasingly promoted meat as a central part of the diet in educational journals, cookbooks and schools of domestic science.[11] Such efforts at reform generally focused on working-class households, because despite the symbolic value of meat, household surveys from the end of the nineteenth century demonstrated that for economic reasons the lower classes could hardly afford any animal proteins from meat. Numerous proposals tried to compensate for the lack of animal protein by recommending cheap and protein-rich foods like legumes, fish, low-fat milk and cheese. However, fish consumption remained low and men continued to disdain milk as suited only for women and children.[12] Surrounded by vegetables and side-dishes, meat remained, whenever affordable, the centrepiece of menus as the main course. This model of the 'proper' meal, the meal that could also be served to guests, continued to dominate for decades, remaining, like other dietary habits, remarkably impervious to change.[13]

Vegetarianism and Life Reform

Vegetarianism thus emerged against a backdrop of rising meat consumption, and the growing centrality of meat to efforts to reform the German diet. Of course, people had abstained from meat long before this time, but by the 1920s and 30s rejecting meat had become a voluntary and deliberate decision for an increasing part of the population. Despite the fact that many working-class people were still unable to afford animal protein, fewer individuals refrained from meat consumption out of economic necessity. In addition, abstaining from meat occurred in the context of a broader 'Lebensreformbewegung' (life reform movement) – a term used to cover various reform movements in Germany and Switzerland that, beginning in the middle of the nineteenth century, were critical of industrialization and urbanization, and called for a return to more natural ways of living – 'Back to Nature'. Convinced vegetarians produced a veritable trove of writings in order to make others join what had become part of this broader social movement.

I am not the first to explore this literature. Beginning in the 1970s, and in part arising from the emerging ecology movement and the renewed interest in oppositional movements and protest, a growing number of historians began to examine these writings; an interest that peaked in the 1990s in conjunction with the 'cultural turn' in history.[14] The majority of these studies focus on the period around the turn of the century, an era of forced industrialization, migration to the cities, and the emerging industrialization of food production. These new challenges and the resulting profound transformations within society and politics created an increasing uncertainty and anxiety, particularly among the middle classes. It was in this context that 'life-reformers' issued their calls for a 'return to nature', and formed a kind of oppositional movement that aimed to change both the conditions of daily existence and the broader social structures in which they were embedded. Although the movement was complex and is difficult to reduce to a single factor, the consensus is that 'life reformers' were at their core a middle-class movement of anti-modernist protest. This interpretation is supported by evidence that suggests that vegetarians chose the structure of the 'Verein' – a form of middle-class association – as their form of institutionalization, just like so many other middle-class groups of the nineteenth century.

The first vegetarian association in Germany was founded in 1867 by Eduard Baltzer. This was followed by the founding of numerous smaller local associations. In 1892, two previously independent associations merged to form the German Vegetarian Union, based in Leipzig. Within ten years, the Union had developed into a supra-regional vegetarian organization of 1,300 members.[15] The smaller local associations ultimately merged in 1918 to form the Federation of German Vegetarian Associations, which conceived itself as an alternative to the Vegetarian Union. The two associations did not cooperate, continuing each to publish their own journals and having a membership that also remained largely separate. Even if the term 'life reform movement' suggests unity in favour of a common goal, vegetarian and 'life reform' movements were by no means homogeneous. A common element, however, was the key importance of charismatic figures, 'prophets' such as Theodor Hahn (1824–83), Eduard Baltzer (1814–87) and especially Fidus (i.e. Hugo Reinhold Karl Johann Höppener, 1868–1948) whose writings provided an impetus to the movement in the nineteenth century. These leading men appeared and reappeared in reform writings over the decades.

The leading reformers did agree on one fundamental principle: that the consumption of meat by humans was unnatural, a violation of the natural and God-given herbivorous human diet and of the peaceful coexistence of humans and animals.[16] Indeed, as the title of Wilhelm Zimmermann's book – *The Path to Paradise: An Illumination of the Central Causes of the Physical and Moral Decline of the Civilized Peoples* – suggests, the abandonment of the naturally and theologically ordained vegetarian diet had broader consequences for civilization as a whole. From such a perspective, vegetarianism thus became a means of staving off decline and degeneration. The 1892 bylaw of the Federation of German Vegetarians defined the purpose of the organization as an 'idealistic, but also an entirely practical' association for the promotion and dissemination of 'the noble and true humanity on the foundation of a meatless diet' in order to 'further the creation of a power that can accomplish more than any individual'.[17]

Vegetarian reformers based their understanding of the inherent aggressiveness of meat on ideas contained within philosophical treatises dating back to antiquity, which constituted a common point of reference among the educated middle classes. Within the tradition of Greek humoural pathology, meat was believed to generate heat and incite the passions. The corresponding choleric temperament was described as bad-tempered and easily angered.[18] By contrast, vegetables were regarded as cool and moist, and associated with a gentle temper. The contrast between meat and plant eaters supposedly expressed itself directly in national character and outward physical appearance, prompting heated debates about whether human dentition was that of a carnivorous animal or, as vegetarians argued, that of herbivorous organisms.

The ways in which diet shaped character were also associated with the life-reformers' tendency to associate meat with spoilage and illness. In a metaphorical sense, this was extended to discussions of putative moral decay, for example in the discussion of the corrupt "carnal disposition" that 'contrasts sharply with what we regard as "nobly human", "spiritual", and "mannerly".'[19] These were not merely medical or academic deliberations, but beliefs that were deeply anchored in daily consciousness. In contrast, advocates of meat typically depicted vegetarians as small, joyless, gaunt and emaciated individuals; a stark difference to their depiction of meat eaters as brimming with strength and zest for life.[20]

Vegetarians conceived hunting and animal slaughter as aggressive acts that damaged the natural and God-given harmony between humans, animals and nature. They believed that the violence inherent in hunting and in animal slaughter extended into society as a whole, since the 'habit of enjoying nourishment acquired through the slaughter of animals also dulls the antipathy toward carnage on the battlefields'. Vegetarians considered that any person willing to 'constantly wade in rivers of animal blood in order to acquire a frivolous and unnecessary foodstuff will not hesitate to instigate a war. The murder of animals is without doubt one of the causes for the killing of men.'[21] Such criticism often helped to explain why men were more violent than women. The male figures of the worker and the soldier were often portrayed as meat eaters.

In addition to ethical and religious reasons, vegetarians also argued that there were nutritional and hygienic reasons for not eating meat. Physicians had long argued that certain 'diseases of civilization' were associated with an overly rich diet and an excess consumption of meat. But for many critics, conventional scientific medicine did not do enough, and the natural health movement, which began to attract ever more followers in the late nineteenth century, attacked it for treating symptoms rather than the entire person in a holistic manner, and, as part of this critique, also attacked medicine for encouraging excess meat consumption. Their critique was buttressed by some conventional medical practitioners who came to acknowledge the positive effect of a meatless diet on the course of certain diseases.[22] And further evidence in support of a vegetarian position came during the course of discussions from the late 1870s on the needs and minimum rations of animal protein, when some researchers conducted self-experiments to prove that it was possible to consume a strictly vegetarian diet without nutritional deficiencies. Yet, none of this seemed to undermine growing German consumption of meat. In spite of the fact that vegetarians demonstrated their physical performance with long-distance running and outstanding athletic feats, the belief that a mixed diet improved performance and resistance to disease persisted.[23] Perhaps in response to the persistence of such carnivorous tendencies, vegetarians with a social reformist bent highlighted an economic aspect of the debate. Since grains needed first to pass through the stomach of an animal in order to make a caloric contribution to humans in the form of meat, the energy derived from meat depended on the consumption of an enormous amount of energy from grain that was then lost to human consumption.[24]

Nineteenth-century vegetarians did not satisfy themselves with critique. They also founded projects like the Eden Orchard Colony in Oranienburg nearby Berlin in order to show the world how it might be possible to live in the modern world without meat, in peaceful harmony with humans and nature, and thus acquire a portion of heaven upon earth, and perhaps a portion of profit.[25] The Eden colony, like many other 'life reform' initiatives, was designed as an economic enterprise. In other instances, vegetarian reformers earned their living by publishing books and pamphlets or as speakers at events. There were also vegetarian restaurants, guesthouses and a number of very successful vegetarian spa resorts.[26] Most notably the producers of vegetarian products were among the first who used modern packaging, branding and marketing practices. Initially these products could be purchased via mail order, but later many became available at the growing number of health-food stores.[27] Today many are supermarket staples, including Kellogg's Cornflakes, fruit juices and Graham crackers.

Meat and its problems might have remained a focal point of the life-reform and vegetarian movement, however, as Eva Barlösius has convincingly argued, this did not mean that vegetarians entirely abandoned meat as a part of their diet. 'In fact', Barlösius writes, 'it can be assumed that many who described themselves as 'vegetarian' did not practice a 'meatless diet' with any consistency, even when they were convinced that the vegetarian diet was ethically superior to a diet that also contained meat'.[28] Rather, vegetarian reformers were concerned primarily with achieving a 'just and proper' life, and were also concerned with a range of alternatives to the contemporary society they believed to be in crisis. But, for most of the movement's members, vegetarianism only appealed to them as long as they were still engaged in their search for answers. Certainly this is what membership lists of the vegetarian associations seem to imply. In most instances, the members of the association remained active on the rolls for only four to eight years, generally in transitional life phases when their status and place in society seemed uncertain or at risk. Membership in a vegetarian association thus appeared to have been a strategy to help determine and delineate one's place in society. It did not necessarily represent an anti-bourgeois protest aiming at political revolution. Instead, it was a movement profoundly shaped by the middle class that was most of all concerned with the idea of practice, with religious (especially Protestant) overtones, and later also with an ability to demonstrate self-discipline and self-control.[29]

Vegetarianism under National Socialism

On the eve of the National Socialist seizure of power, there were twenty-six vegetarian associations in Germany, with a membership that totalled about 200,000.[30] These numbers made them a force to be reckoned with. For their part, the vegetarians greeted the new regime in 1933 with high hopes and expectations. It was well-known that the National Socialists approved of 'life-reform' issues, and vegetarians mistakenly hoped to gain support and recognition under the new regime. Thus, the vegetarian journals greeted the political overthrow for the most part with euphoria. In declarations of loyalty to the new system, their editors expressed the hope that the *Volk* community would 'place humanity above machines and money, and would achieve [for individuals] the right to a wage, bread, and a homeland.'[31] Hitler's vegetarianism was well known,[32] and he was 'adopted' by the movement. The *Vegetarische Presse* even declared Hitler's appointment to the position of Reich Chancellor to be the movement's greatest public success.[33]

In fact, there were clear affinities between vegetarianism and National Socialism, both arguing for the idea of purification and towards a strict policy of health.[34] Leading members of the Eden Orchard Colony were early members of the National Socialist party, and shared the party's *völkisch* and nationalist attitudes. Shaped by the intensely patriarchal quality of the movement, in which (as mentioned above) charismatic leaders played a central role, it was not difficult for the 'life-reformers' to accommodate themselves to the cult of the Führer.[35] Moreover they were well aware of existing commonalities. For example, they emphasized their common esteem for the soil and the fight against 'diseases of civilization' via the propagation of a simpler and more primitive diet.[36] Thus, the vegetarian reform movement soon underwent incorporation or *Gleichschaltung* into the Nazi state. As early as 1933, the Department of National Health (*Volksgesundheit*) in the National Socialist party founded a division for 'life reform.' In that same year, the historic *Vegetarische Warte* journal and the life-reform journal *Die Volksgesundheit* ended publication, with the journal *Lebenskunst* ceasing publication a year later. Certain organizations that were deemed political in nature were banned, like the Mazdanan movement, which was dissolved on 28 February 1933. Others voluntarily disbanded, like the German Vegetarian Union. The Union's governing board arrived at this decision unanimously, noting that under the current state of affairs a 'pressure group' such as their own 'was not permitted by the state to struggle for goals that the state leadership did not endorse'. In addition, the board believed it had been subjected to insults against which they were not able to publicly defend themselves.[37]

In 1934, the associations that still existed were combined under the German Society for Life Reform e.V. (*Deutsche Gesellschaft für Lebensreform e.V.*). This umbrella organization remained under the aegis of the 'life-reform' division of the Department of National Health (*Abteilung Volksgesundheit*), which was also in charge of the individual associations. The *German Life-Reform Movement* (*Deutsche Lebensreform-Bewegung*), which was founded in 1936, turned its attention to addressing the issue of life-reform from a theoretical as well as a practical perspective. It asked for strict loyalty to National Socialism as a key element of its philosophy, was organized according to the strict hierarchical leadership principle of the *Führerprinzip* and accepted only 'pure' 'Aryans' as members.[38] In a sense, the movement did oppose the transformation of a life-world that had become alienated from nature, and placed humans at its centre. However the emphasis was on humans as a biological unit, always conceived as an element within the higher unit of life that was the *Volk*.

The 'Life-reform' also shifted its emphasis after the 1936 Four Year Plan was issued, and the Reich Work Group of New German Medicine (*Reichsarbeits-gemeinschaft für Neue Deutsche Heilkunde*), which was closely associated with 'life-reform', began to wane in power and significance. The life-reform movement thus began to direct its energies toward the enhancement and full realization of natural strength by means of sports medicine, which was conceptualized not as a pleasure for the individual, but as a means to enforce the physical strength of the *Volk*. The indulgence and care for oneself was rejected as strictly as were sectarianism and paternalism.[39] As early as 1935, Hanns G. Müller, head of the life-reform movement and of the German Life-Reform e.V. organization, stated quite frankly that 'We German life-reformers don't believe in an "ethos of love for all living things" ... We don't operate on the assumption of a kind and valuable Self, nor on the basis of an idea somehow grounded in religion or the occult. We root ourselves in simple fashion in the ordinary soil, in the earth, that nourishes us all and that is our homeland (*Heimat*).'[40] While the thought of 'universal love' might have sounded attractive, Müller believed that he had 'spotted the true face behind the mask of pacifism: Marxism!'[41]

Pacifism, a core element of vegetarianism, was complete anathema to the image of the National Socialist soldier. An article entitled 'Life-Reform as Heroic Life-Formation' put forth the following definition: 'The Nordic individual is a man of 'reformation', of constant renewal; he is inspired by a Faustian drive for adventure and the spirit of attack. It is a spirit of attack directed against ideas, objects, and problems. The Viking spirit is the conqueror of new worlds, always exciting, lively, and creating. Someone who lives in this way is a reformer, a destroyer, and a builder, all at once.'[42] Within this view there could not be a peaceful 'return to nature'. Nor would it be possible to eliminate all the harm caused by civilization. Rather these were regarded as 'fundamental to our age and thus unavoidable. We can not change the pace of time and its technological achievements, the telephone, the noise of urban life, urban pollution, automobile exhaust.'[43] The visionary pacifist element was thus circumscribed and curtailed to the practicable and the politically useful. In the end, the movement shifted its focus solely to avoiding harmful alcohol and stimulants, reducing the consumption of meat, and increasing the consumption of vegetables and whole grain products in order to reduce the rate of nutritional disease.[44] The goal was a 'diet rooted in the soil', which was meant quite literally. The diet was to be based on the results of the many historical nutrition studies that were conducted after 1933. These studies were grounded in the idea that humans had optimally adapted to their local dietary conditions over the course of evolution. The result was regional and national differences in dietary habits, which these studies attempted painstakingly to describe. Even the surveys of household budgets, which the German Labour Front (*Deutsche Arbeitsfront*) and the Reich Office of Statistics (*Statistisches Reichsamt*) conducted in 1937, calculated regional differences. According to the idea of biological adaptability to the environment, traditions – which included the consumption of meat – made biological sense, as they embodied the accumulated knowledge of the generations. However, warnings were also issued against the indiscriminate reintroduction of old traditions, since nature and the environment had also meanwhile changed. This was another reason why a simple 'return to nature' was insufficient and could even be harmful. [45]

How then can it be explained that a number of National Socialist Leaders were vegetarians and Heinrich Himmler planned to make vegetarians out of the members of the SS? According to certain sources, there did exist a very small number of NS leaders and elites who, it was claimed, due to their power of will and their outstanding physiognomy, were vegetarians refusing any meat. The triumph of will over the weakness of the flesh would allow them to maintain high levels of performance even without the consumption of meat.[46] However, mentioning this fact in public was considered by NS dignitaries as both arrogant and rude, given that the vast majority of humans were considered as intended by nature to consume a mixed diet.[47]

In practice, registered vegetarians were assigned by the NS regime higher rations of quark, butter and cheese to replace meat.[48] The institutions of the state thus did take the specific needs of a vegetarian diet into account. The nutritional guidelines published in the 1935 *Reichsgesundheitsblatt* declared: 'We do not advocate a strict vegetarian diet, meaning an exclusive reliance upon vegetable products. However, if some individuals decide they want to consume a vegetarian diet, this can be endorsed.'[49] Another publication stated: 'The vegetarian individual should be regarded as a pioneer for necessary dietary changes'[50] – but it was expected, that these ideas needed more time to spread and to become popular. Nonetheless, even though the diet of the Waffen-SS did indeed contain meat, their rations were significantly lower per capita than those of the regular troops. In December 1940 members of the army received 1,000g at home and 1,554g when sent out to the battlefield, whereas the members of those troops of the Waffen-SS were assigned only 660g a week, about fifty per cent less. This was a foretaste of the 'triumph of the will' that was ultimately to apply to wider parts of the population beyond the Führer and his vegetarian followers who headed the state and the party.

While it awaited the day when vegetarianism would be generally accepted, the NS regime only adopted those aspects of vegetarianism that seemed useful from the perspective of food and nutritional policy. To make all Germans follow a vegetarian regime was difficult for economic reasons, because it implied the loss of a distinct feature of Hitler's 'ascetic leadership' useful in propaganda, and because it was perceived as psychologically unfavourable. Above all it was the individualistic perspective of the 'life-reform' movement that was rejected by National Socialism vegetarianism. Subordination of the individual to the NS state meant that 'unnecessary interferences', such as discussion and debate, usual between the numerous small groups and subgroups of the broad life-reform movement, were to be avoided.[51] A look at the photographs taken at the 1932 World Vegetarian Congress held at the already mentioned Garden Orchard Eden helps even better to understand the cultural gap between vegetarians and the Nazis: the photographed men were long haired, had beards and wore unconventional informal costumes, which stressed their individuality instead of melting them in the mass by wearing a uniform.[52]

The NS regime also had reasons to oppose vegetarianism for economic reasons. Germany relied upon imports for its supply of vegetables. This explains state campaigns against raw food diets such as the one advocated by Arthur Scheunert.[53] Furthermore, an increasing number of scientific reports suggested that animal protein enhanced physical performance. For example, researchers who examined the dietary habits of Olympic athletes discovered that some of these athletes consumed massive amounts of meat.[54] The starvation experiments conducted by Heinrich Kraut on prisoners of war and forced labourers and the research conducted by Konrad Lang at the Academy of Military Medicine, also seemed to support the nutritional importance of meat consumption for physical performance.[55] These findings appeared to confirm the standpoint of the largely conservative Reich Department of Health (*Reichsgesundheitsamt*), which argued that both biological law and historical development had conditioned humans to depend on a mixed diet that included meat. This view also had the advantage for the regime that it accorded with most people's beliefs about meat. They expected the regime to satisfy what they regarded as their nutritional need for meat and – what was even more important – insisted on receiving their ration of meat as a sign of their partaking in economic progress. The National Socialist leaders, always concerned about public opinion, were clearly concerned not to alienate the population on the topic of vegetarianism. Thus the regime felt compelled to make allowances, all the more because meat was a traditional part of German food, a strong symbol of status and male power, and was believed to be necessary for physical performance.

National Socialist health and nutritional policy remained focused on human performance and economic autarchy. To achieve this, the regime needed to balance the scientifically recognized healthy diet with people's dietary expectations. It was, in part, the improvement of their material situation, and the fact that the regime managed to keep the food supply more or less stable until 1943, that made the people follow the political line of the Nazi System for so long – perhaps confirmation of Carl von Tyszka's 1934 comment on the importance of food for motivation, will and mental ability to work.[56] As Joachim Drews has shown recently, psychological arguments played an important role in National Socialist nutritional policy from its very beginning.[57] Even the introduction of rationing before the beginning of war followed the psychological calculation that it was important to get the people used to it before real and severe shortages became unavoidable. The impact on the mood of the 'Volk' of every change of the rations was discussed in-depth by the commissions and compensated by increases wherever possible. Had the regime adopted a strict version of vegetarianism, it would have challenged old and deep rooted German traditions, and might have also have undermined Nazi authority by confiscating the very piece of meat the worker had just gained by the successful Nazi economic policy.

This was also the reason why military officers opposed the reduction of the soldier's meat portions, and argued that this would reduce his will to fight. Accordingly soldiers at the front got larger meat portions.[58] Letters to the editors of life-reform publications show that deeply rooted male anxieties also played a role in meat consumption. One reader fearfully asked 'Does a meatless diet lead to impotence?'[59] This was unimaginable to the warrior-soldier, who had been raised to ensure the continuation of his *Volk*. It is impossible to know whether these were actual letters or simply fabrications. In any case, it is apparent that both the regime and nutritional policymakers thought it prudent to take a public stance on these issues.

After 1942 this discussion became increasingly irrelevant as food supplies dwindled over the course of the war. The German diet thus became a largely vegetarian one by default. Heinrich Himmler supposedly still engaged in heated debates on the topic,[60] asking how it was possible that rumours persisted that he hoped to turn the SS into an 'elite troop of vegetarians, teetotallers and non-smokers'.[61]

The status of vegetarianism under National Socialism thus remained ambiguous. Although dignitaries of the NS regime were convinced of the health benefits of a vegetarian diet, they never imposed a purely vegetarian diet on the German people. As was true more generally for the regime, National Socialists paid little apparent heed to ideological consistency, often selecting only those elements that were of immediate use to them. As soon as the general line had been set out clearly, some vegetarian journals were allowed to continue publication. In fact they printed articles about the basic tenets of vegetarianism into the 1940s, justifying vegetarianism with the godliness of the world, which required greater love and respect for animals and plants. Articles that went through NS censors could even suggest that anyone who sullied his hands with the blood of an animal's death would not be in a position to bear witness to the magnificence of God.[62]

Such evident contradictions with NS ideology are hard to understand, but the regime followed its line of picking the useful things from ideologies or convictions not only in the case of vegetarianism, but in other areas of nutrition as well, including artificial vitamins, food colorants and preservatives. In general, these products were condemned by the NS regime. Yet as undesirable as they were, the regime nevertheless tolerated them as indispensable makeshifts for securing the peoples' food supply under the conditions of war economy.[63] Similarly, the Nazi regime also adopted a pick-and-choose inconsistent policy towards organic food and natural medicine: like vegetarianism they were both important to the NS agenda, but the full implementation of policies towards organic food and natural medicine were postponed to the future.[64] In the case of vegetarianism it was believed that nutritional habits changed only slowly and it would take a long time for propaganda to get people used to a meatless diet. Moreover, to Nazi policymakers vegetarianism had to be stripped of its former life-reform associations. The ideals of the middle-class vegetarian movement contradicted the ideology and aims of the proletarian national socialist ideology and were regarded as being dysfunctional in psychological, political and economic matters. What the cultural history of vegetarianism in Germany under the Third Reich shows is that critiques of meat were not only about the supposed unhealthiness of meat, but were also expressions of broader political and ideological concerns, and dependent on social status and class.

9 MAD AND COUGHING COWS: BOVINE TUBERCULOSIS, BSE AND HEALTH IN TWENTIETH-CENTURY BRITAIN

Keir Waddington

Since the 1950s, consumers have come to expect cheap, but safe food. A number of food scares in the 1980s and 90s – E. coli in 1987, Salmonella in 1988, and the furore over GM ingredients – challenged this expectation. Of all these scares Bovine Spongiform Encephalopathy (BSE) or 'mad cow disease', although coming at the end of a decade of food scares, came to embody the fears that had come to surround issues of food safety.

However, the threat from a zoonotic disease and meat are not unique to the late twentieth century. Whereas social scientists have suggested that an obsession with food quality is characteristic of a modern western society, across Europe and North America animal plagues and food safety became important medical, social and political questions in the nineteenth century.[1] In Britain, apprehension about the dangers of consuming adulterated or unwholesome food was present in the mid-nineteenth century, but more was at stake than just questions of quality and composition. After 1850, meat from diseased livestock emerged as a defined danger to health. Regular outbreaks of foot-and-mouth, rabies and pleuro-pneumonia fuelled anxiety, but it was bovine tuberculosis that came to dominate debate about the relationship between animal diseases and human health. In the process, tuberculous meat became symbolic of the dangers represented by meat from diseased livestock. Despite claims that by 1900 food no longer presented a significant threat to public health, the perceived danger of consuming meat from tubercular cattle was an important source of food related anxiety in the Edwardian period.[2] Campaigns to prevent the sale of tuberculous meat and attempts to eradicate the disease in cattle became important components of the 'crusade against consumption'. It was the dismantling of the mechanisms to protect the public from bovine tuberculosis and other animal diseases in the 1980s that has been credited with fostering an environment in which BSE could emerge as a health threat.

This chapter explores the parallels between contemporary responses to BSE and early twentieth-century attitudes to bovine tuberculosis. Historians have drawn attention to questions of food safety, quality and trust and to the similarities between BSE and other animal plagues, but few have considered the zoonotic dimension that proved crucial to constructing debates about both diseases.[3] Both came to embody wider contemporary fears about food and the impact of transformations in the farming industry. Both represented 'invisible' risks that appeared to transcend class, gender, behaviour and geography.

Rather than examining the familiar, often heroic story of milk and tuberculosis, this chapter compares the BSE outbreak with the problem of tuberculous meat in Edwardian Britain. It explores how responses to bovine tuberculosis shaped later efforts against BSE to not only compare two meat-related diseases at different times but also to examine how responses to BSE can be considered in relation to earlier concerns about bovine tuberculosis. By reversing the chronology to emphasize the comparative dimension, the chapter investigates first how BSE and then how bovine tuberculosis were framed as a threat to human health before exploring how science was manipulated to justify policymaking.[4] In examining how both BSE and bovine tuberculosis were framed, the chapter addresses the intersection of policy and the credibility of the various actors involved in defining the dangers from potentially infected meat to explore the interests of stakeholders in policy formation. The chapter goes on to contextualize the responses to the two diseases to address how measures to protect consumers were shaped by a range of competing actors. The ways in which BSE and bovine tuberculosis were defined and managed suggest common patterns in the problems posed by diseased meat in the twentieth century.

Emerging Diseases: BSE and Bovine Tuberculosis

Shortly before Christmas 1984, David Bee, a veterinary surgeon, was called to examine a cow with strange symptoms on Pitsham Farm in West Sussex. Within six weeks, the cow was dead having developed tremors and a loss of coordination; within months, more cows in the same herd showed similar symptoms. The disease was completely unknown and quite unexpected. Studies by neuropathologist Gerald Wells and his colleagues at the Central Veterinary Laboratory (CVL) identified what they believed was a new spongiform encephalopathy in cattle, a disease characterized by small vacuoles in the brain that led to progressive psychomotor dysfunction. Although the CVL had little experience with Transmissible Spongiform Encephalopathies (TSEs), similarities to the sheep disease scrapie led them to attribute the cause of this new disease to scrapie-infected meat and bone meal (MBM) in cattle feed.[5] Scrapie offered a way forward in explaining the new disease and provided an analogy that not only worked but also presented a framework for control. When the Ministry of Agriculture, Fisheries and Food (MAFF) was alerted in 1987, at least four herds had clearly been affected. An epidemic was predicted, but disquiet about the probable effect on exports and the political implications of yet another food scare ensured that details about BSE were held back. It was not until 1988 that BSE was made notifiable and it was this delay between identification and notification that were later to cause problems.[6] Because of the long incubation period, the major phase of the epidemic in terms of the number of cattle infected and public awareness was yet to come.

At first scientists were not overly concerned about the risk to human health: scrapie-infected sheep had entered the food chain for centuries with no damaging effects. This helped frame BSE as an animal health issue. However, scientists in Britain, Europe and North America were puzzled. When BSE was first identified, the nature of the infectious agents causing TSEs was a matter of controversy. However, by defining BSE as a spongiform encephalopath a link was established between BSE and other similar brain diseases, including Creutzfeldt–Jakob disease (CJD) – a disease that had only been properly defined in the early 1960s and that until BSE was considered of little public relevance because of the small number of cases worldwide. Although nobody knew whether BSE was a hazard or not, because the two diseases were related, and because some spongiform encephalopathies (including scrapie) could cross the species barrier, questions were asked about whether BSE could be passed to man. As the number of infected cattle rose to its peak in 1992, media alarm about the dangers from contaminated beef intensified.

Although incidences of BSE in cattle had started to fall by the mid-1990s – a fall that was ironically matched by declining confidence in the Conservative government's ability to cope with the crisis – the death of Stephen Churchill from a new variant of CJD in 1995 suggested a connection between this new disease and BSE.[7] Earlier transmission experiments had hinted at this possibility and in 1990 the Spongiform Encephalopathy Advisory Committee (SEAC) was established to provide a scientifically based assessment of risk from TSEs to public and animal health. Alarm was voiced a few years later when a number of farmers with BSE-infected herds were identified as having CJD, although this proved to be the sporadic form of the disease. In March 1996, epidemiologists and neurologists reported the appearance of a further ten cases. Clinically they showed different symptoms from classical CJD and had a neuropathology similar to patients with Kuru, an encephalopathy found in Papua New Guinea and linked to cannibalism. Not only did these patients have a new variant of CJD but also their neuropathology pointed to a common infective agent: exposure to the BSE agent was considered the most plausible explanation.[8] BSE had become a human disease.

When these findings were announced, a public outcry and media-driven panic ensued as existing anxieties about food safety focused on BSE, vCJD and the dangers of meat. A human epidemic was feared. Although the causal link between vCJD and BSE remained debated, the perceived threat reinforced the public perception of risk associated with contaminated meat. Beef prices dropped as confidence collapsed. Although the crisis proved short-lived, fears about eating infected beef failed to subside.

Just as BSE came to stand at the centre of late twentieth-century debates on food safety, by the Edwardian period bovine tuberculosis dominated professional concerns about zoonoses and public health. Before the mid-nineteenth century, relatively little had been known about the transmission of disease from animals to humans and ideas that meat from diseased livestock might be injurious to health had built on impressionistic evidence and a sense that meat from diseased livestock *should* be hazardous. Veterinarians and sanitary officials found in bovine tuberculosis a concrete threat around which they could articulate growing disquiet about meat and disease, and about the relationship between animal and human diseases. Bovine tuberculosis made diseased meat into a defined threat and pushed the issue into the political arena. Between 1890 and 1911, three royal commissions were appointed to investigate the disease and its effects on man. Added to the publicity created by these commissions was a constant stream of articles in local and national newspapers on the dangers of tuberculous meat and the widespread reporting of the seizure of tuberculous carcasses. Existing public-health measures to prevent the sale of food deemed unfit for consumption were extended as local authorities used the threat from tuberculous meat in their attempts to clean up the meat trade. Campaigns were launched to eradicate the disease in cattle. Responses to BSE nearly 100 years later followed a similar pattern.

Bovine tuberculosis emerged as a public health issue in a different way to BSE. Its history says more about the professional concerns of medical officers and veterinarians, which drove the debate, than about media or public fears about the threat from diseased meat. Unlike the furore surrounding BSE, the popular press played a secondary role in constructing anxiety about bovine tuberculosis. This was not just a simple question of a transformation in the nature of the media, of greater accessibility, or differences in the reporting of alarmist stories or food scares. Concerns about food-borne infections were prominent in both periods. In the early-twentieth century, the growth of 'New Journalism', with its interest in sensation and human-interest stories, and the diversification of the local and national press, expanded news coverage and helped fashion debates about bovine tuberculosis. However, although local and national newspapers reported the dangers of tuberculous meat, shaping public perceptions of the risks from diseased meat and demanding action, the debate surrounding bovine tuberculosis was primarily conducted in the medical and veterinary press. It was evidence from these professional arenas that was reported in the popular press and was used to inform the public. This ensured that the press became a voice for professional, not popular, concern. The reverse was true of BSE. Here the media played a central role in generating national and international alarm and in shaping policy at a time when the Conservative government was highly sensitive and vulnerable on food safety. If media interest in the 1990s was primed to the notion of food 'crisis', BSE was a new and frightening disease that quickly took on a horrific set of meanings as it moved from a veterinary to a human health issue. Uncertainty combined with public scepticism surrounding the science, the Conservative government and British farming methods, and the sense that little was being done, stimulated not only controversy but also media interest. Bovine tuberculosis was neither new, nor dramatic. It was hence less open to sensational reporting, especially when debate was largely framed in the medical and veterinary press. Different values were also assigned to government policy and science. There was less sense that the risks from bovine tuberculosis were being mishandled or that the potential risk to health was being minimized. This combined with different perceptions of food quality at a time when every attempt was made to include meat in meals and when the poor were easily tempted into purchasing anything that looked capable of being converted into a meal. Consequently, the popular press and the public were less actively involved in generating alarm about bovine tuberculosis and in shaping policy.

This is not to underestimate the perceived risks from bovine tuberculosis. A transition in the nature of agriculture, with a shift from cereal production to livestock and dairy farming, combined with farmers' reluctance to stamp out the disease, ensured that bovine tuberculosis was endemic by the 1890s. Estimates of the number of infected cattle varied but even the most conservative suggested that 20 to 30 per cent of all British cattle were tubercular.[9] The economic impact of bovine tuberculosis on the livestock and dairy industry, which was estimated at £1m per annum by 1908, did create unease but it was the connection that was established between tuberculosis in cattle and in man that fuelled alarm. The endemic nature of the disease in cattle was matched to high levels of tuberculosis in the population to suggest that bovine tuberculosis represented a serious threat to human health.[10] Tuberculosis was a feared and stigmatized disease. In the first decades of the twentieth century, it accounted for one death in every eight and conservative estimates suggested that 5 to 10 per cent of these deaths were bovine in origin and due to contaminated meat or milk.[11] The 'crusade against consumption' spearheaded by National Association for the Prevention of Consumption (NAPC) did much to encourage a view that bovine tuberculosis was a major threat to health and that preventing the disease was an important means of combating tuberculosis. Although part of a wider European movement, the NAPC had been established following two royal commissions set up to look at how to protect the public from bovine tuberculosis in the wake of the publicity and uncertainty that had surrounded the 1890 Glasgow trial for the seizure of a tuberculous carcass. Worried that mortality from bovine tuberculosis was not declining at the same pace as the pulmonary form, the Association raised public awareness about the dangers of bovine tuberculosis. By the first decade of the twentieth century, few pronouncements on tuberculosis could ignore the threat from the bovine form of the disease. The position tuberculosis occupied in debates about degeneration and child health deepened these fears. As public apprehension about national deterioration escalated following the Boer War, alarm about bovine tuberculosis as a factor in that deterioration increased. Almost 85 per cent of all deaths of those under five were from non-pulmonary tuberculosis and in the first decade of the twentieth century one third of children between five and sixteen years of age contracted bovine tuberculosis.[12] The disease was blamed for corrupting the health of British children at a time when improvements in child health were considered vital to the enhancement of the nation.

The perceived threats from BSE/vCJD and bovine tuberculosis rapidly exceeded the number of deaths or the actual epidemiological risk of contracting the disease. What mattered was the apparent danger: in BSE this perception was engendered by the media and fuelled by existing concerns about food safety; in bovine tuberculosis it was shaped by sanitary officials and veterinarians but at the same time fed on growing debate about food safety. It was feared that because the diseases were endemic in cattle it was difficult to escape ingesting contaminated meat, hence increasingly the potential to contract a feared disease. Whereas it was acknowledged that a number of animals diseases were directly communicable to man, the dangers presented by bovine tuberculosis and BSE were constructed as 'far in excess of any other disease'.[13] Both diseases quickly provided a focus for existing alarm about food safety.

Understanding Animal Diseases

Questions of aetiology have proved crucial to determining the possible risk of animal diseases to human health. Whether and how a disease might be transmitted from animals to man has over the last two centuries shaped inquiry into potential zoonoses. Studies that examine morphological characteristics and virulence along with feeding and transmission experiments have been essential to this process. If the methods of inquiry have shifted – from microbiological to bacteriological to immunological procedures, for example – the broad question of transmission remained similar for bovine tuberculosis and BSE, with both constructed through the dominant discursive scientific practices of the time. By answering basic science questions about the nature of the pathogen and the mechanism of infection, a framework was created for assessing the risk to health. However, in both cases this was not a straightforward process, revealing how the nature of zoonoses and assessments of risk were frequently contested.

Veterinarians were the first to define what was to become BSE and much of the subsequent research was conducted by a tightly-knit group of MAFF-sponsored researchers. In Britain, medical researchers initially played a marginal role; when they did raise concerns they were dismissed as 'flying in the face of science'.[14] Despite a growing body of research that since the 1940s had pointed to the 'extent and complexity of the interconnections between animal and human disease', few questions were initially asked about the threat to human health.[15] Initial speculations by veterinarians that BSE was a scrapie-like disease were reassuring. It framed BSE as an animal health issue. Although scrapie, BSE and CJD were all spongiform encephalopathies, CJD was not scrapie in man. Only outlying studies pointed to the potential for cross-species transmission. The media drew its own conclusions and raised the spectre of a CJD-type illness affecting humans.[16]

It was the emergence of prions, or self-replicating proteins, as a probable cause of BSE, and the link made with vCJD, which served to recast BSE as a threat to human health. vCJD dispelled the idea that BSE was purely an animal health issue. This reframed the disease. The prion theory was useful, flexible and politically convenient. Support for the idea that TSEs were spontaneously infectious justified the view that no one was to blame. However, prions raised more questions than they answered: they challenged existing ideas of species barriers and accepted experimental and biological precepts.[17] Scientists failed to agree over the origins of BSE, how it was transmitted within and between herds, between cattle and other species, and over the incidence of the disease. Uncertainty existed over the level of risk of animal to human transmission, especially after feeding experiments suggested that the oral route was inefficient.[18] Whether BSE was infectious, contagious or zoonotic continued to be debated. Nearly two decades after the first cases of BSE were reported more questions remained than answers.

As with BSE nearly 100 years later, determining the pathogen responsible and the risk it presented shaped investigations into bovine tuberculosis. The possibility of disease transfer between animals and humans had long been recognized, but it was not until after 1850 that the new sciences of comparative pathology and then bacteriology established clear links and in the process challenged existing ideas about the uniqueness of man. Work on bovine tuberculosis served to break 'the conceptual barrier' that distinguished animal from human diseases, and it was the discovery of the tubercle bacillus by Robert Koch in 1882 that confirmed longstanding prejudices about the threat of animal diseases to human health.[19] The identification of the tubercle bacillus had a similar impact on thinking about bovine tuberculosis as the emergence of prions did in BSE. Both challenged existing ideas of infection, the species barrier and accepted experimental and biological precepts. Koch's announcement that he had identified the tubercle bacillus, and his claim that bovine tuberculosis was identical to tuberculosis in man, gave a rational footing for existing ideas, settling the question of the relationship between tuberculosis in animals and the disease in man and its status as a contagious disease.

Early doubts about the zoonotic properties of the bovine tuberculosis had been swept aside by the start of the twentieth century by a new bacteriological frame of reference. Bacteriology provided the basis for consensus that the disease was 'the most important disease of cows' and 'a substantial risk' to the consumer'.[20] Although hereditary ideas were not entirely displaced – farmers and veterinarians continued to employ hereditary models to explain why certain breeds appeared pre-disposed to tuberculosis – bovine tuberculosis was increasingly constructed within the dominant paradigm of bacteriology. If bacteriological research confirmed the disease's zoonotic properties, investigations into bovine tuberculosis between 1900 and 1914 also helped define and extend bacteriology in much the same way as research into BSE helped shape research into TSEs. A bacteriological and zoonotic understanding of bovine tuberculosis confirmed the idea that 'a very considerable number of what are mainly animal diseases are transmissible to man', reinforcing the role of food and animals in the transmission of disease.[21]

However, just as with BSE at the end of the century, the extent of the danger from bovine tuberculosis to human health remained contested. Although bovine tuberculosis can be seen as the first zoonosis to be clearly identified, different disease models were advanced that suggested that the risk from tubercular livestock might be exaggerated. Experimental studies questioned the virulence of the disease, while bacteriological investigations revealed that the routes of infection were not straightforward.[22] Although doubts about the morphological similarities between tuberculosis in cattle and in man were voiced, Koch challenged the existing consensus at the 1901 London Congress on Tuberculosis. He questioned whether man was susceptible to bovine tuberculosis and asserted that the infection of human beings from the disease was rare. Whether or not tuberculosis could be transmitted from cows to man suddenly became a 'vexed question'.[23] There was an immediate backlash as doctors and veterinarians rushed to defend the existing paradigm. Although the idea that tuberculosis was a zoonosis was defended, the debate stimulated by Koch encouraged a more moderate view to emerge that recognized that the risks from bovine tuberculosis had been overstated.

Uncertainty and conflicting interpretations over the causes of BSE and bovine tuberculosis and their virulence proved crucial in determining how these zoonotic diseases were understood. Ideas of risk and the perceptions of the two diseases shifted as the science proved unstable and a consensus fragile.

'Infectious and Dangerous'? Meat and Disease

Fears about animal diseases can be dated back to the medieval period, but definitions of the risks represented by diseased meat have changed in response to emerging concerns about the capacity of specific animal diseases to cross the species barrier. This is reflected in how ideas of meat safety evolved in response to bovine tuberculosis and BSE. Concerns about meat as a vector for disease replicated contemporary assumptions about the spread of disease and the evolving understanding of the role of specific agents and food safety. Alarm was shaped by fear and uncertainty, and by a complex network of medical, veterinary, political, economic and cultural concerns. With the avoidance of infectious threats often motivated by disgust and fear, meat from obviously diseased livestock generated visceral responses. Where the evidence of disease was less obvious – as was the case in BSE and bovine tuberculosis – concern drew on the intuitively attractive idea that meat from diseased livestock was dangerous until studies confirmed the threat. Commentators at the time did not suggest that there was anything inherently unique about meat as a vector for disease but framed BSE and bovine tuberculosis in a way that served to focus existing unease about meat, food and animal diseases to make contaminated beef into a defined but contested political and health issue.

In 1987, MAFF voiced unease about the possible implications of BSE for human health. However, a policy of reassurance was adopted to prevent an alarmist reaction. Claims that beef was safe were not made on evidence that BSE was not transmissible through food, but on a localized understanding of the disease which suggested that because the portions that might infect were removed from the food chain beef was safe. This was not made clear to the public, who equated statements that beef was safe with claims that BSE presented no risk. Government-funded research supported the idea that BSE was an animal disease and that the risks from BSE-infected cattle were remote, closing 'the door on further research into the human health risks of infected beef'.[24] This was not the view presented in the media, which encouraged a popular perception about the dangers of contaminated beef. After so many food scares, it was easy to believe such claims even if the official line remained that British beef was safe. Popular and government ideas of food and meat safety diverged over BSE.

Studies in the 1990s began to reflect this media and public unease as they pointed to the possibility that beef might cause a BSE-type disease in man.[25]

The government initially played down these concerns, but in 1996 it admitted that the most likely cause of vCJD was eating contaminated beef products. This claim was made against a background of mounting concern about the effectiveness of measures to prevent infected beef entering the food chain. As one writer noted in the *Nutritional Review*, the government's announcement 'alarmed consumers well beyond the borders of the United Kingdom'.[26] Fears were intensified because the extent of the threat was unknown. Uncertainty about incubation periods, age-dependent susceptibility and the level of exposure made beef from BSE-infected cattle an invisible and unknowable risk.

The idea that beef from diseased cattle was a risk to health had already been suggested in the mid-nineteenth century. As the major infectious diseases declined, ideas of risk associated with contagion were modified and food emerged as a source of concern in disease transmission. By the start of the twentieth century, the role of infected foodstuffs in spreading disease was firmly established.[27] A rise in food-borne infections and local food scares combined with evidence of the horrors of the meat trade, which suggested that 'an enormous quantity of diseased and putrid meat' was being sold, saw interest coalesce around the dangers of meat.[28] Tuberculous meat focused this concern and, unlike BSE, no official attempt was made to deny the potential risk to health as it was widely seen as the main source of diseased meat sold. In 1904, for example, identification of tuberculosis accounted for over a quarter of the meat seized in Edinburgh.[29] Lesions were commonest in the cheapest cuts, but with the middle classes consuming more meat, and with children believed to be most susceptible to the disease, attention transcended paternalistic concerns for the poor at a time when the absence of meat in a diet was considered a form of deprivation. However, just as with BSE, the risk to consumers was often invisible. Whereas it was acknowledged that many consumers had 'an aesthetic objection to consuming tubercle bacilli', meat from tubercular cows was often carefully prepared to mask the signs of the disease making it was hard to detect, even for skilled inspectors.[30] Less scrupulous butchers would try other ruses to ensure that the meat they sold had no obvious signs of disease. It was hence widely feared that the public were being duped into buying diseased meat.

A tentative link between meat from tuberculosis cattle and tuberculosis in man was suggested from the 1850s onwards, but it was Koch's discovery of the tubercle bacilli that made the risks from meat into a definable threat. By 1900, few were prepared to deny the risks of contracting tuberculosis from contaminated beef as alarm intensified about the amount of tuberculous meat sold and as meat assumed a more prominent component in urban diets. As the *Text Book of Hygiene* explained, 'as tubercle bacilli entering the digestive tract of man are apt to produce tuberculosis, and also since virulent tubercle bacilli are found in the tuberculous parts of food animals, it follows that all organs and parts of the carcass which are tuberculous must be regarded as infectious and dangerous'.[31] It was feared that because meat juices contained the 'germs of the disease', all meat had to be considered dangerous. As the Mid-Cheshire Farmers Association were informed in 1906, it was 'only non-scientific people who held that there was no such risk' from tuberculous meat.[32]

However, just as the BSE crisis showed that ideas of food safety and the contagious properties of meat could be contested, the extent of the risk from tuberculous meat was equally debated. In the history of concerns about meat and animal diseases, it was never a straightforward issue of 'safe' or 'unsafe'. Where this might suggest similarities with BSE, in the case of bovine tuberculosis the debate was more complex, revealing tensions between veterinarians and butchers on the one hand and the medical profession on the other. Although claims about the properties of cooking in destroying the bacilli were used to downplay the dangers from tuberculous meat, at the heart of the debate were different disease models.[33] It was over the extent of the risk that veterinarians and sanitary officials struggled over definitions of diseased meat and over who was competent to protect the public.

Veterinarians favoured a localized disease model that saw bovine tuberculosis concentrated in the organs affected, a view that reflected late twentieth-century veterinary and government ideas on BSE. This failed to distinguish between the disease and its manifestation, but, just as with BSE, it rendered meat from diseased livestock unproblematic: because the tubercles were located in those parts of the animal that could be removed on butchering. Hence, it was only in acute and advanced cases, where the lesions were widespread, that meat was unfit for consumption. By framing bovine tuberculosis in localized terms, veterinarians sought to limit the role of sanitary officials in meat inspection to the identification and removal of obviously diseased organs. In doing so, they defended their position to determine the degree to which cattle were diseased or not, a move that reinforced their efforts to expand their range of employment and 'establish the scientific and social worthiness of their profession'.[34] Butchers keen to defend their interests wholeheartedly supported this construction of the disease, which was endorsed by the first royal commission on tuberculosis.

Many sanitary officials disagreed. They defended their right to determine the fitness of meat for human consumption. Doctors were sceptical of veterinarians' claims to expertise and actively resisted their encroachment into human medicine, rightly interpreting veterinarians' attempts to define tuberculous meat as a move to gain control over meat inspection. Convinced that tuberculosis was a constitutional disease, sanitary officials framed bovine tuberculosis in a way that exaggerated the danger from diseased meat in much the same way as the media was to play up the threat from BSE-infected cattle. They argued that the localized tubercles concealed a constitutional disease and favoured a generalized model of infection based on the idea that the bacillus circulated through the body through the blood or lymphatic system.[35] As the *Practitioner* revealed, because the tubercle bacilli were scattered throughout the body, they often found 'a temporary lodging in the flesh'.[36] Studies for the third royal commission on tuberculosis justified this stance. The commission's endorsement of a generalized model not only justified the more rigorous control of the meat trade that many local authorities and sanitary reformers were seeking, but also legitimized the risks from contaminated meat.[37]

Disagreements about whether tuberculosis was a localized or generalized disease encouraged a sense that it was 'impossible to lay down any regulations for the partial or total condemnation of carcases on account of tuberculosis'.[38] At a local level these disagreements influenced what meat was seized, prompting complaints from butchers' associations alarmed by the lack of uniformity in inspection practices. Decisions over meat became a frequent source of contention between butchers, traders, sanitary officials and veterinarians. However, if the level of risk remained uncertain, bovine tuberculosis ensured that the idea that meat could transmit disease was already firmly established in the Edwardian period.

Science to the Rescue?

Although the science of BSE and bovine tuberculosis was uncertain, how that science was used presents interesting questions. In the BSE crisis this led to numerous conspiracy theories but the key question is not the science itself but how the advice from scientific experts was manipulated and presented. With both diseases, official narratives based on one reading of the science were constructed that were presented in authoritative terms. Whereas the immediate context of research shifted between bovine tuberculosis and BSE, advice from carefully selected experts was manipulated, scientific pluralism was rejected, and the institutional authority of scientific research was used to justify existing prejudices and policies. In the twentieth-century history of diseased meat, science was employed by policymakers and stakeholders to justify official narratives of safety and assessments of risk.

Throughout the BSE crisis, government ministers repeatedly claimed that policy was shaped by advice from scientific experts. The role of the expert had become well established in the technique of government by the 1920s and scientific expertise was seen to add a seemingly 'disinterested' authority to policy. In an attempt to find answers about the potential risks of BSE to the population, the Conservative government unsurprisingly turned to science for an authoritative view. It established a working party under Richard Southwood, professor of zoology at Oxford University, in 1988 to investigate. Throughout the working party's deliberations, the human health issue was downplayed as the government considered BSE an animal health problem, ensuring that no attempt was made to include anyone who held controversial ideas about BSE. The working party formed part of an international drive to investigate BSE, but with relatively few numbers of cases to draw conclusions from, and with the science of BSE still being developed, it could do little but endorse the assumption that BSE was caused by an agent similar to scrapie. Given the climate of anxiety, the working party feared an overreaction from the public. Its recommendations were therefore ambiguous: the working party concluded that that it was 'most unlikely that BSE would have any implications for human health'. However, because the risk of transmission could not be ruled out it advised that precautions should be based on this possibility. This was not clear in the final report, which was altered by civil servants to satisfy MAFF.[39]

The government manipulated the findings of the Southwood working party 'to try to get the message across that beef was safe' to legitimize the policies already adopted and minimize anxiety. Its report was 'cited as if it demonstrated as a matter of scientific certainty rather than provisional opinion, that any risk to humans from BSE was remote'.[40] Later assessments of BSE continued to repeat the deficiencies of the Southwood working party. Opposing voices were either ignored or quickly dismissed: for example, claims by Richard Lacey, a microbiologist at the University of Leeds, that BSE presented a significant risk to human health were rejected as a 'mixture of science and science fiction'.[41] MAFF restricted access to BSE-infected material and directed support to a few 'trust' sites, which were 'not necessarily those with the most appropriate expertise'.[42] Those researchers it did fund were directed into areas that were likely to confirm the official stance on BSE and at times the Ministry intervened to alter the content of scientific papers.[43] Throughout the BSE crisis, science was employed to confirm government assessments of the disease.

That the views of scientific experts were manipulated and science used to confirm existing policy in the BSE crisis was not unique in the history of food safety. Nor was the process of using scientific committees. Expertise and knowledge had become routinized in the late nineteenth century with science used to serve the public interest through expert advice to parliamentary inquiries. From the 1860s, a number of state-funded studies into pleuro-pneumonia, anthrax, rabies and other contagious animal diseases had been appointed to determine (much like the Southwood working party) the nature and threat from animal diseases. A similar process was repeated for bovine tuberculosis. Disagreement about whether the disease was localized or generalized and hence the grounds on which meat from tuberculous livestock could be condemned had seen the appointment of two royal commissions in the 1890s. Experts were consulted and protracted bacteriological investigations were funded to find answers. In much the same way as the Southwood working party defended existing ideas about

BSE, both commissions drew on expert advice to defend the idea that bovine tuberculosis was a zoonosis. In doing so, they reinforced a particular localized construction of the disease.

However, these claims were quickly upset by Koch's pronouncement at the 1901 Congress on Tuberculosis. His views raised questions 'of no small administrative difficulty' for those sanitary authorities trying to clean up the meat trade and for the Local Government Board (LGB) which was endeavouring to persuade reluctant local authorities to tighten their meat regulation.[44] Amid a flurry of international activity to determine the accuracy of Koch's statements, a third royal commission was established to find answers. However, rather than representing the disinterested authority of science, from the start the commission, much like the Southwood working party, was carefully constructed to justify already accepted policies and to reassure the public. Despite claims that the experts appointed to head the commission had 'unbiased and open minds', most 'were declared hostile critics of Dr. Koch before any experiments were undertaken'.[45] In seeking to refute Koch, they directed bacteriological research to confirm 'the essential identity of the *Tubercle bacillus* and tubercular disease in the cow, in man, and in other animals' and its 'communicability'.[46] Too much had been invested politically and scientifically in proving that bovine and human tuberculosis were connected and that meat was an important source of contagion for any other stance to be taken. It was no surprise therefore that when the commission delivered its final report in 1911, after ten years of extensive bacteriological investigation, that it concluded that it had 'conclusively shown that many cases of fatal tuberculosis in the human subject have been produced by the bacillus known to cause the disease in cattle'. Based on this evidence, the commissioners argued that existing regulations should 'not be relaxed'.[47] The mass of evidence collected by the commission confirmed what policymakers and scientists felt they already knew. The same might be said for BSE.

Making Meat Safe?

How were consumers to be protected from BSE and bovine tuberculosis? A number of interacting and interlocking factors shaped policy and practice. The 'scientific' understanding of both diseases and the perception of risk influenced policy which was also shaped by various networks of actors and interest groups – veterinarians, public health officials, ministers, farming interests and food producers. Financial resources and accepted national and local politics further influenced measures designed to protect the public. The result was a complex series of negotiated compromises that did not substantially challenge business interests even when the dangers of meat became evident.

Because BSE was framed as an animal health issue, and because the science suggested that the risks from beef were negligible, responses to BSE initially focused on mechanisms to halt the spread of the disease in cattle. Efforts to minimize risks to consumers were secondary because few people thought BSE was a risk to human health. Initial reactions hence concentrated on farming through a ban on meat and bone meal feed, the compulsory destruction of affected animals and a ban on certain meat products from entering the food chain. Such policies had been a consistent feature of animal health strategies for the last 200 years. Compulsion was rejected for fear that it would encounter resistance and, following a long tradition of animal disease controls, compensation was paid to encourage compliance. However, the initial precautionary measures were presented in terms that underplayed their importance as public health measures. Many of the regulatory decisions were based on the 'official' science of BSE and were designed to reassure a public increasingly anxious about food safety. At the time, the Common Agricultural Committee praised the government's actions, noting that it was a 'substantial improvement' on its handling of the 1988 salmonella outbreak in eggs.[48]

The announcement in 1996 that vCJD might be linked to BSE resulted in the hasty introduction of further control measures. These included a scheme banning human consumption of meat from cattle more than thirty months old, a subsidy for the slaughter of calves and additional inspections of abattoirs, measures which were designed to restore national and international confidence. Many considered the measures introduced too little, too late.

Reactions to BSE need to be contextualized within longer trends in the control of epizootics and local public health initiatives. Early twentieth-century responses to bovine tuberculosis utilized a similar framework of control and eradication through a combination of mechanisms to prevent the disease in animals and local efforts to minimize risks to consumers. However, as bovine tuberculosis was from the start constructed as a public health issue, and with the science asserting its zoonotoic properties and the role of meat, greater efforts were made to protect consumers.

Attempts to clean up the meat trade and protect the public from purchasing tuberculous meat were shaped by the existing public health framework, which was dominated by local authorities and based on a system of surveillance and identification. Drawing on traditional ideas of nuisances and inspection, and on provisions contained under the 1875 Public Health Act that permitted local authorities to destroy food deemed 'unfit for human consumption', attempts focused on the inspection of markets, slaughterhouses and butchers' shops. As fears about bovine tuberculosis intensified, local authorities invested greater effort in meat inspection and the seizure and destruction of diseased meat. The result was an extension of existing ideas of surveillance and removal that dominated the structure of public health and provided the framework for controlling the meat trade and limiting the sale of diseased meat. Within this system, sanitary officials, veterinarians, butchers and livestock owners competed for authority over what meat to seize. A clear tension existed between veterinarians keen to extend their role and meat traders who sought to limit regulation as they became increasingly worried about the seizure of diseased carcasses. Different constructions of bovine tuberculosis as a localized or generalized disease were voiced to legitimize the competing interests of different groups involved. It was this combination of surveillance mechanisms and tensions between these actors that shaped food policy into the 1940s and 50s.

The idea of surveillance and identification was extended to eradicating the disease in cattle. The possibility that contagious cattle diseases could be stamped out had been established under the 1869 Contagious Diseases (Animals) Act and came to underpin Edwardian attempts to limit epizootics. Although the system of notification, slaughter and compensation established under the 1869 and subsequent acts was beset with problems, the need for 'the detection of disease on the farms and premises where animals are bred and fed, and the concentration of restrictive measures on those centres of disease' remained central to efforts to prevent epizootics.[49] Local measures to eliminate bovine tuberculosis built on these initiatives and utilized a combination of veterinary inspection and testing to identify diseased livestock, an approach that continued to shape responses to zoonotic diseases throughout the twentieth century. However, even though bovine tuberculosis was a risk to public health, because of the scale of the problem the state was reluctant to include the disease under existing slaughter and compensation mechanisms. A mass compulsory surveillance and slaughter programme was hence rejected in favour of voluntary and market-led schemes to create disease-free herds as a step towards eradication. The idea was 'gradual extinction'.[50]

In the postwar period, the systems to prevent the spread of animal diseases and the sale of diseased meat established at a local level in the early twentieth century were curtailed as the emphasis shifted to the farming industry in the control of zoonotic diseases. A bonfire of regulations in the 1980s and Whitehall's belittlement of local government responsibility, allied to a series of funding cuts, made matters worse. Ironically, therefore, the Philips inquiry into BSE concluded that the effective control of animal diseases required the type of surveillance regime that had been implemented to tackle bovine tuberculosis.[51]

Protecting the Consumer

Numerous hypotheses have been put forward to explain why measures to protect the public from BSE evolved in the way they did. Much of the literature views BSE as a 'crisis' that exposed flaws in policymaking or seeks to apportion blame to key participants or departments. Interpretations range from short-termism, to a culture of non-intervention, to faith in market economics, to opportunistic policymaking.[52] However, policy reactions to BSE were multilayered and need to be considered in the historical context of responses to animal diseases, which, since the nineteenth century, have been shaped by the demands of different interest groups (or networks). It was the tensions between and within these groups that shaped policy response to BSE and bovine tuberculosis. In both cases, the needs of consumers were balanced against those of producers.

Government ministers, convinced that BSE represented little danger to the public, were initially preoccupied with preventing an alarmist reaction and the need to be seen to be doing something. They used evidence from their scientific experts to reassure the public that British beef was safe. Ministers tried to balance demands to protect public health with the interests of the farming industry without increasing public expenditure, a juggling act that proved unworkable. Uncertainty and a strong agricultural lobby, which exerted considerable influence over policy, complicated this situation. The Conservative government had a weak parliamentary majority and relied on a combination of Eurosceptics and the agricultural lobby for support. MAFF also staunchly defended farming interests at a time when the government favoured the market.[53] Here the Ministry followed in a long tradition of minimizing the risks of an animal disease to prevent harm to the one of the farming industry's most important products. In the early years of the crisis the Ministry hence openly rejected the need for compulsory or additional precautions, a stance welcomed by senior Conservative politicians, who relied on the agricultural lobby for support, and by those who did not want to pursue BSE with too much vigour for fear of raising the public profile of the disease.

There were also problems at a practical level. Longstanding rivalries between MAFF and the Department of Health led to delays in implementing measures. Measures to exclude MBM from animal feed were considered by certain sections of the agricultural industry as disproportionate to the danger involved and were often initially disregarded. Inadequate compensation further reduced compliance. An incomplete and voluntary ban on MBM permitted an environment in which conditions for disease transfer continued to occur and encouraged the view in the agricultural and food industry that BSE was a non-urgent problem.[54] Nor were measures to protect the public strictly adhered to by the meat industry. When MAFF conducted a spot check of 193 abattoirs in 1995, it found that 48 per cent were failing to remove spinal tissue and offal.[55] Controls were hampered by the need to regulate often messy and chaotic premises; by bureaucratic inertia and political expediency, which was aided by the lack of understanding of how BSE might be transmitted. The scrapie analogy and the findings of the Southwood working party encouraged a false sense of security, while cuts in public funding limited the number of inspectors and hindered the enforcement of the feed and specified bovine offal bans. Those implementing the controls on animal feeds and meat were hence not unduly concerned by breaches of the regulations at a time when the Conservative government was pressing for industrial deregulation.[56] Business interests, governmental rivalries and financial restrictions ensured that in policy reactions to BSE the consumer was often neglected.

Responses to bovine tuberculosis at the start of the twentieth century had already pointed to many of these problems. Attempts to limit the risks from tuberculosis meat conflicted with policymakers' reluctance to interfere with trade. This stance combined with fears that stringent restrictions on the meat trade would force prices up to limit control at a time when a premium was placed on working-class consumption of animal products. MAFF's predecessor, the Board of Agriculture, equally defended farming interests. It was keen to minimize the risks from cattle diseases, fearing that any outcry would damage the livestock industry. It hence wanted sanitary officials to take responsibility on the understanding that the problem would be tackled through measures to improve meat inspection and public education, an approach that was less damaging to farming than a mass slaughter programme. The Board's position was supported by the powerful farming lobby, which feared that the implementation of widespread surveillance would mean ruin. This ensured that what action was taken was only 'a stricter and more general enforcement of the law' and not a concerted attempt to stamp out bovine tuberculosis. Contemporaries found that it was difficult to balance the 'interests of the consumer' whilst 'placing [as] little restriction upon the traders as possible'.[57] The sheer number of infected cattle ensured that neither the state nor stockowners were prepared to meet the high cost of eradicating bovine tuberculosis. Just as MAFF was bound by budgetary restraints during the BSE crisis, so too was the Board of Agriculture and LGB in the Edwardian period. Frequent recessions, a retrenchment in domestic expenditure by a powerful Treasury and the limitations of local government finance created barriers to effective control measures. Even when compensation was introduced under the 1909 Tuberculosis Order awards remained minimal. Many farmers therefore kept cattle until they showed obvious signs of tuberculosis before selling them, ensuring that tuberculous meat continued to enter the food chain.

Further parallels can be detected between BSE and bovine tuberculosis in the implementation of meat control policies. Late twentieth-century food scares have revealed inadequacies with meat control practices and the same concerns were repeatedly voiced between 1900 and 1914. Unease was expressed about how effective meat inspection was conducted and by whom. Tensions emerged between veterinarians and sanitary officials over who was best qualified to inspect meat and what meat should be seized, reflecting the different ways bovine tuberculosis was framed. This had a direct impact on local policy. Most inspections were little more than spot checks and condemnation was based on prejudice or individual assessment rather than firm criteria. This led to protests from the meat industry which not only resented what they saw as the 'harsh proceedings' of medical officers of health who 'confiscate in doubtful cases of tuberculosis animals' but also actively contested prosecutions.[58] If trade associations pressed for regulation and protection to minimize losses, many butchers were known to cheat inspection, with the less scrupulous using various subterfuges to escape seizure. The result was a system of meat inspection in which questions of quality were frequently negotiated between inspectors and butchers, where substantial amounts of tuberculous meat escaped inspection and where seizures frequently relied on voluntary surrender. Many concluded that the system of 'detection has failed to grapple successfully with the problem' of tuberculous meat.[59] A hundred years later the same concerns were to be voiced about BSE and the measures introduced to protect the public.

Conclusions

Although nearly a century has passed between the two meat scares, responses to BSE and bovine tuberculosis highlight continuities in how the risks from animal diseases have been understood and managed in the twentieth century. In both cases, ideas of risk were contested and shaped by different disease constructions that highlight not only the uncertainty that has surrounded the threat from animal diseases and the problems in defining the risk to the public but also how zoonoses are amenable to a number of scientific and political interpretations. There are further continuities. Questions of trust and responsibility repeatedly surfaced in response to BSE and bovine tuberculosis as both diseases came to provide a vehicle for existing concerns about food safety and meat. Likewise, a comparison of BSE and bovine tuberculosis reveals how advice from scientific experts could be manipulated to endorse different paradigms of food safety. Equally, responses to both diseases expose how measures to protect consumers often favoured business interests and how a range of competing agencies and different ways of framing a zoonosis shaped them. At the same time, they illustrate how the surveillance and eradication measures implemented for bovine tuberculosis continued to provide a broad framework for responses to zoonoses throughout the twentieth century. Although much of the regulatory apparatus and inspectorate was scaled down during the 1980s, it was the systems established to protect the public from bovine tuberculosis and other animal diseases that were once more endorsed during the BSE crisis. Bovine tuberculosis had defined the problem of diseased meat, highlighted the risk from animal diseases to human health, and created a framework for protecting the public. Although it was not the Edwardian equivalent of BSE, responses to it demonstrate that food safety and diseased meat are not new 'obsessions' of the late twentieth century.

10 FOOD, DRUG AND CONSUMER REGULATION: THE 'MEAT, DES AND CANCER' DEBATES IN THE UNITED STATES

Jean-Paul Gaudillière

On 26 April 1973, the *Wall Street Journal* announced that the Food and Drug Administration (FDA) had just banned diethylstilbestrol (DES) implants in cattle and other livestock, recalling that one year earlier the FDA had already prohibited the use of DES in animal feeds.[1] Cancer was the official motive for this unusual action, which made a food additive that had been used for more than twenty years as a growth enhancer disappear from the agricultural scene. The industrial and economic significance of the event was not as dramatic as the cattle breeders and the animal-food industry thought it would be when they argued against these administrative measures. As the *Wall Street Journal* failed to point out, other growth-promoting drugs were either already on the market or ready to be introduced as substitutes for DES. The symbolic value of the DES affair should not, however, be underestimated. Controversies over its uses had started fifteen years earlier – as soon as farmers had begun employing DES-enriched premixes – on a massive scale and did not stop with the 1973 ban. The decision was immediately contested in court and even though a federal judge finally approved the FDA ban in 1978, illegal uses of DES remained an issue until the mid-1980s. The DES affair thus lasted for a quarter of a century. Controversies originating in the use of the substance addressed all concerns connected with the domination of industrial practices in US agriculture. In fact, the national DES crisis began in 1971, when it was discovered that DES was not only a potential but an actual carcinogen in humans. Epidemiological studies revealed at the time that DES – in its first function as a gynaecological drug – had caused a wave of cancers in the so-called 'DES daughters', i.e. born from women treated with DES to prevent spontaneous abortion.

The story of DES in the United States has been addressed in many ways. One group of studies has looked at the unfolding of the medical drama and focused on the lessons to be drawn from the affair, either in the perspective of medical practices or from a feminist viewpoint.[2] In parallel, historians and sociologists of medicine have investigated DES to integrate its medical uses into the long history of sex hormones and gynaecology, while more recent studies on gender have analysed the role played in the crisis by the then-emerging Women's Health Movement.[3] Less numerous, analysts of the 'meat and DES' controversy have emphasized two different contexts: the rise of industrial agriculture, and the development of the environmental and consumer movements in the 1960s and 1970s.[4] The literature on agricultural DES all shares a strong interest in the problem of the 'capture', namely the different ways in which political and economic interests have hinged on or even distorted the evaluation of the health risks associated with DES uses. Although the alignments or confrontations between experts and stakeholders, as well as the way they were perceived, are an important element in the DES story, the capture perspective has made the analysis of expertise as process and practice of marginal importance since all the important factors, i.e. social interests and alliances, were in place beforehand.

The aim of this paper is therefore not simply to look at agricultural DES to discuss the rise of consumer politics and its impact on the relations between industrial agriculture, public health and the surveillance of dangerous substances. It is to take the 'meat and DES crisis' as a point of entry into the risk-expertise processes that emerged during the 1960s and 70s and grounded a politics of life that connected individual and collective consumer actions, stakeholder lobbies, citizens' empowerment, precautionary action in the legal sphere and the construction of markets. This politics is still with us and has gained widespread importance in agriculture and medicine, becoming the normal way of handling all sorts of risks beyond the question of how we can objectify and control the dangers possibly posed by health-threatening substances. In other words, the 'meat and DES affair' will be used as a lens into a new 'way of regulating' the industrial uses of life.

The word 'regulation' is often intended to mean an action taken by a government or administration body, or any form of administrative body, to control the marketing of drugs. The trajectories of DES – both agricultural and medical – suggest that it may be worth considering a broader definition. Regulation may then be viewed as a series of *dispositifs*, which aim not only at controlling the marketing of such or such a product, but as well at managing its production and use. Regulation is therefore not exclusively a problem of the state's authority; it is also a problem of standards of action within the laboratory, the production plant, the doctor's office, the newspaper desk and the congressional backroom.

Regulation is therefore not restricted to the actions and tools employed by the FDA or similar agencies. A reasonable assumption based on the current history and sociology of therapeutic agents is that an extended twentieth century, beginning around 1880, has witnessed the emergence of four 'ways of regulating', which may be characterized by the values and aims targeted, the main actors involved, the acceptable forms of evidence, and the legitimate means of intervention (See Table 10.2).[5]

Professional regulation aims at improving the competency of licensed practitioners making or using drugs, as well as at developing patients' compliance. Governance emanates from corporate bodies, medical and pharmaceutical societies, and occasionally from ad hoc committees set up by academic journals or health authorities. Judgements on the benefits of drugs focus on the production of pharmacological knowledge, for instance dose-response curves. The basic concept is that all drugs are potentially poisons if used without care. Regulation thus consists in defining standards of good practice, i.e. appropriate dosage, and lists of indications and contraindications. In addition to the traditional pharmacopoeia, regulatory tools include the many forms of guidelines and recommendations for practice issued by medical-pharmaceutical collectives.

State regulation relies on an alternative set of values and aims. As Harry Marks convincingly demonstrates, it emerged as a means of protecting patients and public health from physicians' credulity and industrialists' tendency to oversell their products. The goal is therefore to control the market by organizing an 'independent', meaning state-based, assessment. The main actors are therefore administrative bodies, where the leading role is played by national regulatory agencies, which were established or developed in Europe and North America after World War II. As the demonstration of both safety and efficacy became the norm, these agencies expanded their internal expertise capabilities and accepted the emphasis placed by elite biomedical scientists on statistical proof. Epidemiological forms of evidence, i.e. randomized trials and case-controlled surveys, first completed, and then superseded the toxicological arsenal of laboratory experimentation. Within this framework, the most important regulatory tools are the mandatory applications for marketing permits. In addition, agencies also organize information networks to collect data on adverse reactions, issue public recommendations on indications, mandate the writing of package inserts, and eventually survey advertising material.

Industrial regulation is rooted in the practices of the producing firms. It aims at maximizing productivity and profit while avoiding liabilities due to accidents and consumer dissatisfaction. Emphasis is placed on quality control and good production practices, which rely on engineering. Standardized assays in animals and sampling are among the basic procedures. Starting in the 1940s, this technical basis was supplemented with an increasing mobilization of managerial knowledge, for instance market research. Regulatory tools therefore focus on the construction of stable markets. They encompass internal quality control protocols, external reporting systems, and the vast array of instruments developed by the firms in the 1950s and 60s to shape prescription practices and drug uses: inserts, brochures, seminars for prescribing physicians and visits by prep representatives.

The more recent consumerist/activist regulation is associated with the escalating role of users' and patients' organizations. It was prompted through two different and often conflicting patterns: on the one hand, by pharmaceutical companies' interest in having a more direct access to users, particularly potential consumers of disease-prevention drugs; on the other, by the critics of paternalistic medicine and the collective empowerment sought by patient groups, inspired for instance by the AIDS movement or the Women's Health Movement. Emphasis is therefore placed on quality of 'service' and on the individual's possibility of making (truly) informed choices. Major attention is given to the risks and potential iatrogenic effects of medical interventions, with observational epidemiology and analysis of routine medical practices playing the leading role. Regulatory tools do not only include administratively organized post-marketing surveillance, but also the precedents set by court decisions, or media campaigns, which may influence regulatory authorities, physicians' prescriptions or users' choices.

Although based on the history of therapeutic agents, this framework has a more general value, especially in the United States where – from the early twentieth century onward – the regulation of drugs was not disconnected from the regulation of food, as shown by the history of the Food and Drug Administration. Veterinary experts or large meatpackers and other large food processors have played a role in the construction and regulation of agricultural markets similar to the one played by physicians and pharmaceutical giants in the drug sector. Moreover, the hypothesis of a new form of regulation rooted in consumer and activist mobilization in public controversies about risks, and in new roles of the courts and the media seems a reasonable assumption when discussing recent 'affairs', ranging from the growth-hormone debates to the mad-cow scandal and the conflicts over GM food.

The 'DES and meat' story is a good test for this latter hypothesis for at least two reasons. First, it reveals a specific moment in the history of regulation characterized by the reinforcement of state interventions gradually articulated with an emerging consumer-activist regulation. Second, the conjunction of debates about agricultural and medical uses of the drug, which developed in the United States among other places, facilitates a broader assessment of regulatory practices beyond the specificities of pharmaceuticals. This paper will therefore approach the question of regulation and risk expertise by focusing on the relations between the two DES crises that characterized the 1970s context.

The argument will be presented in three steps. First, the paper will recall how DES entered into agricultural practice in the 1950s and how its uses rapidly became controversial. The main focus will be, however, on the 1970s crisis as a specific and decisive feature of the US context, namely the conjunction between this agricultural controversy and the medical scandal originating in the cancers and malformations diagnosed in the so-called 'DES-daughters'. The second and third sections will explore the form of public expertise that characterized the US debates and their roots in consumer politics, focusing on the evaluation of DES risks conducted in Congress and in the courts, respectively.

Agricultural DES in the United States: A Contested Growth Enhancer

Charles Dodds first synthesized DES in 1936.[6] Working for the Medical Research Council, the British chemist did not patent the process, even though the molecule revealed promising properties. Although DES did not present a structural similarity with natural sex steroids, the substance proved a potent analogue of oestrogens, mimicking most, if not all the latter's effects in the animal assays then in use for assessing the potency of female hormones. Cheap and easy to produce, DES rapidly became a substitute – and competitor – for industrially made oestrogens, namely those purified by pharmaceutical firms out of the urine of pregnant women or pregnant mares. Initially, DES was used in gynaecology as a therapeutic agent in a variety of indications also handled with oestrogens: infertility, sexual-cycle disorders, uncontrolled bleeding, absence of menses or problematic menopausal symptoms.

The FDA authorized DES for the US market in 1941. As reported by S. Bell, the 'synthetic oestrogen' played an exemplary role in the history of the agency as it was one of the first compounds to be approved according to the procedures defined in the 1938 Food, Drug, and Cosmetic Act. The act partially transferred the burden of proof to the industrialist. A manufacturer seeking authorization was mandated to document the safety of its product, but the new law did not define any type of acceptable evidence or test. Approval was granted for the basic gynaecological indications, i.e. amenorrhea, menopausal symptoms and infertility. DES was however perceived as a potent oestrogen rather than an aromatic compound with an ethylene side chain; 'off label' uses rapidly surfaced in the 1950s. The most important of these – in terms of prescription numbers – was for managing the risk of spontaneous abortion during pregnancy. The idea was widely adopted that DES, a quasi-hormone, could replicate the changes in the concentration of sex steroids occurring during pregnancy. This justified the prescription of the drug as 'replacement' therapy for a condition attributed to oestrogen deficiency.[7] Despite the fact that clinical trials had produced conflicting results, DES use was gradually extended as a reassurance factor to women with no previous experience of abortion. Large uses of DES were never considered trivial. Only a small minority of physicians, however, upheld their concern about the fact that a long time previously, already in the 1930s, laboratory experiments with mice had shown that oestrogens in general, and DES in particular, could induce tumours in healthy animals.

A decade later, in the 1950s, following pioneering work by animal nutritionists at Iowa State College under W. Burroughs's lead, DES use was extended to agriculture. Burroughs and his colleagues discovered that DES given in minute amounts accelerated the growth of cattle animals.[8] The idea of adding DES to industrially prepared premixes was patented by the university and licensed exclusively to the pharmaceutical firm Lilly. The process was a huge success. Lilly sublicensed it to a few dozen companies. As a result, within two years more than 6 million cattle were being fed nutrition containing DES.

FDA approval for the technique was obtained easily. Rather than providing evidence of the non-toxicity of the additive (this was not required for animal drugs), the Iowa nutritionists argued that no residues of DES could be found in the carcasses of animals fed with the growth-enhancing premixes. The risk for the consumer was therefore nil. FDA officials contested the statistical presentation of the results rather than the mere fact of the quick disappearance of the drug. This evaluation left no trace of a comparison with human medicine. To be on the safe side, the FDA simply imposed a withdrawal period of two days between the last treatment and the slaughter. Physicians interested in environmental carcinogens – an issue gaining visibility in the late 1950s – were the first to make a link between agricultural DES and the adverse properties of oestrogens. In 1956, J. Smith – a New York state physician – argued at the congress of the Association of Official Analytical Chemists that DES should be considered as a 'cancer threat' given the massive experimental evidence of its carcinogenic power. Barely taken into account during the meeting, the argument made its way to the *New York Times* and to the US Congress.[9]

The historian Alan Marcus is right to insist that the invention of DES-supplemented feed was a typical event of the postwar transformation of US agriculture, which generalized the model of industrial farms initially used with poultry. Modernity did not only mean scaling up herds, or intensive rather than extensive rearing, it was also synonymous with forms of 'scientific farming' that relied on a controlled input/output balance, which itself implied the use of standardized feed and nutrition supplements in order to increase the productivity of the animal machine or to enhance the health of animals kept in dense populations (sometimes indoors), hence highly susceptible to the spread of contagious diseases. Oestrogens thus entered into the meat chain along with the massive use of vitamins and antibiotics for similar purposes.

This transformation became a matter of concern and an issue of public debate in the 1960s. The trajectory of DES was actually rapidly affected by the emergence of critical voices associated with the consumer movement. Although their origins can be traced back to the 1930s, in the 1960s the heterogeneous organizations targeting 'consumer rights' experienced rapid growth and radicalization, often attributed to the favourable climate generated by the economic expansion of the postwar decades.[10]

The enactment of the so-called Delaney clause in 1958 was a critical event in the polarization of the debates on the quality of food.[11] This amendment to the FDA Act introduced by Congressman Delaney stated that no food additive that had been found to induce cancer either in animals or in humans could be authorized.[12] The measure was adopted despite the FDA's opposition. The FDA considered this broad ban as both prejudicial to the practice of productive agriculture and impossible to enforce. The approval of the clause was not only a symptom of the mounting influence of consumer activism, but – as testified by the parallel drawn between DES and DDT during the Delaney hearings – one of the first legislative consequences of an environmental movement, which was starting to benefit from powerful middle-class constituency and no longer strictly targeted conservation issues but also concerns about the dissemination of chemicals in the environment.[13]

The Delaney clause crystallized the debates in Congress on industrialized food for ten years after it was enacted. Farmers, industrial-feed producers and drug companies joined forces in attempts to repeal the clause, arguing that it would ban all sorts of chemicals that could be used for the betterment, preservation and conservation of food. They claimed that animal tests could not be trusted, upholding that it would always be possible to find models and circumstances under which any chemical could become a carcinogen, and they explored ways of repealing the clause. In 1962, agricultural lobbying succeeded in inserting a short addition to the amended Food and Drug Act, which stated that a substance could be authorized even if proved a carcinogen in the laboratory provided it did not harm the animals and left no residues in the meat for human consumption.[14]

Controversies over the dangers of DES grew in the context of widespread critique of government, industrial capitalism, and established authorities in the 1960s. The public life of DES was to a large extent determined by the power struggle opposing the alliance for industrial agriculture and the loose front connecting the social movements of the 1960s and their Democratic allies. Bestselling books such as *Silent Spring*, *The Poisons in Your Food* and *The Chemical Feast* accompanied the rise of environmental and consumer organizations.[15] These new waves of activism weighed heavily in two different areas. First, some of the reports and studies supporting their positions were given nationwide attention. This was the case, for instance, for the reports circulated by Ralph Nader's Center for Study of Responsive Law, which began to investigate FDA activities in 1968 after a first major success in its indictment of the car industry.[16]

Second, Democratic as well as Republican governments conceded that stronger regulation was necessary to tame market excesses. Although Nixon's institution of the Environmental Protection Agency has received the most historical attention, previous moves were equally important. In the early 1960s, President Kennedy mandated the official recognition of four consumer rights: the right to safety, the right to be informed, the right to choose and the right to be heard. In parallel, he appointed a Citizen's Advisory Committee whose role would be to conduct hearings to reflect on the aims and means of the FDA, and to provide recommendations for its reform, some of these having been incorporated into the 1962 Act that strongly reinforced the agency's role in evaluating both the toxicity and the efficacy of therapeutic agents in human medicine.

Most historical work – Marcus's included – on the relations between the DES affair and this particular context has been articulated in terms of political interests and distrust of scientific expertise. In a nutshell, the argument focuses on uncertainty and capture. Reassuring discourses about the limited nature of the cancer risk involved in the use of food additives did not convince. Paternalistic attitudes towards the 'ignorant lay public' deepened this crisis of confidence: as a consequence of suspicion, the public debate was dominated by wide-ranging generalizations, value-laden evaluations and feelings. Both sides (in favour and against the use of DES) waged a polemical battle, defending their views and interests in the name of science. In this perspective, experts' statements went far beyond the knowledge of the time, which was remarkably uncertain: they need to be understood above all as pleas in favour or against a ban on DES. One side upheld that the social movements proved unable to accept the existing facts regarding the limited dangers of DES in meat; while alternatively, the other side argued that big agro-industrial interests produced ignorance and bad science to mislead the public.

It would however be misleading to limit our reading of the DES affair to the making of these political alliances and their confrontation. The production and discussion of expertise in DES was not merely the expression of entrenched interests, it was a work in its own right, which in turn redefined attitudes and interests. In the following sections, I will contend that it was impossible to dissociate the production of science from political work and public debates. The production of facts was actually inextricably mixed with them, and what characterized the DES debates was the multiplicity of sometimes-conflicting scientific evidence rather than mere distrust of experts or industrially tainted research. In other words, the DES affair may be viewed as a typical example of late twentieth-century biotechnological risk assessment and risk management.

The decisive decade was in this respect not the 1960s but the 70s, when the links between DES as a drug and DES as a food additive were made, bringing in another layer of conflicting and situated scientific discourses. Medical uses of DES were basically unproblematic until 1971, even though feminist authors occasionally made the analogy with the contraceptive pill and targeted gynaeco-logical hormones for their purported carcinogenic properties.[17] The professional 'warning' on DES began locally in 1970, when gynaecologists at the Mas-sachusetts General Hospital reported a surprising series of vaginal tumours.[18] Considered as very rare, this type of cancer had been diagnosed in rapid succes-sion in – which was even more unusual – very young women. Following these early observations, Arthur Herbst and his colleagues reinforced their argument that this was a serious public-health issue by concentrating on the epidemio-logical evidence. They selected a retrospective control group by looking at the records of women admitted the same day as their patients, matching age and social groups. The statistical comparison of their records revealed one single significant difference: the girls suffering from vaginal cancer were born from women who had been treated with DES during their pregnancy. The correla-tion was published in April 1971 in the *New England Journal of Medicine*, after Herbst had sent his data to the FDA.[19] The report alerted the New York Public Health Service, and its cancer-control bureau started to look for similar cases. Having found another five, also correlated with 'DES mothers', they issued a general warning to the state's physicians.[20] It did not take long for the initiative to find its way into the mainstream media. In less than six months, the profes-sional alert had become a national scandal, relayed by public-health authorities and local gynaecologists, widely discussed in the news, a topic for congressional hearings, and an ongoing motive for concern within the FDA.

This alert had two effects on the agricultural scene. First, it gave very concrete meaning to the animal–human translation that had been at the core of all the argu-ments around the carcinogenic risks of the drug. If the correlation evidenced by Herbst and reinforced by the National Cancer Institute survey was accepted, this meant that DES given in therapeutic dosage was inducing tumours in humans, as well as in animals. Second, the medical crisis reinforced doubts about the policy the FDA had implemented since DES had been put on the market. Blind to the doubts raised by a number of physicians regarding the clinical value of the preg-nancy indication, the agency had allied itself with a segment of the gynaecological elite and the DES-producing pharmaceutical firms. A similar scenario might well have taken place within the division of veterinary medicine, leading the agency to support the claims of nutrition scientists and feed producers.

Both crises – on medical DES and on agricultural DES – actually reinforced each other. The medical crisis also benefited from the attention already drawn by agricultural DES in the press, among consumer organizations, and within the administration. Throughout the 1970s, after the FDA had reacted by contrain-dicating pregnancy, other medical uses of DES were questioned. In parallel with its campaigning on the adverse effects of the contraceptive pill, the Women's Health Movement succeeded in drawing attention to the prescription of DES as a morning-after pill. The pill was then regulated to include mandatory risk-warning leaflets in the packages. A second problematic medical application was the use of DES to inhibit lactation and prevent breast engorgement after childbirth. The FDA plain and simply contraindicated it in the late 1970s.

This conjunction of a medical and an agricultural crisis was all the more powerful as links between the two DES uses were at work at various levels, mobilizing texts, objects and persons. First, there were technical links. Toxicological assessment of both usages relied on the same tools: assay procedures and modelling strategies. A mouse test was widely used to reveal the potency of compounds with oestrogenic effects.[21] The same animal model was also central in the study of carcinogenesis: all experiments suggesting that a given dosage of DES induced the formation of tumours were first conducted with mice, which provided the sketchy 'dose-response' relationship then available.[22] Second, there were administrative and institutional links, since the FDA was the agency responsible for the regulation of drugs for human or veterinary uses. FDA Commissioner Charles Edwards issued recommendations, comments and responses for both usages of DES, not always at the same time but in close connection. Even if two separate divisions were in charge of regulating drugs for human medicine on the one hand and veterinary products on the other, the mere existence of a single administrative roof facilitated articulated choices. Given the history of the FDA, controlled use and pharmacological evaluation dominated the discussion in both segments. A peculiar consequence of this administrative unity was the nature of the correspondence the agency received. The hundreds of letters sent to the FDA after 1971 on the subject of DES rarely failed to mention humans and cattle simultaneously as the basis for their concerns.[23] Responses from the FDA initially tried to keep the regulatory issues apart, but this proved increasingly difficult as the controversy developed.[24] Third, the unity of DES was taken as an obvious fact in the public arenas, i.e. the media, and consumer organizations and their statements. Most newspaper articles commenting on agricultural DES thus also reminder their audiences of the carcinogenicity of therapeutic DES (although the opposite was rarely true).[25] The most important arenas for this public conjunction were however Congress and the courts, upon which the rest of our analysis will concentrate, given their role in the making of the 'regulatory science' of DES.

The Regulatory Science of Dangerous Meat, Part 1: The Congressional Hearings

The concept of 'regulatory science' is of current use within regulatory agencies and administrative bodies, where it is usually employed to describe their investments in the development of measurement techniques, methodological tools and decision-making protocols for the standardization, authorization or control of technological goods. By contrast science, technology and society analysts (who look at the regulation of chemicals in the postwar era) have used the concept in a broader sense to include the entire spectrum of expert activities conducted in collaboration among scientists, state officials and politicians; this includes laboratory studies for regulatory purposes, testimonies within political fora such as congressional hearings, as well as court rulings of techno-scientific cases. Within this perspective, 'regulatory science' refers to the production of knowledge for administrative, political, or judicial action, but it also implies the idea that this regulatory perspective 'feeds back' to science, leading to the development of specific forms of knowledge. Toxicology and the environmental regulation of chemicals are among the most frequent examples of this dual relationship.

Looking at the history of the EPA, S. Jasanoff, for instance, stressed the intimate relationship between the assessment of chemicals by the agency's scientists, its participation in the political definition of regulatory rules, and the judicial battles over the resulting decisions.[26] She considered the work on chemical carcinogenesis, which dominated the EPA during the 1970s and 80s, as a form of 'adversarial science' echoing many aspects of the practice of scientific testimony within the courtroom. Comparing the fate of ecotoxicology in the United States, the Netherlands, and the United Kingdom, W. Halffman considers regulatory science as a form of boundary work with two functions: 1) separating the scientific from the political in order to balance legitimate knowledge and bring specific statements to the status of agreed facts, and 2) facilitating negotiations and closure of conflicts by providing an aura of objectivity to decisions.[27] Expert work thus mobilizes boundary entities, i.e. texts, objects and persons, which operate or circulate between the technical arenas linked to or depending on the regulatory agencies and the more administrative arenas of committee and hearing rooms. An essential aspect of the regulatory science produced for the regulation of chemicals has accordingly been the establishment of tests for effects, protocols for measuring damages or concentrations, model systems, limit values or exposure thresholds. The 1970s debate on carcinogens is no exception to this pattern.

The general pattern of expertise within the public debates on DES was not, however, restricted to the polarized production and interpretation of such dose-response curves. The response given to the question of what to do with agricultural DES, i.e. ban it or keep using it under controlled conditions, depended on how a series of issues would be considered, ranging from the relationship – causation or association – between DES and the young patients affected with vaginal cancer, the ability to measure DES residues in carcasses, and the meaning of cancer in mice exposed to low doses of DES, to the benefits of increased productivity and accelerated animal growth for the 'American consumer', and for the economy at large. The sheer number of congressional investigations on one or both uses of DES testifies to the intertwined agricultural and medical debates.

Congressional hearings are worth attention because of the special role they play in the US regulatory machinery. Hearings are parliamentary events, but also events staging expert work in a political context targeting stakeholders. Expert testimonies are gathered to balance, and draw the line between science and politics, between what is reasonably well known and what is not, between sound science and speculation, between the respective merits of various forms of evidence. All of this with a direct angle on the interests such knowledge may serve or disserve. A rather specific feature of US congressional hearings is therefore not the fact that experts are questioned by the members of a bipartisan committee with significant power of investigations, but the agreed-upon concept that all 'interested' parties have to be brought in to present their view of the issues, that these parties have their own expertise, that they are legitimate in exerting some influence in order to craft a reasonable compromise that will balance situated views and power. Political analysts have pointed out that this model of participatory stakeholder democracy emerged during the progressive era as a consequence of the weakness of both Congress and the federal administration, the latter having to negotiate its action with a distrusting 'civil society' beyond the borders of official 'representation'.

Within this theatre of proof, studies of the 1950s on the efficacy of DES in pregnancy, for instance, experienced a new life.[28] It was for instance rediscovered that pregnancy was not among the indications the FDA had initially approved: it was an off-label practice, a matter of collective consensus among women's physicians. The political construction of the affair reinforced the view that the FDA had failed to notice and control market-triggered wrongdoings as its most recent assessment of DES demonstrated. The National Academy of Sciences (NSA), as part of a general review commended by the Reform Act of 1962, had re-examined the evidence of efficacy published in the medical literature or presented in the companies' initial applications and had concluded in 1969 that the prevention of spontaneous abortion was only 'possibly effective'.[29] FDA critics contended that in light of this information, the FDA should have put pressure on the firms to provide new data and, if the firms were unable to comply, should have warned physicians that pregnancy was actually an 'unproven' indication.

The hearings greatly contributed to tightening the link between DES in cattle, residues in meat, and the risk of cancer. The first hearing that followed the Herbst report on vaginal cancer, for instance, took place in the House on 11 November 1971. Although it had been set up to address the medical alert, the investigating committee headed by Representative L. Fountain, a Democrat, repeatedly raised, during the hearings, the question of what the newly discovered human cancers might imply for the agricultural use of DES. Dr Herbst himself was thus directly questioned for his opinion regarding the risks of cattle fed with DES.

Representative L. Fountain (Democrat): Dr. Herbst, I refer to your conclusion on page 5 of your prepared statement, that you do not think you can define with confidence the smallest dose or shortest duration of exposure to DES that might endanger the female foetus. Now I would like to examine the applicability of that conclusion to the use of DES in animal feeds...Would your conclusion that you cannot define with confidence the smallest dose or the shortest duration of exposure that might endanger the female fetus apply to DES residues in liver varying to two to 100 parts per billion?

Dr. Herbst: I do not think we know. I guess that is why I do not feel we can define this with confidence. Certainly the drug was used therapeutically in larger amounts than would be ingested in the dosage you are talking about. But in my opinion, we just do not have enough data or knowledge at the present time...It is quite possible that the amounts you are quoting would have no effect at all. However, they might and, therefore, this would cause me some concern.

Rep. Fountain: I understand that its use in animals, cattle, is primarily an economic one. Bearing in mind the magnitude of DES residues which have been found in livers, and assuming the use of DES results in a saving to the public of approximately $ 3.85 per year per person...in your opinion, does this saving justify the use of this carcinogenic drug in cattle feed?

Dr. Herbst: Well, this is a hard question for me to answer ... I would say, as a physician and one who is interested in the problem I have been discussing, I would certainly feel it prudent that pregnant women not be eating anything that has any stilbestrol in it.[30]

In his testimony, FDA Commissioner Edwards tried to play down both the medical alert and its translation in the agricultural idiom.[31] Having to explain why his agency had not reacted when Herbst had sent his clinical reports in March 1971, before the publication of his article, and had left the issue pending until the eve of the hearings, the head of the FDA argued that a correlation was not a demonstration of causality. Herbst had shown an association, but this association needed to be confirmed in order to rule out the intervention of 'confounding factors'. More science was needed until generalization of the risk could be acknowledged, especially if a bridge was to be made between the effects of high therapeutic dosage and the extremely low concentrations of food additives. Central to Edward's scepticism was the huge difference of doses administered in both contexts.

Given the centrality of the dose–effects relationship in both the pharmacological and toxicological perspective shared by the FDA and specialists in animal nutrition, the question of dosage was addressed in each expert testimony, one after the other. It was addressed directly, with computations of inoculated or ingested quantities. It was also dealt with in a less direct way, when discussing the relationship between DES and natural oestrogens. It is not altogether surprising that feeders and animal nutritionists argued that DES was an oestrogen like any other, thus explaining that its carcinogenic potency was just a manifestation of its ability to mimic the properties of sex hormones. As a consequence of this link, they considered that DES quantities should not be considered in isolation but discussed as a component of a global oestrogenic pool that included much higher quantities of normal oestrogens, both in the bodies of supplemented cows and in women. This position was echoed by the representative of the Middle West participating in the House committees, but also by prominent endocrinologists. For instance, Mortimer Lippset, scientific director at the National Institute of Child Health and Human Development confirmed this parallel.

As the situation evolved, however, the link became looser. During the last hearings, in 1978, the industry adopted another position, separating DES from the other oestrogens. As the former was generally considered as dangerous and was on the verge of being definitely banned, it then became good policy to preserve other oestrogens that could possibly replace DES from an equivalent threat to their use as growth enhancers.

These discussions seem to substantiate the concept of 'capture', i.e. the idea that, once it was caught in the dynamics of stakeholders' politics with its web of conflicting interests, the evaluation – if not the production – of scientific facts was reduced to the status of mere instrument for political and social mobilization. Reading the 1970s series of expert testimonies (both written and oral) presented during the House or Senate hearings, three discursive packages can be identified that link the different levels of the DES controversy. The first is an epidemiological discourse focusing on the gynaecological alert, its meaning, and the surveys organized to stabilize the correlation between vaginal cancer and DES. The latter is seen as a risk factor associated with a high probability of adverse events in certain populations or under specific circumstances. The perspective is to do everything possible to avoid these adverse effects in order to preserve the health of the population. In other words, every 'reasonable precaution' must not only be adopted, but also implemented. The second discourse is pharmacological. It focuses on the experiments conducted with mice and other animals, regarding either the induction of tumours or the fate of DES within the body. It mobilizes statistical tools to draw conclusions regarding the best way of defining thresholds, looking for zones of marginal effects (or better, of no effect) and conditions of relatively safe use. It aims at a controlled use of the substance under investigation. The third discourse focuses on animal physiology and nutrition. Using laboratory animals as well, it takes experiments with natural and artificial hormones as evidence of their identical fate and effects in the body. Nature and artifice being equivalent, the latter will not do more harm than the former. DES, the same as many natural hormones, is rapidly eliminated from the body. Moreover, a consequence of the quasi-biological nature of DES action is that potency and carcinogenicity are two sides of the same coin. This physiological discourse is articulated with nutrition studies focusing on the growth-enhancement effect of DES and its value for agricultural productivity. The more general agricultural-engineering perspective combines this veterinary expertise with economic considerations regarding the positive impact of abundant and cheap meat in balancing costs and benefits. In this perspective, the detection of residues is deemed important since instances of DES in edible meat initially went unnoticed or – according to FDA critics – were not even looked for. The technical answer consisted in seeking a new legal system of chemical measurement that would replace the mouse assay, which was gradually viewed as not sensitive enough. This was not sufficient, however. If controlled use was to be maintained, sanitary inspection and legal action independent of DES producers and users was to be reorganized in order to improve follow-up on cases and assign responsibilities.

Although links and connections between these statements and objects moved during the years of the discussion, this geography of expertise – with 'public health' on one side and 'industrial agricultural management' on the other – roughly matches the opposition between pleas for either a complete ban on DES in farming or a controlled use of the molecule. It also matches the polarity between the 'Democrat-consumer alliance' with allies among the National Cancer Institute (NCI) scientists on one side of the issue, and the 'agro-industrial alliance' led by the American Feed Manufacturers Association or the American Cattlemen's Association on the other.

The idea of capture provides a coherent political understanding of this polarity and of the role of consumers, i.e. in terms of lobbying resulting in increased pressure on a Democratic majority in Congress, which also had its reasons to oppose the lobbying of powerful industrial interests. In this perspective, 'regulatory science' is either (in the worst case) 'biased science' or (in a more positive tone) 'translated science'. The main difficulty of such a reading is however the absence of change: the dynamics of expertise has no effect on the positions taken by the different parties nor on the interests they defend.

The statements of FDA experts and officials are difficult to convey within this frame, as they were contradictory and rapidly changing. As once remarked by Representative Fountain, the Chairman of the House Committee conducting the hearings, there was an underlying conflict of expertise between the US Department of Agriculture (USDA) and the US Public Health Service, but there were also deep divides within the FDA. Tensions were not only related to the form of expertise favoured within the various branches of the administration, they also touched upon the moral economy of the agency and the conception of its role *vis-à-vis* 'the American public'. The positioning of the FDA was dramatically affected by the dynamics of the controversy in general and of the hearings in particular: it shifted gradually from upholding controlled use to implementing a general ban. As a consequence of these shifts affecting both facts and meanings, it became 'scientifically' and 'administratively' inevitable to ban DES. There is not enough room in the context of this paper to analyse all the hearings and the way the FDA, its experts, and their views changed as they went along, but one example will illustrate this point.

The December 1971 hearings had deep consequences on the framing of the dose-response issue. A few days before the hearings, one staff member of the congressional committee received an anonymous phone call from the FDA, mentioning an internal memo written by a certain A. Gross from the Bureau of Drugs and providing a new evaluation of DES risks. Fountain obtained the memo and used it during the hearings to pressure Edwards and the FDA officials (who had not yet examined it). Gross's text was based on the new analysis of an article on DES and the formation of tumours in a peculiar strain of mice called C3H mice, an article that had been 'resurrected' by Ralph Nader's group in a letter published in the *Washington Post* on the risks of agricultural DES. The 1964 article was a typical study of oestrogen effects, except that response was positive with much lower doses than previously thought.[32] Using the so-called Ryan and Mantel (two biometricians at the NCI) statistical approach for 'virtual safety', i.e. a form of computation to estimate thresholds of non-toxicity guaranteeing a very low probability of adverse event, the FDA expert – Gross – had concluded that given the sensibility of existing assays for DES residues, absence of detection could not be equated with absence of risk:

> Although the evaluation procedures always imply assumptions that might be contested, all the calculations result in estimates several order of magnitudes smaller than the 2ppb detection threshold. The analytical methods currently in use therefore do not give any assurance that the absence of detectable quantities of DES in the analyzed material means the absence of carcinogenic quantities of DES.[33]

The memo had been highly criticized within the FDA, especially by the officials in charge of the Bureau of Veterinary Medicine. Internal responses first focused on the abstract, mathematical (and inapplicable) nature of the virtual-safety approach.

Other motives of contention were: *a)* the level of exposure to 'natural' oestrogens in comparison with those added to the food; *b)* the equation DES=natural oestrogens, leading to the conclusion that it is rapidly eliminated (and therefore absent from the meat), which was advanced by officials of the Bureau of Veterinary Medicine.[34]

L. P. Lehmann, head of the FDA bureau of nutrition, felt that:

> 1. FDA is not in a position to set tolerance on a carcinogen. 2. DES is apparently no different than other estrogenic substances, synthetic or natural, with respect to the induction of cancer in sensitive strains in experimental animals. 3. Dr. Gross states conclusions relative to the carcinogenic dose in mice based on an empirical, ultra-conservative model, which, in turn, is based on numerous assumptions (...) 4. Dr. Gross jumps from relationships in mice to relationships in humans without taking

into account the differences in dose per unit of weight, exposure, and the difference in reported carcinogenic dose for mice and man. 5. Dr. Gross comments on the tests in use, their sensitivity, and improvement without a full knowledge of this subject area. 6. When utilizing the Mantel-Ryan model to analyze classical data on zinc and selenium, it is apparent that the calculated 'virtual safety' levels are well below what is contained in normal feedstuffs and the animals' requirement (...).[35]

This internal controversy became the focus of intense written correspondence between the House committee and a number of FDA officials.[36] Pressing the FDA, Representative Fountain obtained copies of several memos, giving them such a visibility that it became impossible to play the card of administrative authority against Gross, turning the memo as well as the responses into legitimate evaluations to be discussed publicly. Although the Mantel-Ryan approach was never endorsed as official policy, discussions in Congress and in the media directly affected the views of high-ranking experts. In the spring of 1972, the Bureau of Veterinary Medicine had rallied to the idea of a ban on some of the agricultural uses of DES.

Two months later the FDA accepted a ban of DES premixes, leaving ear implants as the only authorized form of DES administration in cattle. Although this shift did not formally abolish the 'controlled use' policy, it made it much more difficult to implement, first of all by placing much more significance on the residue-detection issue. First, a new method of detection of DES residues was considered desirable but hopes for a chemical detection by means of gas-liquid chromatography were not (yet) fulfilled. Second, if very small doses could become problematic, then the lack of information to demonstrate that DES actually disappeared from the animal body within the new withdrawal period mandated by the FDA (in November 1971, the FDA extended this period from 48 hours to 7 days) would become a major weakness.

The consequences of this redefined 'no residue' policy became visible a few months later, when the Nader-campaign lawyers announced that: *a)* the USDA consumer service was finding DES residues in statistically significant numbers of carcasses (in less than one year – as the search was reinforced – the percentage of positives shifted from 0.5 per cent to 2 per cent); and *b)* they would sue the FDA for not having done anything about it. In parallel, Fountain circulated proposals for a major reform of the FDA, which would cut its connections with the USDA and reinforce the power of its scientific staff. During the July 1972 hearings, public-health officials, as well as the director of the NCI, insisted on a low-dose carcinogenesis and on the need for caution. Edwards and the head of veterinary medicine thus rediscovered the arguments of agricultural scientists, which pressed for the distinction between DES feeds – which were to be prohibited – and DES implants, which were easier to control and required much lower doses than the former route of administration to obtain allegedly the same nutritional and agricultural benefits.[37] New studies conducted with radioactive DES showed that the FDA-mandated withdrawal period should be extended to 120 days. This plea was taken seriously and became the FDA official requirement by the end of the year. This techno-political reliance on the detection apparatus and its performance was what finally triggered the ban of implants one year later, when it became public knowledge that the number of DES-containing carcasses found by the USDA surveillance system had escalated to 10 per cent of the animals tested.

The Regulatory Science of Dangerous Meat, Part 2: The DES Administrative Trial

The second arena where the regulatory science of DES became a matter of public expertise was the judicial system. Starting in the mid-1970s, DES daughters and victims began to sue the pharmaceutical firms producing DES with the support of the newly created self-help organization, *DES Action*. The DES tort and compensation trials have become a major source of judicial precedents in the United States. The difficulty of identifying the company responsible for the injuries suffered by an individual plaintiff, for instance, resulted in the court's inventing a form of collective responsibility of industrialists called 'market-share liability', which mobilized a probabilistic understanding of guilt with the consequence that financial compensation should be shared among DES producers according to their market shares. Agricultural DES was, however, associated with another layer of legal action, which targeted the FDA.

The 1973 ban on implants was immediately challenged in the court by a coalition of feed producers (the makers of DES followed at arm's length) with the result that the administrative court of the District of Columbia circuit invalidated the FDA decision in 1974 as it had been taken without granting the interested parties preliminary hearings. The court thus mandated a hearing of the case. The procedure started in January 1977 with a final ruling of the judge in September 1978.

S. Jasanoff has insisted on the 'adversarial' type of expertise that characterizes the mobilization of science in the US judicial system. The DES administrative trial thus provided a new arena for the evaluation of DES risks, since: a) experts were cited and associated with the parties; b) the corpus of acceptable documents defining the facts to be taken into account was negotiated between the judge and the parties' lawyers before the hearings; c) each testifying expert was cross-examined by the opposite party with a right to follow up for the citing party; d) one of the aims of the hearings was to include or exclude specific elements or evidence from the corpus that the judge would take into account for his final ruling. This procedure led the trial to stage an open controversy on the effects and risks of agricultural DES, which resulted in much greater focus on the experimental and investigation data than had been given during the congressional hearings (Table 10.1). The judge, for instance, excluded all questions regarding the economic status of DES on the one hand and its medical benefits on the other, to focus the debate on the background for or against a legitimate implementation of the Delaney clause.

Table 10.1: Issues of Expert Testimony: Congressional Hearings (1971–5) versus DES Administrative Trial (1977–8).

Issue	Congressional hearings	Judicial hearings
Meat economy, costs and benefits of production	Central	Excluded
Meat quality	Discussed	Absent
Correlation and causality in Herbst's study	Central	Central
Mice model of low-dose effects, Gass's study	Central	Central
DES relation to natural oestrogens	Discussed	Central
DES effects on the treated mothers	Absent	Discussed
Residue-detection techniques	Peripheral	Central
Metabolic transformation of DES	Absent	Discussed
Therapeutic utility of DES	Central	Excluded
Environmental carcinogenesis, DDT	Mentioned	Absent
Administrative action, reform of the FDA	Central	application of the Delaney clause

The low-dose issue is a good example of the unusual dynamics of these hearings. The hearings repeatedly discussed the above-mentioned 1964 results. The study conducted by G. H. Gass at the University of Illinois with C3H mice was judged to be non-conclusive and non-significant by the feeders' lawyers and was defended as strongly suggestive evidence by those of the FDA. The status of fact or artefact granted to the curve previously published by Gass depended on many questions, beginning with the possibility of using C3H mice for such a study as these had been selected for a very high genetic susceptibility to mammary tumours. The issue most debated was however the nature of dose-response relations and the low-dose data. Gass's curve presented a statistically significant increase of the number of tumours following exposure at doses as low as 6.5 ppb. The controversial nature of the curve, however, originated in the absence of linearity: higher concentrations did not result in more frequent tumours and it was only for concentration higher than 20 ppb that a simple and linear relation between dosage and number of tumours could be observed. As explained by most of the feeders' experts, this 'abnormality' was a strong enough reason to exclude the data. Hardin Jones, a physiologist of the Atomic Energy Commission testifying against the FDA, explained for instance that Gass had simply botched his experiment:

> Jones – In my opinion there is no projectible risk to human beings from exposure to DES in food as far as the mammary cancer is concerned; and to understand my answer I would have to explain the dose-response relationship.
>
> Judge Davidson. Go ahead then, you've finally got your chance.
>
> Jones. Thank you. May I refer to G-22, the studies by Gass, Coates, and Graham? The point of the relationship in mammary cancer from exposure of animals to DES is the dose exposure to DES, which was given in the food and continued over lifetime. I'm sure the audience is generally familiar with this paper, so let me go then to the quantification that have been made by a number of us, including in the first place Gass and his colleagues, in which he showed a tumor response measured in as scale showing probits, which is to be seen on page 973, and a log dose response in the diet, this being a form of dose-response relationship that is customarily shown by toxicologists. Now, in the relationship there is a rather extraordinary response at the 6,25 parts per billion level, which is not significant in elevation from the controls by ordinarily statistical comparison; but nonetheless, it does catch the eye, and it catches the fancy of anyone interested in dose-response relationship as to whether this is an effect or not. The difference is great enough so that one should search in the experiment design for an alternative explanation, other than just random statistical variation although random statistical variation can account for it. In the Gass study, and I refer you to his table 1, involving the time that tumors appear. There is a relationship between dose of DES and latent time: the bigger the dose, the shorter the latent time of the appearance of tumors. Before the experiment was concluded, a large fraction of the animals, all the surviving animals at that time, were killed in a fire. Gass reported his tabulation of these animals as though these animals had in fact been tested for tumorigenic response. In this 55 animals out of the 121 animals in the control group perished in the fire, whereas, in the succeeding intervals of dose there were only 17,17,18, and 18 respectively. One way of proceeding with an analysis is to take these animals out of the study, because in fact they weren't tested. When one does this, you can see that there is a perfectly reasonable explanation as to why the control animals were as low as they were.[38]

The experts cited by the FDA countered with three arguments. First, the article was definitely to be taken into account as it had been published in a prestigious, peer-reviewed journal considered a legitimate source of knowledge. Second, leaving the simplistic requisite of linearity, a more sophisticated statistical modelling of the effects could account for the 'bizarre' decrease in incidence at 10 ppb. Third, updated theories of carcinogenesis shared by NCI specialists concurred in saying that 'one molecular hit' could induce a mutation that would turn one cell into a cancerous one and induce a tumour, thus rationalizing the idea that there was no 'no effect' threshold where proven carcinogens like DES could be considered safe and could be used with marginal risk. Last, a series of mice experiments at the National Center for Toxicological Research commissioned by the FDA potentially (they had not yet been completed) confirmed the Gass data.

The role of the court hearings, with their special dynamics of examination and cross-examination of experts cited by or the other party, was to decide which among such statements would be included in the proceedings, meaning incorporated in the corpus of facts the administrative judge would evaluate for making his final decision. The use Judge Davidson made of Gass's results is highly revealing of the combination of scientific and political considerations involved in a situation of judicial action. He first decided to take the data into account as none of the parties had initially asked for their exclusion. He then defended a balanced, situational approach: the data were not complete proof and could not, taken in isolation, be grounds for a decision, but they were robust enough to suggest that a no-threshold assumption was sound and that low-dose carcinogenesis with DES was a significant risk.

Davidson's final ruling granted the FDA the right to ban all agricultural uses of DES. The conflict of expertise evidenced during the hearings, however, resulted in a new judicial grounding of this choice, which set an administrative DES precedent that completed the idea of collective industrial responsibility. Davidson grounded his evaluation in three elements: a) the chemical and physiological specificity of DES, which he considered different from natural oestrogens; b) its demonstrated toxicity and carcinogenic potency in humans; c) the high probability of low-dose dangerous effects. The legal background for the decision was therefore not the Delaney clause but a public health emergency. The Delaney clause was difficult to invoke because of the additional amendment introduced in 1962 stating that an additive could not be banned if it was absent from the carcasses. During the dispute on DES, the controversy on the detection of data left open the question of the possible disappearance of the artificial hormone within the 120-day quarantine mandated by the FDA. The understanding of a public health alert was clearly rooted in the existence of the medical crisis. It was also – and this proved more important for the future of agricultural biotechnology – grounded in the idea that significant risk commanded 'precautions.'

Robert Proctor in *Cancer Wars* points to the 'political morphology of the dose-response curve' that dominated the 1960s and 70s assessments of chemical carcinogenesis.[39] He distinguishes four types of low dose modelling associated with a group of actors and a specific understanding of risk: a) linear without threshold (environmental and bureaucratic); b) linear with threshold (industrial and apologetic); c) hormetic (beneficial at low doses); d) supralinear (environmental and activist). The 1976–7 trial and its treatment of the toxicological modelling – the Gass results in the first place – actually introduced another type of curve: a U-shape curve with adverse effects both at very low and high doses. The U-shape curve was one among several displacements of the carcinogenesis risk discourse, which took place during the court hearings and originated in the configuration of public expertise created by the agricultural and medical crisis. In spite of weak experimental data, the U-shape was accepted as significant because it could be linked to a physiological scenario that focused on several elements: the difference between chemicals and natural hormones, on the notion that reproduction, development and foetal life provided a 'window of sensibility' to adverse effects, on the existence of multiple exposures and interactions between carcinogenic chemicals, on the necessity of 'banning' some carcinogenic chemicals. These displacements putatively articulated a new way of defining the risks of carcinogenesis, of measuring and modelling them, of organizing their control. Beyond the specific fate of DES implants, the main impact of Davidson's ruling was therefore to transform the problem of low doses and cancer.

Conclusion

The surveillance and control of the dangers associated with the widespread uses of chemicals became major issues in the United States after 1945 when the modernization of agriculture was increasingly based on industrial practices and on the products of techno-science. Centred on quantification, objective experimental testing and controlled use, the ideas of risk, its assessment and its management thus emerged as central features in the handling of the social and political tensions engendered by this transformation. The spread of risk in the domain of food was accompanied by the institution of a large regulatory apparatus comprising a number of state regulatory agencies modelled, to some extent, on medical institutions. Historians as well as law and political-science specialists have tried to understand the mounting importance of risk regulation by focusing their analysis on the status and practices of state bodies such as the FDA or the EPA. The 'meat and cancer' controversy of the 1970s has provided a lens for investigating other aspects of the postwar regulation of 'food and drugs', which takes into account the relations between the main stakeholders, the types of evidence they favour and the regulatory tools they rely on. The controversies that resulted in the final ban of agricultural DES are in effect a privileged entry point into a specific way of regulating, which combined the politics of consumption and a form of regulatory science conducted in political and judicial arenas.

The conjunction of the two DES crises is in this respect an essential dimension of the 'meat and cancer' debates in the United States. As mentioned above, this convergence played a critical role in turning the agricultural use of DES into a major risk and a motive for social mobilization. The relations between the agricultural and the medical DES crisis highlight the contrasted meanings of regulation through the politics of consumption. As other observers have noted, the medical crisis reinforced an emerging women's health movement rooted in

1970s feminism with the institution of powerful DES-daughters organizations that played the card of empowerment, adopted a critical perspective on professional medicine, and sought 'alternative' expertise conducted by and for women's collectives. This approach of regulatory science as 'situated' rather than 'independent' led to singling out DES as another example of medical practices gone wrong for the sake of industry (if not the profession), of medicine that turned risk or women's biology into pathologies to be treated chemically, and of medicine leading to iatrogenic disorders. Agricultural DES reveals another context, which focused on the consumer rather than on the victim and the activist. Even though – as we have seen – 'radical' collectives like the Nader campaign exerted significant influence on the crisis, their role has been to question agro-industrial practices in the name of quality and informed customers.

The politics of consumption visible in the 'meat and DES' crisis is a major feature of US postwar culture. Unlike debates on the quality of drugs, in which the suffering and dependency associated with diseases are essential, debates on the quality of food are linked to taste and choice. Empowerment therefore acquires a different meaning, connected to the individual and the defence of his or her rights as a user. Consumers need to organize in order to balance the power of industrial monopolies and gain influence in the regulatory arenas, but the focus of their action remains the consumer and his or her ability to make informed choices from the market. Fair trade is a key concept here, while practical investments are in the tests, information campaigns and judicial actions claiming compensation for torts. It would be misleading to consider this consumer regulation as simply the outcome and reflection of consumer organizations' postwar developments. The 'meat and cancer' controversy shows that other actors in the regulatory system, from administrative agencies to industrial firms, have adopted various aspects of this way of regulating, beginning with the emphasis on certified quality, information, risk assessment, and a costs-benefit analysis.

As illustrated in the congressional hearings, the latter proved a powerful instrument for bringing together heterogeneous social, economic and professional interests under the umbrella of numerical reasoning. The consumer way of regulating is in this respect closely related to forms of political management that rely on the lobbying capabilities and organized participation of stakeholders.

Stakeholders' politics and consumer regulation have reinforced the role of public expertise more generally (See Table 10.2). Associated with controversies waged in public arenas, assessment of the health-related risks engendered by the chemicals used in agriculture was not only conducted in 'closed' experimental settings, whether academic or depending on the administration. As revealed by the dynamics of DES expertise, court hearings were even more important as directly political arenas for the production of legitimate evidence regarding the nature of risks, their magnitude and the measures necessary to control them.

The final ban of DES is less the result of social activism than the direct product of a judicial assessment that set a both legal and a scientific precedent. The DES administrative trial accordingly reinforced a 'precautionary' approach of cancer risks with considerable attention to the effects of low doses.

Table 10.2: Four Ways of Regulating Food and Drugs.

Way of regulating	Professional	Administrative	Industrial	Consumerist
Aims, values	Compliance, competency	Public health, efficacy, access	Productivity, profit, quality	Individual choices, quality of life
Forms of evidence	Pharmacology, Animal models, Dosage, indications	Statistical, Controlled trials	Animal testing, Market-research, Cost-benefit analysis,	Observational epidemiology, Risk-benefit analysis
Main actors	Corporations, scientific associations	Agencies, governmental committees	Firms, business associations	Patient or consumer groups, The media
Regulatory tools	Pharmacopoeia, Codex alimentarius, Prescription, Guidelines	Marketing permits, Public statements, Labelling	Quality control, Scientific publicity, Package inserts	Post-marketing surveillance, Court decisions

NOTES

Cantor and Bonah, 'Introduction'

1. Quoted in C. Doering, 'US to List Retailers Getting Recalled Meat, poultry', Friday (11 July 2008), http://www.reuters.com/article/email/idUSN1133797820080712 (accessed 18 July 2008).

2. While our focus is on Europe and North America, there is a growing historical literature on the relations of meat and health in other parts of the World, which is beyond the scope of this book. For a survey of the international trade in meat and its intersections with concerns about animal health and food hygiene see R. Perren, *Taste, Trade and Technology: The Development of the International Meat Industry Since 1840* (Aldershot: Ashgate, 2006). See also S. Freidberg, *Fresh: A Perishable History* (Cambridge, MA: Belknap Press of Harvard University Press, 2009), esp. ch. 2 'Beef: Mobile Meat.' P. H. Smith, *Politics and Beef in Argentina: Patterns of Conflict and Change* (New York: Columbia University Press, 1969). J. Bourdieu, L. Piet, and A. Stanziani, 'Crise sanitaire et stabilisation du marché de la viande en France, 18e–20e siècles', *Revue d'Histoire Moderne et Contemporaine*, 51 (2004), pp. 121–56.

3. See Naomi Pfeffer's paper this volume. On cortisone see D. Cantor, 'Cortisone and the Politics of Drama, 1949–55', in J. V. Pickstone (ed.), *Medical Innovations in Historical Perspective* (Basingstoke and London: Macmillan, 1992), pp. 165–84. D. Cantor, 'Cortisone and the Politics of Empire: Imperialism and British Medicine, 1918–1955', *Bulletin of the History of Medicine*, 67 (1993), pp. 463–93. V. Quirke, 'Making British Cortisone: Glaxo and the Development of Corticosteroids in Britain in the 1950s and 1960s', *Studies in the History and Philosophy of the Biomedical Sciences*, 36 (2005), pp. 645–74.

4. H. Kamminga and A. Cunningham, 'Introduction', in H. Kamminga and A. Cunningham (eds), *The Science and Culture of Nutrition, 1840–1940* (Amsterdam/Atlanta, GA: Rodopi, 1995). M. R. Finlay, 'Quackery and Cookery: Justus Von Liebig's Extract of Meat and the Theory of Nutrition in the Victorian age', *Bulletin of the History of Medicine*, 66 (1992), pp. 404–18. W. Gratzer, *Terrors of the Table: the Curious History of Nutrition* (New York: Oxford University Press, 2005). J. W. Dickerson, 'Aspects of the History of Nutrition since 1876', *Journal of the Royal Society for the Promotion of Health*, 121 (2001) pp. 79–84. V. J. Knapp, 'The Democratization of Meat and Protein in Late 18th- and 19th-Century Europe', *Journal of History*, 59 (1997), pp. 541–51. K. J. Carpenter, 'A Short History of Nutritional Science: Part 1 (1785–1885)', *Journal of Nutrition*, 133 (2003), pp. 638–45. K. J. Carpenter, 'A Short History of Nutritional Science: Part 2 (1885–1912)', *Journal of Nutrition*, 133 (2003), pp. 975–84. K. J. Carpenter, 'A Short History of Nutritional Science: Part 3 (1912–1944)', *Journal of Nutrition*, 133

(2003), pp. 3023–32. K. J. Carpenter, 'A Short History of Nutritional Science: Part 4 (1945–1985)', *Journal of Nutrition*, 133 (2003), pp. 3331–42. D. F. Smith and J. Phillips (eds), *Food, Science, Policy and Regulation in the Twentieth Century: Comparative and International Perspectives* (London and New York: Routledge, 2000).

5. A. Stanziani, *Histoire de la Qualité alimentaire* (Paris: Seuil, 2005).

6. P. Zylberman, 'Making Food Safety an Issue: Internationalized Food Politics and French Public Health from the 1870s to the Present', *Medical History*, 48 (2004), pp. 1–28.

7. See for example, J-L. Flandrin and M. Montanari (eds), *Food: A Culinary History from Antiquity to the Present* (New York: Columbia University Press, 1999). L. Moulin, *L'Europe à table: Introduction à une psychosociologie des pratiques alimentaires en Occident* (Paris and Bruxelles: Elsevier Séquoia, 1975). D. J. Oddy, 'A Nutritional Analysis of Historical Evidence: The Working Class Diet 1880–1914', in D. Oddy and D. S. Miller (eds), *The Making of the Modern British Diet* (London: Croom Helm, 1976), pp. 214–31. M. Schaffner, *Brot, Brei und was dazugehört. Über sozialen Sinn und physiologischen Wert der Nahrung* (Zurich: Chronos Verlag, 1992). U. Schultz (ed.), *Speisen, Schlemmen, Fasten. Eine Kulturgeschichte des Essens* (Frankfurt a.M./Leipzig: Insel Verlag, 1993). H. Schwartz, *Never Satisfied: A Cultural History of Diets, Fantasies and Fat* (New York and London: Free Press, 1986). R. I. Rotberg and T. K. Rabb (eds), *Hunger and History. The Impact of Changing Food Production and Consumption Patterns on Society* (Cambridge: Cambridge University Press, 1983).

8. L. Bergeron, 'Approvisionement et consommation' Paris sans le Premier Empire: Paris et Ile de-France', *Memoires*, 14 (1964), pp. 197–232. F. Braudel, *Civilization and Capitalism, 15th–18th Century, Volume 3* (London: Collins, 1981) pp. 108–43 and 187–227. J.-J. Hémardinquer, 'Du nouveau sur le ravitaillement de Paris a la fin du XVIIIe diècle et au debut du XIXe', in J.-J. Hémardinquer (ed.), *Pour une histoire de l'alimentation* (Paris: Armand Colin, 1970), pp. 68–9; M. Morineau, 'Revolution agricole, revolution alimentaire, revolution demographique', *Annales de Demographie Historique*, 9 (1974), pp. 335–71; E. N. Todhunter, 'Some Aspects of the History of Dietetics', *World Review of Nutrition and Dietetics*, 18 (1973), pp. 1–46; H. J. Teuteberg, 'The General Relationship between Diet and Industrialization', in E. Forster and R. Forster (eds), *European Diet from Pre-Industrial to Modern Times* (New York: Harper and Row, 1975), pp. 58–73. B. H. Slicher van Bath, *The Agrarian History of Western Europe, ad 500–1500* (London: Edward Arnold, 1963), pp. 278–99; V. J. Knapp, 'Major Dietary Changes in Nineteenth-Century Europe', *Perspectives in Biology and Medicine*, 3 (1988), pp. 188–93.

9. L. Heyberger, 'L'Evolution des niveaux de vie en France, de la fin de l'Ancien régime à la Seconde Guerre mondiale, approche anthropométrique' (Thèse d'histoire, Université Marc Bloch, Strasbourg, 2004). For a general presentation to the methodological approach of anthropometrical history see: J. Baten, *Ernährung und wirtschaftliche Entwicklung in Bayern (1730–1880)* (Stuttgart: Franz Steiner Verlag, 1999). J. Komlos, *Nutrition and Economic Development in the Eighteenth-century Habsburg Monarchy: An Anthropometric History* (Princeton, NJ: Princeton University Press, 1989). J. Komlos (ed.), *Stature, Living Standards, and Economic Development: Essays in Anthropometric History* (Chicago, IL: Chicago University Press, 1994). J. Komlos, *The Biological Standard of Living in Europe and America, 1700–1900: Studies in Anthropometric History* (Aldershot: Variorum, 1995).

10. For discussions of the transformation of American meat production see M. Walsh, *The Rise of the Midwestern Meat Packing Industry* (Lexington: University Press of Kentucky, 1982). M. Yeager, *Competition and Regulation: The Dynamics of Oligopoly in the Meat*

Packing Industry, 1870–1920 (Greenwich, Connecticut: JAI Press, 1981). On refrigeration see M. Yeager Kujovich, 'The Refrigerator Car and the Growth of the American Dressed Beef Industry', *Business History Review*, 44 (1970), pp. 460–82. D. Fink, *Cutting into the Meatpacking Line: Workers and Change in the Rural Midwest* (Chapel Hill, NC: University of North Carolina Press, 1998). R. Horowitz, *Putting Meat on the American Table: Taste, Technology, Transformation* (Baltimore, MD: Johns Hopkins University Press, 2006). J. M. Pilcher, 'Empire of the "Jungle": The Rise of an Atlantic Refrigerated Beef Industry, 1880–1920', *Food, Culture and Society*, 7 (2004), pp. 63–78. L. A. Craig, B. Goodwin, and T. Grennes, 'The Effect of Mechanical Refrigeration on Nutrition in the United States', *Social Science History*, 28 (2004), pp. 325–36. See also Freidberg, *Fresh*, esp. ch. 2.

11. Schwartz, *Never Satisfied*. According to one survey, average per capita meat consumption in America peaked at about 150lbs each year by the nineteenth century, and apart from a drop during the Great Depression of the 1930s, Americans continued to consume this level of meat until the 1960s, when consumption role to 200lbs per person per year. Horowitz, *Putting Meat on the American Table*, pp. 1–2. For other discussions of the quantity of meat in the American diet see H. Levenstein, *Revolution at the Table: The Transformation of the American Diet* (New York: Oxford University Press, 1988), pp. 23–4; S. Williams, *Savory Suppers and Fashionable Feasts: Dining in Victorian America* (Knoxville, TN: University of Tennessee Press, 1996), esp. pp. 98–102; W. Root and R. de Rochemont, *Eating in America: A History* (Hopewill, NJ: Ecco Press, 1976), pp. 189–212; E. N. McIntosh, *American Food Habits in Historical Perspective* (Westport, CT: Praeger, 1995).

12. Rima Apple (this volume).

13. His official French titles were Médecin consultant de l'Empereur, Inspecteur de santé de l'armée, Directeur de l'Ecole Impériale d'application de médecine et de pharmacie militaires (Val de Grâce).

14. M. Lévy, *Traité d'hygiène publique et privée* (Paris: Baillière, 1869), pp. 581–2.

15. Ibid., p. 580.

16. For later food inquiries see F. Verzar (ed.), *Gegenwartsprobleme der Ernährungsforschung*, Symposium Basel 1.–4. Oktober 1952 (Unter dem Patronat der Internatioinalen Union der Ernährungswissenschaften) (Basel and Stuttgart: Birkhäuser, 1953).

17. A. Newsholme, *The Prevention of Tuberculosis* (London: Methuen, 1908). A. Newsholme, *The Elements of Vital Statistics in their Bearing on Social and Public Health Problems* (London: George Allen and Unwin, 1923). T. McKeown and R. G. Record, 'Reasons for the Decline of Mortality in England and Wales during the Nineteenth Century', *Population Studies*, 16 (1962), pp. 94–122. T. McKeown, *The Modern Rise of Population* (London: Edward Arnold, 1976). A. Mitchell, 'Obsessive Questions and Faint Answers: The French Response to Tuberculosis in the Belle Époque', *Bulletin of the History of Medicine*, 62 (1988), pp. 215–35. L. G. Wilson, 'The Historical Decline of Tuberculosis in Europe and America: Its Causes and Significance', *Journal of the History of Medicine and Allied Sciences*, 45 (1990), pp. 366–96. A. Mitchell, 'An Inexact Science: The Statistics of Tuberculosis in Late-Nineteenth-Century France', *Social History of Medicine*, 3 (1990), pp. 387–417. D. Barnes, 'The Rise and Fall of Tuberculosis in Belle-Époque France: A Reply to Allan Mitchell', *Social History of Medicine*, 5 (1992), pp. 279–90. A. Mitchell, 'Tuberculosis Statistics and the McKeown Thesis: A Rebuttal to David Barnes', *Social History of Medicine*, 5 (1992), pp. 291–6. D. S. Barnes, *The*

Making of a Social Disease: Tuberculosis in Nineteenth-Century France (Berkeley, CA: University of California Press, 1995).

18. A. I. Marcus, *Cancer from Beef: DES, Federal Food Regulation, and Consumer Confidence* (Baltimore, MD: Johns Hopkins University Press, 1994).

19. Jacqueline Tavernier-Courbin, 'The Call of the Wild and *The Jungle*: Jack London's and Upton Sinclair's Animal and Human Struggles', in D. Pitzer (ed.) *The Cambridge Companion to American Realism and Naturalism: Howells to London* (Cambridge: Cambridge University Press, 1995), pp. 236–62. H. Bloom (ed.), *Upton Sinclair's the Jungle* (Chicago, IL: Chelsea House Publishers, 2001). A. F. Kantor, 'Upton Sinclair and the Pure Food and Drugs Act of 1906. "I Aimed at the Public's Heart and by Accident I hit it in the Stomach"', *American Journal of Public Health*, 66 (1976), pp. 1202–5. J. H. Young, 'The Pig that Fell into the Privy: Upton Sinclair's The Jungle and the Meat Inspection Amendments of 1906', *Bulletin of the History of Medicine*, 59 (1986), pp. 467–80. C. Phelps, 'Welcome to the Jungle: Meatpacking Then and Now', *Canadian Dimension*, 39 (2005), p. 25. W. Parmenter, 'The Jungle and its Effects', *Journalism History*, 10 (1983), pp. 14–17 and 33–4. For the changes in the sort of injuries found in meat packing plants since the publication of *The Jungle* see R. Horowitz, '"That Was a Dirty Job!" Technology and Workplace Hazards in Meatpacking over the Long Twentieth Century', *Labor: Studies in Working-Class History of the Americas*, 5 (2008), pp. 13–25.

20. J. Rifkin, *Beyond Beef: The Rise and Fall of Cattle Culture* (New York: Dutton, 1992). E. Schlosser, *Fast Food Nation: The Dark Side of the All-American Meal* (Boston, MA: Harper Perennial, 2001). S. Striffler, *Chicken: The Dangerous Transformation of America's Favorite Food* (New Haven, CT and London: Yale University Press, 2005).

21. F. Moore Lappé, *Diet for a Small Planet* (New York: Ballantine Books, 1971). For a history of such ecological concerns see also W. J. Belasco, *Meals to Come: A History of the Future of Food* (Berkeley, CA: University of California Press, 2006).

22. An exception is the paper by Stull and Broadway this volume, which explores changes in working conditions in the meat industry and their impact on human health.

23. Kamminga and Cunningham (eds) *The Science and Culture of Nutrition*.

24. R. Pillsbury, *No Foreign Food: The American Diet in Time and Place* (Boulder, CO: Westview Press 1998), pp. 71–3.

25. P. Young Lee (ed.), *Meat, Modernity, and the Rise of the Slaughterhouse* (Durham, NH: University of New Hampshire Press; Hanover: published by University Press of New England, 2008).

26. See for example the American Meat Institute's resistance in the 1980s to FDA proposals to ban or restrict the use of nitrites: R. J. Smith, 'Ever So Cautiously, the FDA Moves Toward a Ban on Nitrites', *Science*, 201 (1978), pp. 887–91. R. J. Smith, 'Nitrites: FDA Beats a Surprising Retreat Nitrites: FDA Beats a Surprising Retreat', *Science*, 209 (1980), pp. 1100–1. 'Diet, Cancer and the American Meat Institute', *Washington Post*, 10 July 1982, p. 22. See also General Accounting Office, *National Academy of Sciences' Reports on Diet and Health – Are They Credible and Consistent?* GPO No. O-421-843/287 (21 August 1984), pp. 18, 61, 62.

27. Striffler, *Chicken*. Pillsbury, *No Foreign Food*, pp. 71–3.

28. For a recent example of this see 'Why do the French Call the British "The Roast Beefs"?', http://news.bbc.co.uk/2/hi/2913151.stm (accessed 22 February 2010).

29. Perren, *Taste, Trade and Technology*, c. 6.

30. R. Perren, 'The Retail and Wholesale Meat Trade, 1880–1939', in D. J. Oddy and D. S. Miller (eds), *Diet and Health in Modern Britain* (London: Croom Helm, 1985), pp. 46–65.

F. Capie, 'The Demand for Meat in England and Wales Between the Two World Wars', in Oddy and Miller (eds), *Diet and Health in Modern Britain*, pp. 66–80.

31. R. Perren, *The Meat Trade in Britain 1840–1914* (London: Routledge and Kegan Paul 1978), p. 172.

32. F. B. Smith, *The People's Health: 1830–1910* (London, Weidenfeld and Nicholson, 1990).

33. Perren, *The Meat Trade in Britain*, p. 88.

34. 'Experimental central slaughterhouses', U.K. National Archives, MAF 31/47.

35. See the essays by C. Otter, I. MacLachlan, and R. Perren in Young Lee (ed.) *Meat, Modernity, and the Rise of the Slaughterhouse*.

36. R. Horowitz, J. M. Pilcher, and S. Watts, 'Meat for the Multitudes: Market Culture in Paris, New York City, and Mexico City over the Long Nineteenth Century', *American Historical Review*, 109 (2004), pp. 1055–83. Young Lee (ed.) *Meat, Modernity, and the Rise of the Slaughterhouse*.

37. For a general history of the German food industry see K.-P. Ellerbrock, *Geschichte der deutschen Nahrungs- und Genussmittelindustrie: 1750–1914* (Stuttgart: Steiner, 1993).

38. E. Reeck, *Frankfurter Würstchen. Der Stolz der Frankfurter Schweinemetzger und der Weltruhm der Stadt des Deutschen Handwerks* (Frankfurt: Henrich, 1939).

39. B. Jussen (ed.), *Liebig's Sammelbilder: Vollständige Ausgabe der Serien 1 bis 1138 auf CD-ROM Atlas des Historischen Bildwissens 1* (Berlin: Directmedia Publishing GmbH, 2002). H.-J. Teuteberg, *Die Rolle des Fleischextrakts für die Ernährungswissenschaften und den Aufstieg der Suppenindustrie. Kleine Geschichte der Fleischbrühe* (Stuttgart: Steiner, 1990). M. A. Ginor, M. Davis, A. Coe, J. Ziegelman, *Foie Gras: A Passion* (New York: Wiley, 1999). This account of a French 'passion' for liver might be compared Susan Lederer's account of American reactions to liver diet in this volume. On the commercialization of other foodstuffs in twentieth century France see for example P. Boisard, trans. R. Miller, *Camembert: A National Myth* (Berkeley, CA and London: University of California Press, 2003).

40. The German language distinguishes between food substances ingested for nutritional reasons and in response to hunger and foods ingested for reasons of pleasure and taste such as coffee, tea, sugar, alcohol, tobacco and spices. 'Genussmittel' lie at the frontier between foods (Nahrungsmittel) and addictive substances (Suchtmittel).

41. For a history of food advertising in Germany see K. Schlegel-Matthies, 'Anfänge der modernen Lebens und Genußmittelwerbung, Produkte und Konsumgruppen im Spiegel von Zeitschriftenannoncen', in H. J. Teuteberg (ed.) *Durchbruch zum modernen Massenkonsum: Lebensmittelmärkte und Lebensmittelqualität im Städtewachstum des Industriezeitalters* (Münster: Coppenrath, 1987), pp. 277–308. More generally B. Selter, 'Der 'satte' Verbraucher. Idole des Ernährungsverhaltens zwischen Hunger und Überfluß 1890–1970', in P. Borscheid and C. Wischermann (eds) *Bilderwelt des Alltags. Werbung in der Konsumgesellschaft des 19. und 20. Jahrhunderts* (Stuttgart: Franz Steiner Verlag, 1995), pp. 190–221.

42. A. Guerrini, *Obesity and Depression in the Enlightenment: The Life and Times of George Cheyne* (Norman, OK: University of Oklahoma Press, 1999). R. Porter and G. S. Rousseau, *Gout: The Patrician Malady* (New Haven, CT: Yale University Press, 1998). J. C. Whorton, *Inner Hygiene: Constipation and the Pursuit of Health in Modern Society* (Oxford and New York: Oxford University Press, 2000).

43. J. C. Turner, *Reckoning with the Beast: Animals, Pain, and Humanity in the Victorian Mind* (Baltimore, MD and London: Johns Hopkins University Press, 1980), pp. 15–38.

In general on 'ethical vegetarianism' see R. Preece, *Sins of the Flesh: A History of Ethical Vegetarian Thought* (Vancouver: UBC Press, 2008).

44. Preece, *Sins of the Flesh*, ch. 11. J. Twigg, 'The Vegetarian Movement in England, 1847–1981: A Study in the Structure of its Ideology' (Unpublished PhD Thesis, London School of Economics, London University, 1981). T. Stuart, *The Bloodless Revolution: A Cultural History of Vegetarianism from 1600 to Modern Times* (New York: W.W. Norton and Co., 2007). For other histories of vegetarianism see K. Iacobbo and M. Iacobbo, *Vegetarian America: A History* (Westport, CN: Praeger, 2004). J. Gregerson, *Vegetarianism: A History* (Fremont, CA: Jain Pub. Co., 1994). The first French vegetarian society (the short-lived Société Végétarienne de Paris) was created in 1878, followed by the Société Végétarienne de France (founded 1884), which published the journal *La Reforme Alimentaire*, which, after a period of inactivity, was re-established under the same name in 1897, jointly publishing a new series of *La Reforme Alimentaire* with the Societé Belge pour l'étude de la Réforme alimentaire. The Société Végétarienne de France was eclipsed after World War I, and the number of vegetarian societies multiplied and diversified during the interwar years with the creation of Jacques Demarquette's Trait d'Union, Paul Carton's Société Naturiste de France, and a new version of the Société Végétarienne de France that continued its activities after World War II. On Paul Carton and the interwar period see: A. P. Ouédraogo, 'Food and the Purification of Society: Dr Paul Carton and Vegetarianism in Interwar France', *Social History of Medicine*, 14 (2001), pp. 223–45.

45. Preece, *Sins of the Flesh*, p. 306.

46. On vegetarianism in the twentieth century see Preece, *Sins of the Flesh*, ch. 12. See also Iacobbo and Iacobbo, *Vegetarian America: A History*, esp. ch. 9 and 10. Twigg, 'The Vegetarian Movement in England, 1847–1981'. Stuart, *The Bloodless Revolution: A Cultural History of Vegetarianism*, esp. epilogue.

47. J. C. Whorton, '"Tempest in a Flesh-Pot": The Formulation of a Physiological Rationale for Vegetarianism', *Journal of the History of Medicine and Allied Sciences*, 32 (1977), pp. 115–39. On vitamins see R. D. Apple, *Vitamania: Vitamins in American Culture* (New Brunswick, NJ: Rutgers University Press, 1996).

48. In this we build on a growing literature that has emerged in the last ten years following the publication by Harmke Kamminga and Andrew Cunningham of one of the rare historical monographs devoted to 'the science and culture of nutrition.' Like Kamminga and Cunningham's volume, the essays in our collection highlight the intersection of nutritional science with state formation and the rise of the meat industry, and how various critics of meat came to adopt science as a rationale for their critiques. Kamminga and Cunningham, 'Introduction'. See also D. F. Smith (ed.), *Nutrition in Britain: Science, Scientists, and Politics in the 20th Century* (London: Routledge, 1997). Smith and Phillips (eds), *Food, Science, Policy and Regulation in the Twentieth Century*.

49. J. Tanner, *Fabrikmahlzeit: Ernährungswissenschaft, Industriearbeit und Volksernährung in der Schweiz, 1890–1950* (Zurich: Chronos, 1999), esp. ch. 2 'Menschlicher Motor', 'Muskeldynamo' und 'Körperfabrik': Wissenschaftliche Körperbilder und produktivistische Metaphern', pp. 53–88.

50. N. Mani, 'Die wissenschaftliche Ernährungslehre im 19. Jahrhundert', in E. Heischkel-Artelt (ed.) *Ernährung und Ernährungslehre im 19. Jahrhundert* (Göttingen: Vandenhoek Ruprecht, 1976), pp. 22–75.

51. Lévy, *Traité d'hygiène publique et privée*, p. 580.

52. Tanner distinguishes between 'Volksernährung' as a discourse about rational nutrition for the collective body of the 'Volk' and 'food supplies for the nation' which referred to

the empirical question what people did eat indeed and what nutritional problems they faced. Tanner, *Fabrikmahlzeit*, p. 93. See also. M. Rubner, *Volksernährungsfragen* (Leipzig: Akademische Verlagsgesellschaft, 1908). M. Rubner, *Deutschlands Volksernährung* (Berlin: Springer, 1930).

53. Tanner, *Fabrikmahlzeit*, p. 53.

54. Ibid., p. 72.

55. *A Practical Treatise on How to Preserve Perfect Nutrition in Health and Disease by Natural Means; Bovinine* (New York: Bovinine Company, 1888). Bovinine Company, New York, *A Provisional Hand Book of Haematherapy, or Auxiliary Blood Supply in Medicine and Surgery ... Comp. and reprinted from numerous medical journals and correspondents, including the 'entire records', up to date, of Sound View Hospital, Stamford, Conn.* (New York: Bovinine Company 1898). On Richet see Löwy this volume.

56. J. L. W. Thudichum, *On the Origin, Nature, and Uses of Liebig's Extract of Meat; with an Analytical Comparison of other Essences and Preparations of Meat* (London: J. Churchill and Sons, 1869). For a historical analysis see M. R. Finlay, 'Early Marketing of the Theory of Nutrition: The Science and Culture of Liebig's Extract of Meat', in Kamminga and Cunningham (eds), *The Science and Culture of Nutrition*, pp. 48–74. M. R. Finlay, 'Quackery and Cookery: Justus Von Liebig's Extract of Meat and the Theory of Nutrition in the Victorian Age', *Bulletin of the History of Medicine*, 66 (1992), pp. 404–18.

57. K. J. Carpenter, 'A Short History of Nutritional Science: Part 2 (1885–1912)', *Journal of Nutrition*, 133 (2003), pp. 975–84.

58. See for example Ilana Löwy this volume. More generally, Heischkel-Artelt (ed.) *Ernährung und Ernährungslehre*. E. von Leyden (ed.), *Handbuch der Ernährungstherapie und Diätetik*, 2nd edition (Leipzig: Thieme, 1903–4).

59. Papers by Ilana Löwy, Susan Lederer, and Naomi Pfeffer this volume.

60. M. Rubner, *Die Gesetze des Energieverbrauchs bei der Ernährung*, Leipzig/Wien: Deuticke, 1902. M. Rubner, 'Physiologie der Nahrung und Ernährung', in E. von Leyden (ed.), *Handbuch der Ernährungstherapie und Diätetik*, Volume 1 (Leipzig: Thieme, 1903).

61. R. L. Kremer, *The Thermodynamics of Life and Experimental Physiology, 1770–1880* (New York and London: Garland, 1990).

62. See for example, J. Amar, *Le moteur humain et les bases scientifiques du travail professionnel* (Paris: Dunod et Pinat, 1914). A. Rabinbach, *The Human Motor: Energy, Fatigue and the Origins of Modernity* (Berkeley, CA and Los Angeles: University of California Press, 1990).

63. Tanner, *Fabrikmahlzeit*, pp. 71–6.

64. See for example, Bureau International du Travail, *L'alimentation des travailleurs et la politique sociale* (Geneva: 1936). For the reference to the human body as engine see p. 14.

65. Tanner, *Fabrikmahlzeit*, p. 76.

66. For meat's association with some of these values see M. Montanari, 'Peasants, Warriors, Priests. Images of Society and Styles of Diet', in J-L. Flandrin and M. Montanari (eds), *Food: A Culinary History from Antiquity to the Present* (New York: Columbia University Press, 1999), pp. 178–85, esp. pp. 178–80.

67. *Die Bedeutung der Vitamine als Nahrungsstoff und Heilmittel* (Geneva: Veröffentlichung des Vereinigten Hilfswerks vom Internationalen Roten Kreuz, 1943). B. Bächi, *Vitamin C für alle! Phamazeutische Produktion, Vermarktung und Gesundheitspolitik (1933–1953)* (Zurich: Chronos, 2009). B. Bächi, 'Natürliches oder künstliches Vitamin C? Der prekäre Status eines neuen Stoffes im Schatten des Zweiten Weltkriegs', *N.T.M.*, 16 (2008), pp. 445–70. Rabinbach, *Human Motor*.

68. S. M. Horrocks, 'The Business of Vitamins: Nutrition Science and the Food Industry in Inter-war Britain', in Kamminga and Cunningham (eds), *The Science and Culture of Nutrition*, pp. 235–58.

69. M. Teich, 'Science and Food during the Great War: Britain and Germany', in Kamminga and Cunningham (eds), *The Science and Culture of Nutrition*, pp. 213–34.

70. Tanner, *Fabrikmahlzeit*, p. 81–3, and ch. 3 and 4. See also Apple, in this volume.

71. Kamminga and Cunningham (eds), *The Science and Culture of Nutrition*.

72. For a more general argument along this line see P. Sarasin and J. Tanner (eds), *Physiologie und Industrielle Gesellschaft. Studien zur Verwissenschaftlichung des Körpers im 19. und 20. Jahrhundert* (Frankfurt a.M.: Suhrkamp, 1998).

73. See for example David Cantor this collection.

74. Tanner, *Fabrikmahlzeit*, pp. 273–332.

75. See for example Apple this volume. Also Tanner, *Fabrikmahlzeit*, ch. 2, pp. 89–126.

76. A. Hardy, 'Animals, Disease, and Man: Making Connections', *Perspectives in Biology and Medicine*, 46 (2003), pp. 200–15.

77. D. Berdah, 'Innovation biologique, expertise et crise sanitaro-agricole. La lutte contre la tuberculose bovine et la fièvre aphteuse en France et en Grande-Bretagne du milieux du 19e siècle aux années 1960' (PhD thesis, Paris EHESS, 2010). A. Woods, *A Manufactured Plague? The History of Foot-and-Mouth Disease in Britain* (London: Earthscan, 2004). Smith and Phillips (eds) *Food, Science, Policy and Regulation in the 20th Century*.

78. On veterinarian medicine in France and UK see Berdah, 'Innovation biologique, expertise et crise sanitaro-agricole.' Woods, *A Manufactured Plague?*. For the USA see Susan D. Jones, *Valuing Animals: Veterinarians and Their Patients in Modern America* (Baltimore, MD: The Johns Hopkins University Press, 2003).

79. Jones, *Valuing Animals*.

80. Stuart, *The Bloodless Revolution: A Cultural History of Vegetarianism*, p. 376.

81. J. Barkas, *The Vegetable Passion: A History of the Vegetarian State of Mind* (London: Routledge and Paul, 1975). Stuart, *The Bloodless Revolution: A Cultural History of Vegetarianism*.

82. Stuart, *The Bloodless Revolution: A Cultural History of Vegetarianism*, p. xxiv.

83. Ibid. T. Stuart, *The Bloodless Revolution: Radical Vegetarians and the Discovery of India* (London: HarperPress, 2006).

84. Stuart, *The Bloodless Revolution: A Cultural History of Vegetarianism*. See also Thoms's paper in this volume.

85. Tanner, *Fabrikmahlzeit*, pp. 78–81.

86. Ibid., pp. 89–126.

87. For a useful survey of McDonaldization see J. M. Pilcher, *Food in World History* (London and New York: Routledge, 2006), ch. 12.

88. J. Forero, 'Day of the Gaucho Waning in Argentina. Cattle Being Moved Off Plains and Into US-Style Feedlots', *Washington Post*, 10 September 2009, http://www.washingtonpost.com/wp-dyn/content/article/2009/09/09/AR2009090903211.html?referrer=emailarticle (accessed 19 December 2009). C. Piette, 'Argentina's Solitary Cowboy – The Gaucho Under Threat', 28 November 2009, http://news.bbc.co.uk/2/hi/europe/8383927.stm (accessed 19 December 2009). The point about the tastiness beef from of grass-fed cows was made to one of us (DC) by Juan Manuel Juaire, a veterinarian at the estancia La Trinidad, Departamento de Chascomús, Provincia de Buenos Aires on 6/7 August 2009.

89. Stuart, *The Bloodless Revolution: A Cultural History of Vegetarianism*, p. 401.
90. Ibid.

1 Löwy, 'Zomine'

1. C. Richet, 'L'emploi de la viande crue dans le traitement de la tuberculose', *La Semaine Médicale* (18 July 1900) pp. 203–6; Richet told the story of his early experiments in his book *La Nouvelle Zomothérapie* (Paris: Masson, 1924), pp. 22–30.

2. The studies of Richet and his collaborators until 1909 are summed up in six volumes of collected works of his laboratory. *Travaux du Laboratoire de physiologie de Charles Richet* (Paris: Alcan, 1888–1909).

3. M. R. Finlay, 'Cookery and Quackery: Justus von Liebig's Extract of Meat and the Theory of Nutrition in the Victorian Age', *Bulletin of the History of Medicine*, 66 (1992), pp. 404–18; M. R. Finlay, 'Early Marketing of the Theory of Nutrition: The Science and Culture of Liebig's Extract of Meat', in A. Cunningham and H. Kamminga (eds), *The Science and Culture of Nutrition, 1840–1940* (Amsterdam and Atlanta, GA: Rodopi ,Clio Medica Series, 1995), pp. 48–74; W. H. Brock, *Justus von Liebig: The Chemical Gatekeeper* (Cambridge: Cambridge University Press, 1997).

4. The only biography of Richet is Stuart Woolf's book, *Brain, Mind and Medicine: Charles Richet and the Origins of Physiological Psychology* (New Brunswick and London: Transaction Publishers, 1992). Wolfe's book is a rich source of data on Richet's life, but if does not analyze Richet's scientific studies. Another sources on Richet's life and work are Pierrette Estingoy's DEA thesis, 'Charles Richet, 1850–1935: Esquisse biographique et bibliographie' (DEA d'Histoire, Université Lyon III, Jean Moulin, 1993). See also, A. Mayer, 'Notice Nécrologique sur M. Charles Richet', Académie de Médecine, séance du 14 janvier 1936; *Bulletin de l'Académie Nationale de Médecine*, 101 (1936), pp. 51–64; Gustave Roussy, 'Eloge de Charles Richet', Académie de Médecine, séance du 18 décembre 1945, *Bulletin de l'Académie Nationale de Médecine*, 129 (1945), pp. 725–31; W. H. Schneider, 'Charles Richet and the Social Role of Medical Men', *Journal of Medical Biography*, 9:4 (2001), pp. 213–19. Richet's autobiography, *Souvenirs d'un physiologiste* (Paris; J. Peyronnet and Cie, 1933) is a personalized and subjective narrative.

5. Richet, *Souvenirs d'un physiologiste*, pp. 38–41.

6. Richet had won in 1913 the Academy of Science poetry prize for the best 'éloge' to celebrate the 100th anniversary of Pasteur's birth. C. Richet, *La gloire de Pasteur* (Paris: Académie des Sciences, 1914).

7. Charles Richet, unpublished manuscript, *Mémoires sur moi et sur les autres*, vol. 6, p. 5, Archives of the Académie de Médecine, Paris. I'm grateful to Charles Richet's grandson, professor Gabriel Richet, for the permission to consult this manuscript.

8. Richet, *Souvenirs d'un physiologiste*, pp. 33–5. Tuberculosis was chosen, among other things, because it is not very contagious, and therefore did not put the life of laboratory aides in danger. J. Héricourt, 'Vaccination et thérapie anti-tuberculeuse: quelques points d'histoire', in *Livre jubilaire du Professeur Richet* (Paris: Alcan, 1912), pp. 191–9.

9. Richet, 'L'emploi de la viande crue dans le traitement de la tuberculose', A. Josias and J. C. Roux, 'Essais sur le traitement de la tuberculose pulmonaire chez les enfants par le sérum musculaire', in *Travaux du Laboratoire de physiologie de Charles Richet*, 7 vols (Paris: Alcan, 1902), vol. 5, pp. 300–9.

10. J. Héricourt, 'Observations de la zomothérapie anti- tuberculeuse', *Travaux du Laboratoire de physiologie de Charles Richet* (Paris: Alcan, 1902), vol. 5, pp. 310–44; J. Héricourt,

'Trente et une observations de zomothérapie anti-tuberculeuse', *Revue de la tuberculose*, 2 (1901), pp. 165–200. On Richet's view of specificity, see I. Löwy, 'On Guinea Pigs, Dogs and Men: Anaphylaxis and the Study of Biological Individuality', *Studies in History and Philosophy of Medicine and Biomedical Sciences,* 34 (2003), pp. 399–423.

11. C. Richet, 'Ration alimentaire dans quelques cas de la tuberculose humaine' *Revue de Médecine,* 25:2 (1905), pp. 22–7.Richet, *La Nouvelle Zomothérapie,* p. 151.

12. Richet, *Mémoires sur moi et sur les autres*, volume 7, p. 74.

13. Josias and Roux, 'Essais sur le traitement de la tuberculose pulmonaire'.

14. This regime may be compared to the drastic therapy of pernicious anaemia with high intake of raw liver, proposed in 1926 by George Minot and William Murphy. From 1927 on, Eli Lilly marketed the raw liver extract. K. Wailoo, *Drawing Blood: Technology and Disease Identity in Twentieth Century America* (Baltimore, MD: The Johns Hopkins University Press, 1997), pp. 99–133. In the 1920s, some researchers proposed to treat diabetes with ingestion of raw pancreas. M. Eduards, 'Good, Bad or Offal? The Evaluation of Raw Pancreas Therapy and the Rhetorics of Control in the Therapeutic Trial, 1925', *Annals of Science,* 61 (2004), pp. 79–98. I'm indebted to Christiane Sinding for indicating this reference. See also Susan Lederer in this volume.

15. Richet, 'Ration alimentaire dans quelques cas de la tuberculose humaine'. Later Richet admitted, however, that patients could not stand this cure for a long time: the only exception was a patient that took such linking to meat juice that could not live without it. Richet, *La Nouvelle Zomothérapie*, p. 37.

16. Richet, *Souvenirs d'un physiologiste*, p. 98; Charles Richet, *Mémoires sur moi et sur les autres*, vol. VI. pp. 8–9. The dispensary was at Paris's 20th arrondissement, at the corner of Stendhal and Pyrenees streets.

17. Richet, 'Ration alimentaire dans quelques cas de la tuberculose humaine'.

18. Report of the administration council of the Jouve-Rouves-Taniers dispensary, 15 December, 1905. Richet's papers, Archives of the Académie de Médecine, Paris (hereafter Richet's papers). Richet was aware of the fact that patients who improved thanks to zomotherapy, often relapsed.

19. In the early twentieth century, Albert Calmette opened a model anti-tuberculosis dispensary in Lille, the 'Preventorium Emile Roux' destined mainly to treat tuberculous miners and their families. Calmette did not propose a miracle treatment, but only rest, food and teaching of hygiene principles. The 'preventorium' was highly successful, and similar institutions were opened in other cities in the north of France: Douai, Cambrai and Valenciennes. On the other hand, it was judged, in fine, insufficiently cost-efficient: its public was not composed exclusively from tuberculosis patients and the – modest – improvement in health it produced was attributed mainly to material help provided to patients. N. Bernard and L. Nègre, *Albert Calmette, Sa vie et son œvre* (Paris: Masson and Cie, 1939); N. Bernard, *La vie et l'œuvre de Albert Calmette* (Paris: La Colombe, 1961); N. Rougeaux, 'La Lutte contre le tuberculose à Lille, 1895–1940, discours et réalités' (Thèse de l'Ecole des Chartres, 1992); L. Murad and P. Zylberman, *L'Hygiène dans la République* (Paris, Fayard, 1996), pp. 505–25.

20. Richet, *La Nouvelle Zomothérapie*, pp. 97–100. Richet did not comment on the vast difference between zomotherapy for the affluent and the poor.

21. Richet, *La Nouvelle Zomothérapie*, pp. 44–6.

22. Ibid., p. 43.

23. Ibid., p. 42.

24. 'Dans ce vaste édifice entrons. Des salles claires
    Aux parois qui tapisse un glorieux décor

Microscopes, creusets, balances, filtres, verres
Là l'ouvre de Pasteur se continue encore!'
Richet, *La Gloire de Pasteur*.

25. H. Paul, 'Louis Pasteur', in W. Bynum and H. Bynum (eds), *Dictionary of Medical Biography* (London: Greenwood Press, 2007), vol. 4, pp. 978–83, quotation p. 983. The 'proper' medical staff, is attributed to Asclepius, the son of Apollo and the nymph Coronis, trained in medical science and art by the centaur Cheiron. On the commercial aspects of Pasteurian enterprise see, I. Löwy, 'On Hybridizations, Networks and New Disciplines: The Pasteur Institute and the Development of Microbiology in France', *Studies in the History and Philosophy of Science*, 25:5 (1994), pp. 655–88; M. Cassier, 'Appropriation and Commercialization of the Pasteur Anthrax Vaccine', *Studies in the Philosophy and History of Biology and Biomedical Sciences*, 36 (2005), pp. 722–42.

26. Richet, *Mémoires sur moi et sur les autres*, volume VI, p. 16.

27. Richet, *La Nouvelle Zomothérapie*, pp. 48–9.

28. Ibid., pp. 50–6.

29. Richet, *Mémoires sur moi et sur les autres*, vol. 6, pp. 17–18.

30. Ibid., vol. 7, p. 28. Richet did not provide information on the sources of meat used by Latham, but he stressed that zomine was prepared from fresh beef muscles of good quality.

31. Richet, *La Nouvelle Zomothérapie*, p. 57–60. Richet describes, however, a case of a soldier who ingested zomine either in a broth, or in wine. One may assume that other soldiers also received this preparation. Richet, *La Nouvelle Zomothérapie*, p. 76.

32. Richet, *Mémoires sur moi et sur les autres*, volume 7, pp. 74–6; Richet, *La Nouvelle Zomothérapie*, pp. 107–50.

33. Richet, *Mémoires sur moi et sur les autres*, volume 7, p. 76.

34. Ibid., p. 76. After the war, Regaud became the director of the Curie Foundation dispensary and a pioneer of radium therapy of cancer.

35. Richet, *Mémoires sur moi et sur les autres*, volume 7, p. 83–6; C. Richet, P. Brodin and F. de Saint-Girons 'Survie temporaire et survie définitive après les hémorragies graves ', *Comptes rendus de l'Académie des Sciences*, 167 (1918), pp. 574–9.

36. Richet, *La Nouvelle Zomothérapie*, pp. 63–6.

37. Ibid., pp. 166–90. Richet Jr provided full names of the Russian soldiers, while French soldiers were designed by their initials only.

38. Richet, *Mémoires sur moi et sur les autres*, vol. 6, p. 17–18.

39. Ibid., p. 16.

40. Publicity leaflet for zomine of Laboratoire Longuet, 34 rue Sedane, Paris, Richet papers.

41. Richet, *Mémoires sur moi et les autres*, vol. 7, p. 36.

42. Richet, *La Nouvelle Zomothérapie,* pp. 12–21. Richet proposed the same explanation in a short autobiographic sketch that closes his memoirs. Richet, *Mémoires sur moi et les autres*, vol. 7, p. 33. Richet stresses that when he and Héricourt first described therapeutic virtues of raw meat juice, vitamins and hormones were not known yet.

43. Richet, *La Nouvelle Zomothérapie,* p. 49. Richet also stressed that the chemical process used to produce zomine was the same that was employed in fabrication of glandular extracts.

44. l'aliment réparateur par excellence'. Richet, *La Nouvelle Zomothérapie*, p. 218.

45. P. Portier and C. Richet, 'De l'action anaphylactique de certains venins', *Comptes rendus de la Société de Biologie*, 54 (1902), pp. 170–2.

46. P. Estingoy, *Charles Richet (1850–1935) et la découverte de l'anaphylaxie*, mémoire d'Histoire de la Médicine, 1994, Université de Lyon I; K. Krocker, 'Immunity and Its Others: The Anaphylactic Selves of Charles Richet', *Studies in the History and Philosophy of the Biological Sciences*, 30c (1999), pp. 273–96; Löwy, 'On Guinea Pigs, Dogs and Men'.

47. C. Richet, *L'Anaphylaxie* (Paris: Felix Alcan, 1911), pp. 195–8. C. Richet, 'Anaphylaxis', Nobel Lecture, 11 December 1913, in *Nobel Lectures: Physiology or Medicine* (Amsterdam and London: Elsevier Publishing Company, 1967), vol. 1, pp. 473–92, on pp. 487–8. Richet attempted to integrate his view of anaphylaxis with the one of allergy as 'modified reactivity', developed by Clemens Von Pirquet. C. Von Pirquet, 'Allergie', *Münchner Medizinische Wochenschrift*, 53 (1906), pp. 1457–63.

48. C. Richet, 'De l'anaphylaxie alimentaire par la crépitine', *Annales de l'Institut Pasteur*, 8 (1911), pp. 580–93. C. Richet, 'Introduction', in G. Laroche, C. Richet fils and F. Saint Girons, *Anaphylaxie alimentaire* (Paris: Libraire J.B Ballière, 1925), pp. 1–9. The majority of physiologists denied the possibility of adsorption of intact protein from the digestive tract. Only from the 1970s on did scientists return to systematic studies of trans-parietal passage of proteins or their fragments, and its role in immunity. G. Richet, 'Les débuts de l'anaphylaxie alimentaire', *Alim'Inter: Le Journal de l'allergie alimentaire*, 4 (1999), pp. 3–8.

49. Richet, 'Anaphylaxis', Nobel Lecture.

50. Richet, *La Nouvelle Zomothérapie*, p. 20.

51. C. Richet, 'Les réflexes psychiques', in *Travaux du Laboratoire de physiologie de Charles Richet*, vol. 5, pp. 373–475; C. Richet, Ancient humorists and modern humorism', *British Medical Journal*, 2 (1910), pp; 921–6; Richet, 'Anaphylaxis', Nobel Lecture.

52. Richet, *La Nouvelle Zomothérapie*, p. 152; p. 212. Richet's understanding of 'solidarity between systems' mediated by small quantities of active compounds may be seen as related – but not identical to – the ulterior concept of regulatory substances.

53. Richet, *La Nouvelle Zomothérapie*, pp. 19–20.

54. T. Kuhn, *The Structure of Scientific Revolutions* (Chicago, IL: Chicago University Press, 1962).

55. L. Fleck, *Genesis and Development of a Scientific Fact*, trans. F. Bradley and T. Trenn (Chicago, IL: Chicago University Press, 1979), pp. 125–36.

56. L. Fleck, 'W sprawie artykulu Izydory Dambskiej w Przegladzie Filozoficznym rocznik 40, zeszyt III' ('On Izydora Dambska's paper in Przeglad Filozoficzny 40, n°III'), *Przeglad Filozoficzny*, 41 (1936), pp. 192–5.

57. On the other hand, some scientists today also blur the boundaries between immunizing substances and aliments. A paper on oral vaccination published in July 2007 issue of *Expert Opinion on Drug Delivery* starts with the statement: 'the Nobel laureate, Charles Richet, demonstrated in 1900 that feeding raw meat can cure tuberculous dogs – an approach he termed zomotherapy', for the authors, a proof of the validity of *per os* administration of vaccines. D. S. Silin, O. V. Lyubomska, V. Jirathitikal, A. S. Bourinbaiar, 'Oral vaccination: where we are?', *Expert Opinion on Drug Delivery*, 4:4 (2007), pp. 323–40.

2 Lederer, 'Treat with Meat'

1. P. de Kruif, *Men Against Death* (New York: Harcourt Brace, 1932), p. 88.

2. 'Conquest of Anemia One of Medicine's Great Epics', *Science News Letter*, 3 November 1934, p. 275. In Toronto, the public health department reported a 45 per cent reduction in deaths due to pernicious anaemia in the city; see 'Pernicious Anemia in Toronto,

Canada, 1923–1926 and 1928–1931', *American Journal of Public Health*, 22 (1932), pp. 1295–6.

3. De Kruif, *Men Against Death*, pp. 88–9.
4. W. P. Murphy, *Anemia in Practice* (Philadelphia, PA: W. B. Saunders, 1939), p. 78.
5. E. A. Miner, *Living the Liver Diet* (St. Louis, MO: C.V. Mosby, 1931), p. 18.
6. For the transformation of diabetes into a chronic disease, see C. Feudtner, *Bittersweet: Diabetes, Insulin, and the Transformation of Illness* (Chapel Hill, NC: University of North Carolina Press, 2003).
7. 'Conquest of Anemia', p. 275.
8. Murphy, *Anemia in Practice*, p. 69.
9. L. Kass, *Pernicious Anemia* (Philadelphia, PA: W.B. Saunders, 1939), p. 7.
10. W. Osler, 'Clinical Lecture on Idiopathic or Pernicious Anemia', *Canadian Journal of Medical Sciences*, 6 (1881), pp. 35–41.
11. W. Osler and T. McCrae, *Principles and Practice of Medicine* 10th edn (New York: D. Appleton, 1925), pp. 747–53. (This edition appeared after Osler's death in 1919, but T. McCrae had assisted Osler on the textbook since the eighth edition published in 1912.) For the role of splenectomy and the pharmaceutical construction of the disease, see K. Wailoo, *Drawing Blood: Technology and Disease Identity in Twentieth-Century America* (Baltimore, MD: Johns Hopkins University Press, 1997). For other historical treatments, see W. B. Castle, 'The Conquest of Pernicious Anemia', in M. M. Wintrobe (ed.) *Blood, Pure and Eloquent* (New York: McGraw-Hill, 1980); and 'A History of Pernicious Anaemia', *British Journal of Haematology*, 2000, 111, 407–15.
12. R. C. Cabot, 'Pernicious and Secondary Anemia, Chlorosis and Leukemia', in W. Osler (ed.), *Modern Medicine: Its Theory and Practice*, 3rd edn (Philadelphia, PA: Lea and Febiger, 1925), p. 33.
13. Obituary, *New York Times*, 25 July 1890, p. 5.
14. 'Death of George H. Scripps', *Washington Post*, 14 April 1900, p. 3; 'Senator Hughes Dead', *Washington Post*, 12 January 1911, p. 1; 'Governor Da Baca Dead', *New York Times*, 19 February 1917, p. 10; 'Gives His Blood to Peary', *New York Times*, 10 April 1918, p. 13; 'Anna Held Died After Brave Fight', *New York Times*, 13 August 1918, p. 9.
15. 'End Comes To Maj-Gen. Bell', *Los Angeles Times,* 29 October 1926, p. 4; 'Gen. Robert M'Coy Dies in Wisconsin', *New York Times*, 6 June 1926, p. 2; 'George Siegmann, Film Actor', *New York Times,* 24 June 1928, p. 27 'Chaney Slowly Improves', *New York Times*, 26 August 1930, p. 27.
16. G. Minot and W. P. Murphy, 'Treatment of Pernicious Anemia by a Special Diet', *JAMA*, 87 (1926), pp. 470–6, on p. 471. The doctors offered *Henry IV*, act 2, scene 3.
17. T. S. Chen and P. S. Chen, *Understanding the Liver: A History* (Westport, CT: Greenwood Press, 1984), p. 181.
18. L. Barker and T. P. Sprunt, 'The Treatment of Some Cases of So-Called 'Pernicious' Anemia', *JAMA*, 69 (1917), pp. 1920–7.
19. G. H. Whipple and F. S. Robscheit-Robbins, 'Blood Regeneration in Severe Anemia. I. Standard Basal Ration Bread and Experimental Methods', *American Journal of Physiology*, 72 (1925), pp. 395–407.
20. G. W. Corner, *George Hoyt Whipple and His Friends: The Life-Story of a Nobel Prize Pathologist* (Philadelphia, PA: J.B. Lippincott Company, 1963), p. 182.
21. See F. M. Rackemann, *The Inquisitive Physician The Life And Times Of George Richards Minot, A.B. M.D. D. Sc.* (Cambridge, MA: Harvard University Press, 1956).
22. Minot and Murphy, 'Pernicious Anemia', p. 472.

23. Murphy, *Anemia in Practice*, p. 81.
24. Ibid., p. 120.
25. J. Bordley, 'Pernicious Anemia and Liver Therapy', *American Journal of Nursing*, 30 (1930), pp. 1481–8, on p. 1487.
26. D. O'Hara and J. S. Grewal, 'An Unusual Case of Pernicious Anaemia', *Boston Medical and Surgical Journal*, 197 (1927), pp. 129–31.
27. B. M. Wood, 'The Therapeutic Value of Diet in Anemia', *American Journal of Nursing*, 27 (1927), pp. 811–14.
28. L. H. Peters, 'Diet and Health: Liver Cocktail in Pernicious Anemia', *Atlanta Constitution*, 1 May 1928, p. 17.
29. Advertisement, *New York Times*, 15 December 1926, p. 30. For earlier references to shrimp, lobster, and crabmeat cocktails, see I. C. B. Allen, *Mrs. Allen's Cooking, Menus, Service* (Garden City, New York: Doubleday, Doran and Co., 1924), pp. 112–13.
30. For Castle's work, see A. Karnad, *Intrinsic Factors: William Bosworth Castle and the Development of Hematology and Clinical Investigation at Boston City Hospital* (Boston, MA: Harvard University Press, 1997).
31. W. B. Castle, 'Observations on the Etiologic Relationship of Achlyia Gastrica to Pernicious Anemia', *American Journal of the Medical Sciences*, 178 (1929), pp. 748–77, on p. 755.
32. W. B. Castle and M. Bowie, 'A Domestic Liver Extract for Use in Pernicious Anemia', *JAMA*, 92 (1929), pp. 1830–2.
33. 'Nobel Prizeman Simplifies Liver Treatment of Anemia', *Science News Letter*, 3 November 1934, p. 276.
34. Bordley, 'Pernicious Anemia and Liver Therapy', p. 1487.
35. Murphy, *Anemia in Practice*, p. 192. A. Tuchman, 'Diabetes: A Cultural History' (paper delivered at Yale School of Medicine, October 2006).
36. J. H. Lewis, *Biology of the Negro* (Chicago, IL: University of Chicago Press, 1942), pp. 227–8.
37. Miner, *Living the Liver Diet*, p. 22.
38. Ibid., *Diet*, p. 19.
39. 'Forego the Liver', *Los Angeles Times*, 21 April 1928, p. A4.
40. Dr. W. Brady, 'Eat Liver and Live to Eat More', *Atlanta Constitution*, 18 December 1928, p. 10.
41. W. A. Evans, 'The High Cost of Liver', *Chicago Tribune*, 2 May 1928, p. 10.
42. H. M. Conner, 'The Treatment of Pernicious Anemia with Swine Stomach', *JAMA*, 94 (1930), 388–90.
43. C. C. Sturgis and R. Isaacs, 'Treatment of Pernicious Anemia with Desiccated, Defatted Stomach', *American Journal of Medical Sciences*, 180 (1930), pp. 597–602, on p. 598.
44. 'Blow To', *Los Angeles Times*, 20 September 1929, p. 1.
45. 'Finds Mother Love Dies as Manganese is Lost from Diet', *New York Times*, 28 March 1931, p. 8.
46. 'Interprets Radio Words', *New York Times*, 20 April 1930, p. 30.
47. Murphy, *Anemia in Practice*, p. 110.
48. L. S. P. Davidson, 'The Treatment of Pernicious Anaemia with Fish-Liver Extract', *British Medical Journal*, 2 (1932), pp. 347–50.
49. Advertisement, Nason's Cod Liver Oil, *Hygeia*, 7 (1929), p. 1159.
50. Murphy, *Anemia in Practice*, p. 175.

51. See Wailoo, *Drawing Blood*, for the commodification of pernicious anaemia and the corporate culture of liver extract.
52. W. Brady, 'Here is Bad News for the Butcher', *Los Angeles Times*, 1 June 1932, p. A6.
53. Quoted in B. Wansink, 'Changing Eating Habits on the Home Front: Lost Lessons from World War II Research', *Journal of Public Policy and Marketing*, 21 (2002), pp. 90–9.

3 Pfeffer, 'How Abattoir "Biotrash" Connected the Social Worlds of the University Laboratory and the Disassembly Line'

1. J. M. Skaggs, *Prime Cut: Livestock Raising and Meatpacking in the United States, 1607–1983* (College Station, Texas: A & M University Press, 1986); D. Fitzgerald, *Every Farm a Factory: the Industrial Ideal in American Agriculture* (New Haven, CT: Yale University Press, 2003).
2. V. C. Medvei, *The History of Clinical Endocrinology: a Comprehensive Account of Endocrinology from earliest times to the present day. Revised and updated edition* (Dordrecht: Kluwer Academic Publishers, 1993) p. 123.
3. F. G. Young, 'The Evolution of Ideas about Animal Hormones', in J. Needham (ed.), *The Chemistry of Life: Lectures on the History of Biochemistry* (Cambridge: Cambridge University Press, 1970), pp. 125–55.
4. E. A. Doisy, *Sex Hormones: Porter Lectures Delivered at the University of Kansas School of Medicine* (Lawrence, KS: University of Kansas, 1936), pp. 3–5.
5. D. L. Hall and T. F. Glick, 'Endocrinology: a Brief Introduction', *Journal of the History of Biology*, 9:2 (1976), pp. 229–33.
6. A. S. Parkes, *Sex, Science and Society* (Newcastle upon Tyne: Oriel Press, 1966), p. 43.
7. W. Cronon, *Nature's Metropolis: Chicago and the Great West* (New York: W. W. Norton and Co, 1991), p. 251.
8. J. Russell Ives, *The Livestock and Meat Economy of the United States* (Chicago, IL: AMI Center for Continuing Education American Meat Industry, 1966), p. 213.
9. M. Borell, 'Organotherapy, British Physiology, and the Discovery of the Internal Secretions', *Journal of the History of Biology*, 9:2 (1976), pp. 232–68.
10. Skaggs, *Prime Cut*, p. 77.
11. Ibid., p. 8.
12. R. M. Aduddell and L. P. Cain, 'The Consent Decree in the Meatpacking Industry, 1920–1956', *Business History Review*, 55:3 (1981), pp. 359–78.
13. C. E. Dillon, *Meat Slaughtering and Processing* (St Louis, MO: Meat Merchandising Inc., 1947), p. 63.
14. M. Borell, 'Brown-Sequard's Organotherapy and its Appearance in America at the end of the Nineteenth Century', *Bulletin of the History of Medicine*, 50 (1976), pp. 309–20.
15. W. Karmfert, 'Hormone Balance', *The New York Times*, 31 October 1943.
16. M. Bliss, *The Discovery of Insulin* (Boston, MA: Faber and Faber, 1988).
17. J. H. Madison, *Eli Lilly: a Life, 1885–1977* (Indianapolis, IN: Indiana Historical Society 1989), p. 63.
18. H. E. Dale, 'The Chemistry of the Sex Hormones', *Pharmaceutical Journal* (29 April 1939), pp. 432–40.
19. A. Clarke, *Disciplining Reproduction: Modernity, American Life Sciences and the 'Problem of Sex'* (Berkeley, CA: University of California Press, 1998), pp. 233–58.

20. M. Fishbein, 'Glandular Physiology and Therapy: Introduction', *JAMA*, 104:6 (1935), p. 463.

21. P. E. Smith, 'General Physiology of the Anterior Hypophysis', *JAMA*, 104:7 (1935), pp. 548–53.

22. Dillon, *Meat Slaughtering and Processing*, p. 58.

23. R. Horowitz, *Putting Meat on the American Table: Taste, Technology, Transformation* (Baltimore, MD: The Johns Hopkins University Press, 2006), p. 89.

24. R. Horowitz, '"Where Men Will Not Work": Gender, Power, Space and the Sexual Division of Labor in America's Meatpacking Industry, 1890–1990', *Technology and Culture*, 38:1 (1997), pp. 187–213.

25. N. Wade, *The Nobel Duel: Two Scientists' 24 year Race to win the World's Most Coveted Research Prize* (New York: Anchor Press/Doubleday, 1981), pp. 64–5.

26. G. Corner, *The Seven Ages of a Medical Scientist: an Autobiography* (Philadelphia, PA: University of Pennsylvania Press, 1981), p. 247.

27. A. Oakley, *The Captured Womb: A History of the Medical Care of Women* (Oxford: Basil Blackwell, 1986), pp. 194–204.

28. Armour Company Advert, *The Chemist and Druggist Year-Book 1930* (London: Chemist and Druggist), p. 247.

29. A. S. Parkes, 'Herbert Evans: an Interview', *Journal of Reproduction and Fertility*, 19 (1969), pp. 1–49; E. C. Amoroso and G. W. Corner, 'Herbert Evans, 1882–1971', *Biographical Memoirs of Fellows of the Royal Society*, 18 (1972), pp. 83–186; L. L. Bennett, 'Herbert Evans: a Rare Spirit', *Perspectives in Biology and Medicine*, 22 (1978), pp. 90–103; L. L. Bennett, 'His Future Foretold – the 1904 Address by Herbert Evans', *Perspectives in Biology and Medicine*, 29 (1985), pp. 153–63.

30. Clarke, *Disciplining Reproduction*, p. 223.

31. D. C. Aron, 'The Path to the Soul: Harvey Cushing and Surgery of the Pituitary Gland and its Environs in 1916', *Perspectives in Biology and Medicine*, 37:4 (1994), pp. 551–65.

32. A. F. W. Hughes, 'A History of Endocrinology', *Journal of History of Medicine and Allied Sciences*, 32 (1977), pp. 292–313; L. G. Wilson, 'Internal Secretions in Disease: the Historical Relations of Clinical Medicine and Scientific Physiology', *Journal of the History of Medicine and Allied Sciences*, 39 (1984), pp. 263–302.

33. H. M. Evans and J. A. Long, 'The Effect of the Anterior Lobe of the Hypophysis Administered Intraperitoneally on Growth, Maturity and the Oestrus Cycles of the Rat', *Anatomical Record*, 21 (1921), p. 61.

34. Development of Vascular System File, Box 38, The Herbert McLean Evans Papers, History of Science and Technology Collection, The Bancroft Library, University of California, Berkeley (hereafter The Evans Papers).

35. Skaggs, *Prime Cut*, p. 3.

36. Applications, 1922–3 File, Box 13, The Evans Papers.

37. N. P. Christy, 'Faculty Remembered: Philip E. Smith, 1884–1970', *P & S Journal*, 17:1 (1997), http://healthsciences.columbia.edu/news/journal (accessed July 2007).

38. Clarke, *Disciplining Reproduction*, p. 86.

39. R. Greep, 'The Saga and the Science of Gonadotrophins', *Journal of Endocrinology*, 39 (1967), pp. ii–ix.

40. W. Engelbach, 'The Growth Hormone: Report of a Case of Juvenile Hypopituitarism Treated with Evans' Growth Hormone', *Endocrinology*, 81 (1932), pp. 1–19.

41. 'Letter of Dr W. A. Reilly, Department of Pediatrics, University of California at Los Angeles Medical School to Herbert Evans', May 1935, April–September 1935 File, Box 1, The Evans Papers.

42. E. Edelson, 'The Remarkable Dr Li: Master of the Master Gland', *Family Health* (August 1971), pp. 15–18.

43. N. Rasmussen, 'Steroids in Arms: Science, Government, Industry, and the Hormones of the Adrenal Cortex in the United States, 1930–1950', *Medical History*, 46 (2002), pp. 299–324.

44. N. Rasmussen, 'Of "Small Men", Big Science and Bigger Business: the Second World War and Biomedical Research in the United States', *Minerva*, 40 (2002), pp. 115–46.

45. G. Moritz, 'Coupons and Counterfeits: World War II and the US Black Market', www.gtexts.com/college/fc.html, accessed April 2003.

46. C. H. Li and H. Evans, 'The Isolation of Pituitary Growth Hormone', *Science*, 99 (1944), p. 183.

47. Letter of the Editor, *Jersey Journal*, to Herbert McLean Evans, 7 August 1946, Fl File, Box 6, The Evans Papers.

48. Editorial, 'Hormone to Aid Growth Isolated, But It is Too Costly for Wide Use', *New York Times*, 8 March 1944.

49. 'Letter of Armour Laboratories to Herbert Evans', 26 August 1946. Bra-Bri File, Box 1, The Evans Papers.

50. United Packing Company 1945–6 File, Box 22, The Evans Papers.

51. R. F. Escamilla and L. Bennett, 'Pituitary Infantilism Treated with purified Growth Hormone, Thyroid and Sublingual Methyltestosterone: A Case Report', *Journal of Clinical Endocrinology*, 11 (1951), pp. 221–8.

52. 'Proposal from Doctor John R. Mote of Armour and Company, sent 21 July 1948 to Doctor Joseph H. Barach', US Metabolism and Endocrinology Study Section File, Box 28, The Evans Papers.

53. D. Cantor, 'Cortisone and the Politics of Drama, 1949–55', in J. Pickstone (ed.), *Medical Innovations in Historical Perspective* (Basingstoke: Macmillan, 1992), pp. 165–84; D. Cantor, 'Cortisone and the Politics of Empire: Imperialism and British Medicine, 1918–1955', *Bulletin of History of Medicine*, 67 (1993), pp. 463–93.

54. Anon., 'Making the Hormone for Growth', *Medical World News*, 21 February 1969, pp. 32–5.

55. G. W. Gray, 'Cortisone and ACTH', *Scientific American*, 182 (1950), pp. 30–6.

56. Anon., 'New Drug, ACTH, Curbs Diseases', *San Francisco Chronicle*, 29 July 1950.

57. W. L. Laurence, 'ACTH is Reported Swift Aid in Gout', *New York Times*, 22 October 1949.

58. R D. Cole, 'Choh Hao Li', National Academy of Sciences', Biographical Memoirs, http://stills.nap. edu/html/biomems/cli.html (accessed June 2007).

59. Editorial, 'Structure of ACTH; First Step Toward Synthesis of the Drug Is Taken', *New York Times*, 19 June 1955, p. E9.

60. Editorial, 'Apparatus for Hormone Research', *New York Times*, 25 January 1953, p. F6.

61. J-P. Gaudillière and I. Löwy, 'General Introduction', in, J-P Gaudillière and I. Löwy (eds), *The Invisible Industrialist: Manufacturers and the Production of Scientific Knowledge* (Basingstoke: Macmillan Press, 1998), pp. 3–15.

62. N. M. Rockafellar, *Conversations with Dr Leslie Latty Bennett: The Research Tradition at UCSF* (San Francisco, CA: University of California, San Francisco Oral History Program, Department of History and Health Sciences, 1992), p. 21.

63. N. Oudshoorn, *Beyond the Natural Body: An Archaeology of Sex Hormones* (London: Routledge, 1994).

4 Stull and Broadway, 'What's Meatpacking Got to Do with Worker and Community Health?'

1. N. Vialles, *Animal to Edible* (Cambridge: Cambridge University Press, 1994).
2. U. Sinclair, *The Jungle* (1906 New York: Penguin, 1985).
3. The most comprehensive discussion of our research is presented in: D. D. Stull and M. J. Broadway, *Slaughterhouse Blues: The Meat and Poultry Industry in North America* (Belmont, CA: Wadsworth, 2004).
4. R. Halpern, *Down on the Killing Floor: Black and White Workers in Chicago's Packinghouses, 1904–1954* (Urbana, IL: University of Illinois Press, 1997).
5. Stull and Broadway, *Slaughterhouse Blues*, pp. 16, 35.
6. D. D. Stull, 'Knock 'Em Dead: Work on the Killfloor of a Modern Beefpacking Plant', in L. Lamphere, A. Stepick and G. Grenier (eds), *Newcomers in the Workplace: Immigrants and the Restructuring of the US Economy* (Philadelphia, PA: Temple University Press, 1994), pp. 44–77. I. MacLachlan, *Kill and Chill: Restructuring Canada's Beef Commodity Chain* (Toronto: University of Toronto Press, 2001).
7. *Newsweek*, 'Color it Green', 8 March 1965, p. 76.
8. L. A. Duewer and K. E. Nelson, 'Beefpacking Costs are Lower for Larger Plants', *Food Review*, 14:4 (1991), pp. 10–13.
9. US Department of Labor, '1994 Employment Hours and Earnings' (Washington, DC: US Government Printing Office, 1994). US Department of Labor, 'Employment and Earnings' (Washington, DC: US Government Printing Office, various dates).
10. L. Gouveia and D. D. Stull, 'Dances With Cows: Beefpacking's Impact on Garden City, Kansas, and Lexington, Nebraska', in D. D. Stull, M. J. Broadway and D. Griffith (eds), *Any Way You Cut It: Meat Processing and Small-Town America* (Lawrence, KS: University Press of Kansas, 1995), pp. 85–107.
11. D. D. Stull, M. J. Broadway, and K. C. Erickson, 'The Price of a Good Steak: Beef Packing and its Consequences for Garden City, Kansas', in L. Lamphere (ed.), *Structuring Diversity: Ethnographic Perspectives on the New Immigration* (Chicago, IL: University of Chicago Press, 1992), pp. 35–64.
12. Stull and Broadway, *Slaughterhouse Blues*, p. 80.
13. M. A. Grey and A. C. Woodrick, 'Unofficial Sister Cities: Meatpacking Labor Migration Between Villachuato, Mexico, and Marshalltown, Iowa', *Human Organization*, 61:4 (2002), pp. 364–76. L. Fink, *The Maya of Morgantown: Work and Community in the Nuevo New South* (Chapel Hill, NC: University of North Carolina Press, 2003).
14. M. E. Whitcomb, 'The Challenge of Providing Doctors for Rural America', *Academic Medicine*, 80 (2005), pp. 715–16.
15. D. D. Stull fieldnotes on workers' compensation hearings, Garden City, Kansas, 15–21 May 1989, author's files.
16. J. R. Barrett, *Work and Community in the Jungle: Chicago's Packinghouse Workers 1894–1922* (Urbana, IL: University of Illinois Press, 1987), pp. 69–71.
17. Stull and Broadway, *Slaughterhouse Blues*, pp. 75–6.

18. US Department of Labor, Bureau of Labor Statistics, 'Occupational Injuries and Illnesses in the United States by Industry' (Washington, DC: US Government Printing Office, n.d.).
19. Stull and Broadway, *Slaughterhouse Blues*, p. 153.
20. US Department of Labor, Occupational Safety and Health Administration, *Ergonomics Program Management Guidelines for Meatpacking Plants* (Washington, DC: US Government Printing Office, 1993).
21. C. C. Gjessing, T. F. Schoenborn and A. Cohen, 'Participatory Ergonomic Interventions in Meatpacking Plants' (US Department of Health and Human Services, Washington, DC: US Government Printing Office, 1994).
22. M. E. Personick and K. Taylor-Shirley, 'Profiles in Safety and Health: Occupational Hazards of Meatpacking', *Monthly Labor Review*, 112:1 (1989), p. 5.
23. J. Brooks, *Here's the Beef: Underreporting of Injuries, OSHA's Policy of Exempting Companies from Programmed Inspections Based on Injury Records, and Unsafe Conditions in the Meatpacking Industry.* Forty-Second Report by the Committee on Government Operations together with additional views (Washington, DC: US Government Printing Office, 1988), p. 13.
24. Personick and Taylor-Shirley, 'Profiles in Safety and Health: Occupational Hazards of Meatpacking', p. 5.
25. US Department of Labor, OSHA Office of Communications, 'Statement of Assistant Secretary Charles N. Jeffress on Effective Date of OSHA Ergonomics Standard' (2001), at http://www.osha.gov/pls/oshaweb/owadisp. show_document?p_table=NEWS_RELEASES&p_id=1368.
26. Center for American Progress; OMB Watch, *Special Interest Takeover: The Bush Administration and the Dismantling of Public Safeguards* (Washington, DC: Reece Publishing, 2004).
27. US Department of Labor, Bureau of Labor Statistics, 'Occupational Injuries and Illnesses in the United States by Industry' (Washington, DC: US Government Printing Office, n.d.).
28. Human Rights Watch, *Blood, Sweat, and Fear: Workers' Rights in US Meat and Poultry Plants* (New York: Human Rights Watch, 2005).
29. J. P. Boyle, 'In Meatpacking, Progress to Be Proud Of', *Washington Post,* 31 August 2005, p. A23.
30. American Meat Institute, 'American Meat Institute Establishes Cooperative Alliance with Occupational Safety and Health Administration', 22 October 2002 at http://www.meatami.com/Template.cfm?Section=Archive [accessed 3 August 2006).
31. The research at Running Iron Beef was conducted by Stull, Ken Erickson, and the late Miguel Giner over eight months during 1994. All quotes concerning Running Iron Beef, unless otherwise indicated, come from Stull's fieldnotes. For a fuller discussion of this research, see Stull and Broadway, *Slaughterhouse Blues*, pp. 82–98.
32. D. D. Stull interview with shop steward, Running Iron Beef, 6 June 1994, p. 10.
33. Stull and Broadway, *Slaughterhouse Blues*, pp. 63, 107.
34. Royal Canadian Mounted Police, Brooks Detachment, 'Reported Crimes and Crimes Per Officer, Brooks', undated one-page typescript, Broadway's files.
35. Brooks Bulletin (Alberta, Canada), 'Year in Review: What did 1997 Bring to Brooks (31 December).
36. M. J. Broadway fieldnotes, Brooks, Alberta, 6 January 1998, author's files.

37. D. McKenzie, *Canadian Profile: Alcohol, Tobacco and Other Drugs* (Ottawa: Centre on Substance Abuse, 1997).
38. M. J. Broadway fieldnotes, Brooks, Alberta, 6 January 1998, author's files.
39. M. Nicholson, 'Canadian Beef Plant Looks Overseas for Workers', Reuters, 24 August 2006, at http://www.ellinghuysen.com/news/articles/38112.shtml [accessed 24 August 2006].
40. M. J. Broadway fieldnotes, Brooks, Alberta, 5 February 2006, author's files.
41. Ibid.
42. M. J. Broadway fieldnotes, Brooks, Alberta, 16 January 2006, author's files.
43. M. J. Broadway fieldnotes, Brooks, Alberta, 17 January 2006, author's files.
44. I. Hyman, N. Vu and M. Beiser, 'Post Migration Stresses Among Southeast Asian Youth in Canada: A Research Note', *Journal of Comparative Family Studies*, 31 (2000), pp. 281–93.
45. Statistics Canada, 'National Population Health Survey 1996' (Ottawa, 1999).
46. Statistics Canada, 'Profile of Census Divisions and Subdivisions in Alberta', Catalogue No. 95-190-XPB. Ottawa, 1999). Statistics Canada, 'Profile of Census Divisions and Subdivisions in Alberta', Catalogue No. 95-223-XPB (Ottawa, 2004).
47. M. J. Broadway fieldnotes, Brooks Alberta, 14 February 2006, author's files.
48. M. J. Broadway, 'Meatpacking and its Social and Economic Consequences for Garden City, Kansas', in the 1980s, *Urban Anthropology*, 19:4 (1990), p. 339.
49. Personal communication, Dr Choung Le, 8 September 1985.
50. R. A. Hackenberg and G. Kukulka, 'Industries, Immigrants, and Illness in the New Midwest', in D. D. Stull, M. J. Broadway, and D. Griffith (eds), *Any Way You Cut It: Meat Processing and Small-Town America* (Lawrence, KS: University Press of Kansas, 1995), p. 195.
51. Authors' fieldnotes, Garden City, Kansas, 2004, authors' files. Penney Schwab, MAM executive director, personal communication, 14 January 2005.
52. Kansas Department of Social and Rehabilitation Services, 'Program Statistics' (County Packet Information, n.d.), at http://www.srskansas.org/admin/mapprogram.html.
53. Stull and Broadway, *Slaughterhouse Blues*, p. 155.

5 Pilcher, 'Is Refrigerated Meat Healthy?'

1. L. A. Craig, B. Goodwin, and T. Grennes, 'The Effect of Mechanical Refrigeration on Nutrition in the United States', *Social Science History*, 28:2 (Summer 2004), pp. 325–36.
2. U. Sinclair, *The Jungle* (New York: W. W. Norton, 2003), p. 97; R. Horowitz, *Putting Meat on the American Table: Taste, Technology, Transformation* (Baltimore, MD: Johns Hopkins University Press, 2006), pp. 59–60; J. Rifkin, *Beyond Beef: The Rise and Fall of Cattle Culture* (New York: Dutton, 1992); E. Schlosser, *Fast Food Nation: The Dark Side of the All-American Meal* (Boston, MA: Harper Perennial, 2001).
3. S. J. Hale, *Early American Cookery: 'The Good Housekeeper' (1841)* (Mineola, NY: Dover Publications, Inc., 1996), p. 37.
4. University of California, Berkeley, Bancroft Library, Manuel Gamio Book Notes, Microfilm 2322, reel 2, page 437, Luis Felipe Recinos, 'Vida del Sr. José Rocha', 8 April 1927.
5. This difference might tempt the reader to an environmentally determinist conclusion that tropical climates forced Spanish and Latin American cooks to forego the pleasures of aged meat. In fact, owing to its altitude, Mexico City has an average summer high tem-

perature of about 24oC (75oF), while temperate Argentina shares this same preference for freshly slaughtered meat.

6. M. Bruegel, 'How the French Learned to Eat Canned Food, 1809–1930s', in W. Belasco and P. Scranton (ed.), *Food Nations: Selling Taste in Consumer Societies* (New York: Routledge, 2002), pp. 113–30.

7. J. M. Pilcher, 'Empire of the "Jungle": The Rise of an Atlantic Refrigerated Beef Industry, 1880–1920', *Food, Culture and Society*, 7:1 (Autumn 2004), pp. 63–78.

8. M. Harner, 'The Ecological Basis for Aztec Sacrifice', *American Ethnologist*, 4:1 (February 1977), pp. 117–35; M. Harris, *Good to Eat: Riddles of Food and Culture* (New York: Simon and Schuster, 1985), p. 232; M. Sahlins, 'Culture as Protein and Profit', *New York Review of Books*, 23 November 1978, pp. 45–53; B. R. Ortiz de Montellano, *Aztec Medicine, Health, and Nutrition* (New Brunswick, NJ: Rutgers University Press, 1990).

9. F. Chevalier, *Land and Society in Colonial Mexico: The Great Haciendas* (Berkeley, CA: University of California Press, 1966), p. 106; A. W. Cosby, Jr, *The Columbian Exchange: Biological and Cultural Consequences of 1492* (Westport, CT: Greenwood Press, 1972); J. C. Super, *Food, Conquest, and Colonization in Sixteenth Century Spanish America* (Albuquerque, NM: University of New Mexico Press, 1988); E. G. K. Melville, *A Plague of Sheep: Environmental Consequences of the Conquest of Mexico* (Cambridge: Cambridge University Press, 1997).

10. W. H. Dusenberry, 'The Regulation of Meat Supply in Sixteenth-Century Mexico City', *Hispanic American Historical Review*, 28:1 (February 1948), p. 45. Admittedly, preserved beef, known as *tasajo* and *cecina* in the south and *carne seca* along the northern frontier, was an important rural industry that had markets in Mexico City.

11. G. Pérez San Vicente (ed.), *Recetario de doña Dominga de Guzmán, siglo XVIII: Tesoro de la cocina mexicana* (Mexico: Consejo Nacional para la Cultura y las Artes, 1996), p. 110; J. L. Curiel Monteagudo (ed.), *Libro de cocina de la gesta de Independencia: Nueva España, 1817* (Mexico: Consejo Nacional para la Cultura y las Artes, 2002), p. 40; Elisa Vargas Lugo (ed.), *Recetario Novohispano: México, siglo XVIII* (Mexico: Consejo Nacional para la Cultura y las Artes, 2000), pp. 27, 88.

12. *La cocinera poblana y el libro de las familias* (Puebla: N. Bassols, 1881), p. 60; W. Ayguals de Izco, *Manual del cocinero y cocinera, tomado del periodico literaria* La Risa (Puebla: Imprenta de José María Macías, 1849), p. 93; *El cocinero mejicano: Refundido y considerablemente aumentado en esta segunda edición*, 3 vols (Mexico: Imprenta de Galvan a cargo de Mariano Arevalo, 1834), vol. 2, p. 253.

13. V. Torres de Rubio, *Cocina michoacana* (Zamora: Imprenta Moderna, 1896), pp. 45, 110; J. Anduiza, *El libro del hogar* (Pachuca: Imprenta 'La Europea', 1893), p. 198.

14. A. García Cubas, *El libro de mis recuerdos* (Mexico City: Porrúa, 1986 [1904]), p. 251.

15. W. Barret, 'The Meat Supply of Colonial Cuernavaca', *Annals of the Association of American Geographers*, 64:4 (December 1974), p. 527; Archivo General de la Nación, Mexico City (hereafter AGN), Abasto, vol. 8, exp. 16, fo. 266.

16. Quote from I. González-Polo (ed.), *Reflexiones y apuntes sobre la ciudad de México (fines de la colonia)* (Mexico City: Departamento del Distrito Federal, 1981), p. 27. See also AGN, Abasto, vol. 8, exp. 16, fo. 266.

17. AGN, Abasto, vol. 8, exp. 10, fo. 186, 191, quote from exp. 16, fo. 280; Archivo Histórico de la Ciudad de Mexico (hereafter AHCM), vol. 8, exp. 256, 260, vol. 3768, exp. 7. By 1814, supplies of mutton had recovered from their earlier slump in 1812 and 1813 at least briefly, although it is impossible to draw similar conclusions about beef because cattle butchers had largely abandoned the rastro and seldom paid municipal taxes. Certainly

after 1815 and the abolition of customs duties on meat, the statistics are too sporadic to draw any firm conclusions. See AHCM, vol. 8, exp. 273, 280.

18. AHCM, vol. 3758, exp. 22, Ramón Rayón to council, 17 March 1839.

19. AHCM, vol. 3622, exp. 8, Commission report, 2 May 1844.

20. AHCM, vol. 3768, exp. 1, various rent statements, exp. 23, Francisco Carbajal report, 29 August 1849.

21. P. Saucedo Montemayor, *Historia de la ganadería en México*, vol. 1 (Mexico: UNAM, 1984), p. 249.

22. J. Swabe, *Animals, Disease and Human Society: Human-Animal Relations and the Rise of Veterinary Medicine* (London: Routledge, 1999), pp. 85–94; C. Schwabe, *Cattle, Priests, and Progress in Medicine* (Minneapolis, MN: University of Minnesota Press, 1978), pp. 156–7.

23. Archivo Histórico de la Secretaría de Salubridad y Asistencia (hereafter AHSSA), Inspección, box 1, exp. 15, Health Board report, 5 October 1894, R. Mancerola to Secretary of Interior, 9 October 1894; *Gil Blas*, 28 September 1894.

24. *La Patria*, 8 September 1897.

25. *El Imparcial*, 18 February 1902. For a fuller discussion of Porfirian nutritional discourse, see J. M. Pilcher, *¡Que vivan los tamales! Food and the Making of Mexican Identity* (Albuquerque, NM: University of New Mexico Press, 1998), pp. 77–84, 93–7.

26. Quoted in S. Giedion, *Mechanization Takes Command: A Contribution to Anonymous History* (New York: Oxford University Press, 1948), p. 213.

27. Ibid., pp. 211–24; M. Yeager, *Competition and Regulation: The Development of Oligopoly in the Meat Packing Industry* (Greenwich, CT: JAI Press, Inc., 1981), pp. 58–63.

28. *Boletín del Consejo Superior de Salubridad*, 20 September 1880.

29. AHCM, vol. 3763, exp. 25.

30. *El Economista Mexicano*, 3 May 1902. See also *El Imparcial*, 17 February 1902.

31. AHCM, vol. 1279, exp. 5, Padilla and Fernández petition, 20 March 1905.

32. *El Tiempo*, 15 April and 25 August 1905. AHCM, vol. 1279, exp. 5, Interior Secretary report, 27 May 1905.

33. AHSSA, Inspección, box 1, exp. 24, Dr. Jesús E. Monjarás to Veterinary Inspector Francisco López Vallejo, 21 September 1907.

34. *El Imparcial*, 30 July and 2 October 1907; M. Wasserman, *Capitalists, Caciques, and Revolution: The Native Elite and Foreign Enterprise in Chihuahua, Mexico, 1854–1911* (Chapel Hill, NC: University of North Carolina Press, 1984), p. 58.

35. Yeager, *Competition and Regulation*, pp. 67–77.

36. *Mexican Herald*, 13 January, 23 February and 12 March 1908.

37. *El Obrero Mexicano*, 5 November 1909, 14 and 28 January 1910; J. Lear, *Workers, Neighbors, and Citizens: The Revolution in Mexico City* (Lincoln: University of Nebraska Press, 2001), pp. 118–23. See also W. E. French, *A Peaceful and Working People: Manners, Morals, and Class Formation in Northern Mexico* (Albuquerque, NM: University of New Mexico Press, 1996); S. B. Bunker, "Consumers of Good Taste': Marketing Modernity in Northern Mexico, 1890–1910', *Mexican Studies/Estudios Mexicanos*, 13:2 (Summer 1997), pp. 227–69.

38. Archivo José Yves Limantour (hereafter AJYL), Centro de Estudios de Historia de México, Condumex, Mexico City, roll 55, carp. 24/30, British Mexican Trust Company report, 27 February 1908.

39. AJYL, roll 54, carp. 24/30, DeKay to Limantour, 17 February 1908.

40. *Mexican Herald*, 15 April 1908; *El Imparcial*, 18 April 1908.

41. *Mexican Herald*, 24 May 1908. AHCM, vol. 1280, exp. 25, Hinkle to Corral, 26 March 1908.
42. AJYL, roll 54, carp. 24/30, DeKay memorandum, 14 March 1908, and D. A. Holmes to Limantour, 21 August 1908; Archivo Porfirio Díaz, Universidad Iberoamericana, Mexico City, leg. 33, no. 8039, Wiseman to Porfirio Díaz, 17 June 1908.
43. *El Imparcial*, 14 June 1908; *Boletín Oficial del Consejo Superior de Gobierno del Distrito Federal*, 31 January 1908.
44. *Mexican Herald*, 23 October 1908. On the size of the American colony, see W. Schell, Jr, *Integral Outsiders: The American Colony in Mexico City, 1876–1911* (Wilmington, DE: Scholarly Resources, 2001), p. 51.
45. AHCM, vol. 1279, exp. 10, Hinkle petitions, 7 December 1908, 11 February 1909; vol. 1280, exp. 27, DeKay petition, 29 July 1909; vol. 3773, exp. 448, Serrano et al. petition, 26 June 1890.
46. *Mexican Herald*, 12 and 13 September 1909; Washington National Record Center (hereafter WNRC), Claims, RG 76, entry 125, agency 4850, DeKay Memorial, 20.
47. *Mexican Herald*, 29 September 1909.
48. AHCM, vol. 1280, exp. 29, DeKay to Zakany, 11 October 1909, exp. 31, H. P. Chesley, 2 November 1909.
49. Schell, *Integral Outsiders*, pp. 164–8.
50. J. M. Pilcher, 'Mad Cowmen, Foreign Investors, and the Mexican Revolution', *Journal of Iberian and Latin American Studies*, 4:1 (July 1998), pp. 1–15.
51. Pilcher, 'Empire of the "Jungle"', pp. 63–78.
52. S. A. Sanderson, *The Transformation of Mexican Agriculture: International Structure and the Politics of Rural Change* (Princeton, NJ: Princeton University Press, 1986), pp. 124–7, 171; *El Universal*, 22 November 1946; E. Alanis Patiño, 'La industria de la carne en México', *Problemas Agrícolas e Industriales de México*, 4:3 (Julio–Septiembre 1952), p. 250; Secretaría de Agricultura y Ganadería, *Reglamento de la Industrialización Sanitaria de la Carne. Inspeccion Federal* (Mexico City: N.p., 1953).
53. *La Jornada*, 14 March 1992.
54. Comisión Económica para América Latina, *La industria de la carne de ganado bovino en México: Análisis y perspectivas* (Mexico City: Fondo de Cultura Económica, 1975), p. 165; F. Schyer, *Ethnicity and Class Conflict in Rural Mexico* (Princeton, NJ: Princeton University Press, 1990), pp. 152–6.
55. W. J. Belasco, *Appetite for Change: How the Counterculture Took on the Food Industry* (Ithaca, NY: Cornell University Press, 1993), p. 40.

6 Cantor, 'Confused Messages'

1. W. R. Williams, *The Natural History of Cancer with Special Reference to Its Causation and Prevention* (London: W. Heinemann, 1908), p. 350.
2. Ibid., p. 332.
3. Ibid., p. 333.
4. Ibid., p. 64.
5. D. Cantor, 'The Frustrations of Families: Henry Lynch, Heredity and Cancer Control, 1962–1975', *Medical History*, 50 (2006), pp. 279–302.
6. W. H. Woglom, 'Does Meat Cause Cancer?', *Hygeia*, 1 (1923), pp. 23–4, at p. 23.

7. This is not to say that the ASCC never provided any public discussion of research on diet and cancer, but reports tended to be rare, and to be cautious about their applicability to humans. See 'Studies on Cancer and Diet', *Hygeia*, 5 (February 1927), p. 99.

8. This search was for the keywords 'diet' and 'cancer' in Indexcat at http://www.indexcat. nlm.nih.gov/ accessed (22 January 2009).

9. S. Monckton Copeman and Major Greenwood, *Reports on Public Health and Medical Subjects No.36. Diet and Cancer with Special Reference to the Incidence of Cancer upon Members of Certain Religious Orders* (London: HMSO), 1926, p. 1.

10. F. L. Hoffman, *Cancer and Diet, with Facts and Observations on Related Subjects* (Baltimore, MD: Williams and Wilkins, 1937), pp. 115–16, and 655–66.

11. H. C. Saltzstein, 'Newspaper Publicity in the Control of Cancer', in American Society for the Control of Cancer, *Cancer Control: Report of an International Symposium Held under the Auspices of the American Society for the Control of Cancer, Lake Mohonk, New York, USA., September 20–24, 1926* (Chicago, IL: Surgical Publishing Co. of Chicago, 1927), pp. 299–307. E. H. Rigney, 'A Practical Program in Cancer Publicity', *Bulletin of the American Society for the Control of Cancer*, 13:11 (November 1931), pp. 5–6. M. R. Lakeman, 'Cancer Education in Massachusetts', in G. H. Bigelow and H. L. Lombard (eds), *Cancer and Other Chronic Diseases in Massachusetts* (Boston and New York: Houghton Mifflin, 1933), pp. 147–59.

12. W. S. Bainbridge, 'The Cancer Campaign Quaternary; The Problem; The Public; The Patient; The Physician', *American Journal of Surgery*, 31 (1917), pp. 107, 136–7, and 162–6, quotation at p. 107.

13. W. P. Graves, 'The Cancer Problem in Gynaecology', *The Journal of Obstetrics and Gynaecology of the British Empire*, 34 (1927), pp. 224–43, quotation at pp. 229–30.

14. Hoffman, *Cancer and Diet*, p. 116.

15. Ibid., p. 259 and 466.

16. Williams, *Natural History of Cancer*, pp. 43 and 46. Hoffman, *Cancer and Diet*, pp. 444–5 and 467–80. But for a criticism – based on studies of Eskimos and North American Indians – of the idea that that meat was a cause of cancer see H. Gilford, *Tumors and Cancers: A Biological Study* (London: Selwyn and Blount, 1925), pp. 28 and 375. For early Western interest in vegetarianism and health among non-Europeans see T. Stuart, *The Bloodless Revolution: A Cultural History of Vegetarianism from 1600 to Modern Times* (New York: W.W. Norton and Co., 2007).

17. 'Cancer and the Meat Eater', *Current Literature*, 43:5 (November 1907), p. 560.

18. For a survey of such arguments see Hoffman, *Cancer and Diet*.

19. E. E. Ziegler, *The Nutritional Origin of Cancer* (Boise, ID: The author, 1934).

20. The review of Zeigler's book is in *Journal of the American Medical Association,* 104:22 (1 June 1935), p. 2022.

21. Hoffman, *Cancer and Diet*, pp. 106–9, 602–3, and 656.

22. On food faddism, see L. M. Barnett, '"Every Man His Own Physician": Dietetic Fads, 1890–1914', in H. Kamminga and A. Cunningham (eds), *The Science and Culture of Nutrition, 1840–1940* (Amsterdam/Atlanta: Rodopi, 1995), pp. 155–78. On Hippocratism and holism see D. Cantor (ed.), *Reinventing Hippocrates* (Aldershot: Ashgate, 2002) and C. Lawrence and G. Weisz (eds), *Greater than the Parts: Holism in Biomedicine, 1920–1950* (New York and Oxford: Oxford University Press, 1998).

23. J. T. Patterson, *The Dread Disease: Cancer and Modern American Culture* (Cambridge, MA: Harvard University Press, 1987). B. H. Lerner, *The Breast Cancer Wars: Fear, Hope and the Pursuit of a Cure in Twentieth-Century America* (New York: Oxford University

Press, 2003). K. E. Gardner, *Early Detection: Women, Cancer, and Awareness Campaigns in the Twentieth-Century United States* (Chapel Hill, NC: University of North Carolina Press, 2006). On the 'do not delay message' see R. A. Aronowitz, 'Do Not Delay: Breast Cancer and Time, 1900–1970', *Milbank Quarterly*, 79 (2001), pp. 355–386. R. A. Aronowitz, *Unnatural History: Breast Cancer and American Society* (Cambridge: Cambridge University Press, 2007), ch. 6. L. Breslow, D. Wilner, L. Agran, et al., *A History of Cancer Control in the United States, with Emphasis on the Period 1946–1971*, 4 vols, prepared by the History of Cancer Control Project, UCLA School of Public Health, pursuant to Contract no. N01-CN-55172 (Bethesda, MD: Division of Cancer Control and Rehabilitation, National Cancer Institute, Bethesda; Dept. of Health, Education, and Welfare, Public Health Service, National Institutes of Health, National Cancer Institute, Division of Cancer Control and Rehabilitation, 1977).

24. For the ASCC's general position on diet and cancer see 'Studies on Cancer and Diet', *Hygeia*, 5 (February 1927), p. 99.

25. For meat industry attacks on faddism see A. C. Schueren, *Meat Retailing* (Chicago, IL: Vaughan Company, 1927), pp. 479–80 'Further Success Won in Stopping Untruths About Meat', *Annual Report, National Live Stock and Meat Board*, 1923, p. 40. C. R. Moulton and E. B. Wilson, *Meat and the Well-balanced Diet* (Chicago, IL: Institute of American Meat Packers, Dept. of Nutrition, 1930), p. 9.

26. J. H. Kellogg, *The Natural Diet of Man* (Battle Creek, Michigan: The Modern Medicine Publishing Co, 1923), pp. 145–8. See also J. H. Kellogg, *Colon Hygiene* (Battle Creek, MI: Good Health Publishing, 1916), p. 349.

27. L. D. Bulkley, *Cancer and its Non-Surgical Treatment* (New York: W. Wood and Co., 1921). Bulkley was Senior Physician to the New York Skin and Cancer Hospital. As alternatives to surgery he advocated dietetic, hygienic and medicinal measures, a recommendation criticized by one reviewer: 'His [Bulkley's] opinion that his method is more efficient than surgery in the treatment of such cancers as can be removed surgically is wrong. His teaching in this respect is heresy; his book should be burned at the stake' Anon., *Boston Medical and Surgical Journal*, 186:4 (26 January 1922), pp. 119–20. Many of the popular writers were British medical practitioners including William Roger Williams mentioned above, Sir Arbuthnot Lane, Ernest Tipper and John Cope. See A. Dally, *Fantasy Surgery, 1880–1930: With Special Reference to Sir William Arbuthnot Lane* (Amsterdam: Rodopi, 1997). E. Tipper, *The Cradle of the World and Cancer: A Disease of Civilization* (London: Faber and Faber, 1927), pp. 10, 53 and 137. J. Cope, *Cancer: Civilization: Degeneration. The Nature, Causes and Prevention of Cancer, Especially in its Relation to Civilization and Degeneration* (London: H. K. Lewis, 1932), pp. 26, 116–7, and 229.

28. Bainbridge, 'The Cancer Campaign Quaternary', esp. pp. 165–6.

29. Ibid., p. 165.

30. Ibid., p. 165.

31. American Society for the Control of Cancer, *Essential Facts about Cancer. A Handbook for the Medical Profession* (New York: ASCC, 1927), pp. 25–6. The quotation can also be found in an earlier edition American Society for the Control of Cancer, *Essential Facts about Cancer. A Handbook for the Medical Profession* (New York: ASCC, 1924), p. 21. However, it is not present in the 1918 edition: American Society for the Control of Cancer and American Medical Association, *What We Know about Cancer: A Handbook for the Medical Profession, Prevention of Cancer Series* Pamphlet No. 10 (Chicago, IL: AMA, 1918).

32. Barnett, 'Every Man His Own Physician'.
33. 'Medical Broadcast for the Week', *Journal of the American Medical Association*, 91 (10 November 1928), p. 1467 'Medical Broadcast for the Week', *Journal of the American Medical Association*, 93 (27 July 1929), p. 288.
34. F. A. R. Russell, *Preventable Cancer: A Statistical Research* (New York: Longmans, Green, 1912). J. E. Barker, *Cancer: How it is Caused, How it can be Prevented* (New York: E. P. Dutton, 1924).
35. J. Ewing, 'The Prevention of Cancer', in American Society for the Control of Cancer, *Cancer Control*, pp. 165–84, p. 173. On the history of constipation see J. C. Whorton, *Inner Hygiene: Constipation and the Pursuit of Health in Modern Society* (Oxford and New York: Oxford University Press, 2000).
36. See for example the portrayal of the fictional quack, Maurice Maxwell, in the ASCC's educational movie, *Reward of Courage* (1921), who is portrayed as an unscrupulous dandy. This movie is discussed in D. Cantor, 'Uncertain Enthusiasm: The American Cancer Society, Public Education, and the Problems of the Movie, 1921–1960', *Bulletin of the History of Medicine*, 81 (2007), pp. 39–69, esp. pp. 42–4.
37. J. F. Hall-Edwards, *Cancer: Its Control and Prevention* (Birmingham: Cornish Brothers, 1926), p. 64.
38. J. Ewing, *Neoplastic Diseases: A Treatise on Tumors*, 2nd edn (Philadelphia, PA and London: W. B. Saunders, 1922), p. 104.
39. H. J. Deelman, 'The Mortality from Cancer among People of Different Races', in American Society for the Control of Cancer, *Cancer Control*, pp. 247–72, p. 249.
40. G. A Soper, 'Discussion', in American Society for the Control of Cancer, *Cancer Control*, p. 273.
41. S. Monckton Copeman, Paper for the Ministry of Health's Departmental Committee on Cancer cited in Copeman and Greenwood, *Reports on Public Health and Medical Subjects No.36. Diet and Cancer*, p. 1. M. Hindhede, 'Cancer Statistics – Cancer and Diet', *Acta Medica Scandinavica*, 62 (1925), pp. 379–391.
42. W. S. Bainbridge, *The Cancer Problem* (New York: Macmillan, 1914), p. 82.
43. Woglom, 'Does Meat Cause Cancer?', p. 23.
44. Copeman and Greenwood, *Reports on Public Health and Medical Subjects No.36. Diet and Cancer*.
45. A. Hardy and M. E. Magnello, 'Statistical Methods in Epidemiology: Karl Pearson, Ronald Ross, Major Greenwood and Austin Bradford Hill, 1900–1945', *Sozial- und Präventivmedizin*, 47 (2002), pp. 80–9. E. Magnello, 'The Introduction of Mathematical Statistics into Medical Research: The Roles of Karl Pearson, Major Greenwood and Austin Bradford Hill', in E. Magnello and A. Hardy (eds), *The Road to Medical Statistics* (Amsterdam and New York: Rodopi, 2002), pp. 95–123. J. R. Matthews, 'Major Greenwood versus Almroth Wright: Contrasting Visions of 'Scientific' Medicine in Edwardian Britain', *Bulletin of the History of Medicine*, 69 (1995), pp. 30–43.
46. Copeman and Greenwood, *Reports on Public Health and Medical Subjects No. 36. Diet and Cancer*, p. 2.
47. Russell, *Preventable Cancer*.
48. Copeman and Greenwood, *Reports on Public Health and Medical Subjects No. 36. Diet and Cancer*, p. 3.
49. Copeman and Greenwood, *Reports on Public Health and Medical Subjects No. 36. Diet and Cancer*, p. iv.

50. H. M. Marks, *The Progress of Experiment: Science and Therapeutic Reform in the United States, 1900–1990* (New York: Cambridge University Press, 1997).

51. See for example American Medical Association. Council on Health and Public Instruction. American Society for the Control of Cancer. *Prevention of Cancer Series*, Pamphlets 1–10 (Chicago, IL: American Medical Association, 1915–24).

52. For a general discussion of the different meanings of prevention see D. Cantor, 'Cancer Control and Prevention in the Twentieth Century', *Bulletin of the History of Medicine*, 81 (2007), pp. 1–38.

53. W. L. Rodman, *Cancer of the Breast, Prevention of Cancer Series*, Pamphlet No. 5 (Chicago, IL: American Medical Association, 1917), p. 3. J. C. Bloodgood, *The Cancer Problem, Prevention of Cancer Series*, Pamphlet 6 (Chicago, IL: American Medical Association, 1917), p. 5. The surgeon James Ewing, another member of the ASCC, argued elsewhere that a rational basis for the prevention of cancer lay in the fact that the major forms of the disease were the result of some from of chronic irritation, and he cited especially cancer of the intra-oral group – cancers of the lip, mouth, tongue and tonsil, which were due to bad teeth, tobacco and syphilis – hygiene in the case of external genitals; skin removal of suppressed hair follicles; cervix inflammation and infection gastric cancer – habitual over eating. Ewing, 'The Prevention of Cancer'.

54. Hoffman, *Cancer and Diet*.

55. W. Arbuthnot Lane, *New Health for Everyman* (London: Geoffrey Bles, 1932), p. 100.

56. G. Soper quoted in 'The Importance of Answering Letters', *Campaign Notes of the American Society for the Control of Cancer*, 5:11 (November 1923), [1–4] quotation p. [2].

57. Ewing, 'The Prevention of Cancer', p. 173. The following letter written by the ASCC to a member of the public was quoted by George Soper: 'A sedentary life, meat eating, and wearing corsets are not especially dangerous, but should not be carried to excess for general health reasons. It is impossible to say with accuracy whether vegetarian nations have as much cancer as do others, for the reason that the methods of diagnosis and reporting in vegetarian countries are not such as to make a fair comparison possible.' Soper quoted in 'The Importance of Answering Letters', pp. [2–3].

58. For a discussion of the problem of mistaking the fact that a starvation diet might reduce the size of tumours for a favourable therapeutic result see Ewing, *Neoplastic Diseases*, p. 59.

59. C. Moreschi, 'Beziehungen Zwischen Ernährung und Tumorwachstum', *Zeitschrift f. Immunitätsforschung. Originale*, 2 (1909), pp. 651–75. P. Rous, 'The Rate of Tumor Growth in Underfed Hosts', *Proceedings of the Society for Experimental Biology and Medicine*, 8 (1910–11), pp. 128–30. P. Rous, 'The Influence of Diet on Transplanted and Spontaneous Mouse Tumors', *Journal of Experimental Medicine*, 20 (1914), pp. 433–51. E. V. N. Van Alstyne and S. P. Beebe, 'Diet Studies in Transplantable Tumors I', *Journal of Medical Research*, 29 (1913–1914), pp. 217–32. J. E. Sweet, E. P. Corson-White and G. J. Saxon, 'The Relation of Diets and of Castration to the Transmissible Tumors of Rats and Mice', *Journal of Biological Chemistry*, 15 (1913), pp. 181–91. J. E. Sweet, E. P. Corson-White and G. J. Saxon, 'On the Influence of Certain Diets upon the Growth of Experimental Tumors', *Proceedings of the Society for Experimental Biology and Medicine*, 10 (1912–13), pp. 175–6.

60. Hoffman, *Cancer and Diet*, p. 664.

61. Ibid., p. 466.

7 Apple, 'What's for Dinner?'

1.   A note on the use of the word American: strictly speaking, American describes all the peoples of the western hemisphere. Many of those in the south refer to those in the north as North Americans, a category that includes people living in Canada, the United States and Mexico. Most Canadians are willing to call people in the United States 'Americans', because they term themselves as Canadians. For the purposes of this chapter, American refers to the United States.

2.   R. D. Apple, *Perfect Motherhood: Science and Childrearing in America* (New Brunswick, NJ: Rutgers University Press, 2006).

3.   K. J. Carpenter, *Protein and Energy: A Study of Changing Ideas in Nutrition* (New York: Cambridge University Press, 1994); L. Shapiro, *Perfection Salad: Women and Cooking at the Turn of the Century* (New York: Farrar Straus Giroux, 1986); J. C. Whorton, 'Muscular Vegetarianism: The Debate over Diet and Athletic Performance in the Progressive Era', in J. W. Berryman and R. J. Parks (eds), *Sport and Exercise Science: Essays in the History of Sport Medicine* (Urbana, IL: University of Illinois Press, 1992), pp. 297–318.

4.   For more on the role of scientific advice in mothering in the twentieth century, see Apple, *Perfect Motherhood: Science and Childrearing in America*. N. Tomes, '"Skeletons in the Closet": Women and "Rational Consumption" in the Inter-War American Home', in M. Jackson (ed.), *Health and the Modern Home* (New York: Routledge, 2007), pp. 177–95 discusses women's increasingly important role as the domestic consumer responsible for the health of the family.

5.   C. E. Beecher and H. B. Stowe, *The American Woman's Home* (New Brunswick, NJ: Rutgers University Press, 1869 [2002]; reprint, Edited with an introduction by Nicole Tonkovich), p. 95.

6.   Beecher and Stowe, *American Woman's Home*, p. 104.

7.   H. Levenstein, *Revolution at the Table: The Transformation of the American Diet* (New York: Oxford University Press, 1988), pp. 23–4; S. Williams, *Savory Suppers and Fashionable Feasts: Dining in Victorian America* (Knoxville, TN: University of Tennessee Press, 1996), esp. pp. 98–102; W. Root and R. de Rochemont, *Eating in America: A History* (Hopewill, NJ: Ecco Press, 1976), esp. pp. 189–212; E. N. McIntosh, *American Food Habits in Historical Perspective* (Westport, CT: Praeger, 1995), passim.

8.   *Cornell Bulletin of Homemakers*, Part I (no. 10) (1903), p. 7. See also C. B. Burrell, 'Mother's Responsibility in Regard to Diet', *The Child Welfare Manual: A Handbook of Child Nature and Nurture for Parents and Teachers* (New York: University Society, 1916), pp. 218–20.

9.   L. T. Dudgeon, 'Food Makes a Difference', *Cornell Extension Bulletin 775*, (November 1949). See also M. H. Abel, *Successful Family Life on the Moderate Income* (Philadelphia, PA: J. B. Lippincott Company, 1921); 'Child Welfare and Economics', *American Food Journal* (December 1919), p. 8; 'Improving Your Family's Health', *Parents* (October 1941), pp. 54, 59, 61; L. G. Shouer, 'Is Your Family Well Fed?' *Ladies' Home Journal* (December 1941), pp. 114–15.

10. For more on women and nutrition in general, see R. D. Apple, 'Science Gendered: Nutrition in the United States, 1840–1940', in H. Kamminga and A. Cunningham (eds), *The Science and Culture of Nutrition, 1840–1940* (Amsterdam and Atlanta, GA: Rodopi, 1995), pp. 129–54.

11. 'Food for the Farmer's Family', *Cornell Reading-Course for Farmers' Wives*, February 1903.

12. J. Putnam and S. Gerrior, 'Trends in US Food Supply, 1970–1997', in Elizabeth Frazao (ed.), *America's Eating Habits: Changes and Consequences* (Washington, DC: USDA-ERS Agriculture Information Bulletin-750, 1999), p. 136.

13. USDA Economic Research Service, *Briefing Rooms: Food Consumption Overview* (2007); available from http://www.ers.usda.gov/Briefing/Consumption/, accessed 7 May 2008.

14. A. Pierce, 'Meat in the Child's Dietary', *Parents* (April 1930), p. 30; J. Plant and F. Berg, 'Healthy Eating, Happy Kids' (*Parents*, January 2007), pp. 103–04, 106, 109.

15. 'What the American Eats', *American Food Journal*, 15:2 (1920), pp. 37–8.

16. 'Our Diet Changing', *American Food Journal*, 15:3 (1920), p. 7.

17. K. Iacobbo and M. Iacobbo, *Vegetarian America: A History* (Westport, CT: Praeger, 2004), p. 158.

18. R. Horowitz, *Putting Meat on the American Table* (Baltimore, MD: Johns Hopkins Press, 2006), pp. 13–17.

19. W. H. Jordan, *Principles of Human Nutrition: A Study in Practical Dietetics* (New York: Macmillan Co., 1912).

20. Jordan, *Principles of Human Nutrition*, pp. 247–8.

21. Ibid., pp. 255–6. Jordan was not alone in drawing comparison between meat-eating societies and those that ate less meat. See, for example, M. Rubner, 'The Nutrition of the People', *Journal of Home Economics*, 5:1 (1913), pp. 1–25.

22. Jordan, *Principles of Human Nutrition*, p. 257.

23. Iacobbo and Iacobbo, *Vegetarian America: A History*, pp. 131–2.

24. 'What About Meat?', *Hygeia*, 17 (1939), pp. 1062–3 and 'Meat and the authority behind it ...', advertisement, *Journal of Home Economics*, 33:6 (1941), p. 19.

25. P. Baird, 'The Diet Women Need Most', *Redbook* (April 1992), pp. 123–6; D. Eller, 'Should You Eat Meat?' *Redbook* (March 1993), pp. 130, 34; C. Krucoff, 'Exercise and Iron', *Saturday Evening Post*, September–October 1996, p. 21; J. Storm, 'Did Mother Know Best?' *Women's Sports and Fitness*, January–February 1991, pp. 18–26.

26. A. Davis, *Let's Eat Right to Keep Fit* (New York: New American Library, 1954, 1970), p. 29. Amino acids had been a point of discussion for many decades before Davis, see, for example, B. W. Gardner, 'Value of Meat in the Diet', *Consumers' Research Bulletin*, 11 (1943), pp. 15–17; C. Robert Moulton, 'The Value of Meat in the Diet', *American Food Journal*, December 1923, pp. 559–61, 90; Elsie Fjelstad Radder, 'The Growing Child Eats Meat', *Hygeia* 6 (1928), pp. 343–4; P. Rudnick, 'The Nutritive Values of Meats', *American Food Journal* (September 1921), pp. 12–13. See also M. S. Chaney, *Nutrition*, 5th edn (Boston, MA: Houghton Mifflin Co., 1954); C. M. Taylor and Grace Macleod, *Foundations of Nutrition*, 5th edn (New York: Macmillan, 1956) for widely used home economics textbooks.

27. Davis, *Let's Eat Right to Keep Fit*, p. 30.

28. Ibid. Vegetarians of this period accepted the need for complete protein in the diet and constructed complicated recipes and meal plans that ensured the consumption of all necessary amino acids at the same meal without the inclusion of meat. See, for example, E. B. Ewald, *Recipes for a Small Planet: The Art and Science of High Protein Vegetarian Cookery* (New York: Ballantine Books, 1973); F. M. Lappe, *Diet for a Small Planet* (New York: A Friends of the Earth/Ballantine Book, 1971).

29. 'The High Priestess of Nutrition', *Time*, 18 December 1972; D. Yergin, 'Supernutritionist: "Let's Get Adelle Davis Right"', *New York Times Magazine*, 20 May 1973. For a less positive perspective on Davis, see J. C. Whorton, *Crusaders for Fitness: The History of*

American Health Reform (Princeton, NJ: Princeton University Press, 1982), pp. 339–41.

30. By auto-intoxication, commentators meant that the body poisoned itself through the absorption of toxins, usually from the large intestine. The concept has a long history and the introduction of the germ theory in the late nineteenth century strengthened its saliency, providing a mechanism that could explain how intestinal bacteria gave rise to internal putrefaction. J. C. Whorton, *Inner Hygiene: Constipation and the Pursuit of Health in Modern Society* (New York: Oxford University Press, 2000), esp. pp. 22–7.

31. M. D. Swartz, 'How Much Meat?' *Good Housekeeping*, January 1910, pp. 106–9. Other examples include: G. F. Butler, 'Why So Much Meat? One Importance Aspect of the Big Problem of the High Cost of Living', *Ladies' Home Journal*, October (1912), p. 30; C. C. Greer, *School and Home Cooking* (Boston, MA: Allyn and Bacon, 1920); 'Meat – Its Uses and Abuses', *Delineator* (1906), pp. 360–2; S. T. Rorer, 'Do We Eat Too Much Meat?', *Ladies' Home Journal*, January 1898; S. T. Rorer, 'Why I Do Not Believe in Much Meat', *Ladies' Home Journal* (April 1905), p. 39.

32. As it turned out, Girdner had his facts wrong. The Japanese military was not vegetarian at this time. In the late nineteenth century, milk and meat had been added to its dietary of polished rice and fish in an effort to stem the problem of beriberi. This fact, however, did not stop Girdner and other vegetarians from proudly proclaiming the superiority of a vegetarian militia. Iacobbo and Iacobbo, *Vegetarian America: A History*, pp. 130–1.

33. J. H. Girdner, 'Why Eat Meat?' *Cosmopolitan* (March 1907), pp. 571–4.

34. 'How Much Food Do We Need', *American Food Journal* (July 1919), pp. 15–16. For more on the impact of vitamin discoveries, see R. D. Apple, *Vitamania: Vitamins in American Culture* (New Brunswick, NJ: Rutgers University Press, 1996).

35. For examples, see Butler, 'Why So Much Meat?'; 'How Much Food Do We Need'.

36. A. Pierce, 'Meat Cookery', *Parents*, November 1930, p. 44.

37. J. Seligmann and et al., 'America's Nutrition Revolution', *Newsweek*, 19 November 1984, p. 111.

38. E. B. Forbes, 'The Nutritive Value of Meat and Its Place in the Diet', *American Food Journal* 17:4 (1922), p. 10; W. H. Lipman, 'Exploded Fallacies About Meat', *American Food Journal* 16:8 (1921), pp. 9–12; Moulton, 'The Value of Meat in the Diet'; W. D. Richardson, 'The Value of Meat in the Diet', *American Food Journal*, 16:9 (1921), pp. 11–12; Rudnick, 'The Nutritive Values of Meats'.

39. Forbes, 'The Nutritive Value of Meat and Its Place in the Diet'.

40. Ibid.

41. These advertisements appeared frequently in the *Journal of Home Economics*. For examples, see 'New Chart Tells Story of B Vitamins in Meat', advertisement, *Journal of Home Economics*, 33:1 (1941), p. 11, 'Meat and the Summer diet', advertisement, *Journal of Home Economics*, 33:4 (1941), p. 16; 'A Short Lesson on the Economy of Meat', advertisement, *Journal of Home Economics*, 33:2 (1941), p. 12.

42. M. Nestle, *Food Politics: How the Food Industry Influences Nutrition and Health* (Berkeley, CA: University of California Press, 2002), p. 34. See also, C. Davis and E. Saltos, 'Dietary Recommendations and How They Have Changed over Time', in E. Frazao (ed.), *America's Eating Habits: Changes and Consequences* (Washington, DC: USDA-ERA Agriculture Information Bulletin–750, 1999), pp. 33–50, http://www.ers.usda.gov/Publications/AIB750/ accessed 27 June 2008.

43. M. Henry and D. Monroe, *Low Cost Food for Health, Cornell Bulletin for Homemakers No. 236* (Ithaca, NY: New York State College of Home Economics at Cornell University, 1932), pp. 3, 6.

44. 'The Better Way: Is Your Family Eating Sensibly?' *Good Housekeeping* (September 1968), pp. 169–71; 'Everyday Nutrition', *Parents* (April 1957), p. 97; G. McCarthy, 'What It Takes to Feed Your Family Well', *Parents* (November 1966), pp. 94–5, 152.; *Nutrition and Healthy Growth* (Washington, DC: US Department of Health, Education, and Welfare, Children's Bureau, 1955).

45. C. G. King, 'Nutrition Research Is Vital to Family Health', *Parents* (October 1961), pp. 100–3, 149–50, 152.

46. Agricultural Research Service Consumer and Food Economics Research Division, *Family Fare: A Guide to Good Nutrition*, Home and Garden Bulletin No. 1 (Washington, DC: US Department of Agriculture, 1970), p. 7.

47. Agricultural Research Service Consumer and Food Economics Research Division, *Family Fare*.

48. Agricultural Research Service Consumer and Food Economics Research Division, *Family Fare*, p. 8.

49. 'The ABC's of Family Meal Planning', *Parents* (February 1970), pp. 72–3.

50. On creating your own food pyramid, see C. A. Rinzler, *Nutrition for Dummies* (Foster City, CA: IDG Books Worldwide, 1999), pp. 207–8.

51. *What's in a Meal? Resource Manual for Providing Nutritious Meals in the Child and Adult Care Food Program* (Chicago, IL: US Department of Agriculture, Food and Nutrition Service, [1994]).

52. 'If You Want to Do without Meat', *Ladies' Home Journal* (August 1918), p. 26. A typical advice column is Maria Lincoln Palmer's, 'Meats That We Should Use: And Those That We Shouldn't – and Why', *Delineator* (1917), p. 35.

53. 'If You Want to Do without Meat'.

54. 'The Patriotic Food Show', *American Food Journal*, 13:1 (1918), pp. 9–15.

55. See, for example, A. Barrows, 'The Lesson of the "Meat Map"', *Harper's Weekly*, 19 February 1910, pp. 13–14; A. Barrows, 'Making a Little Meat Go a Long Way', *Ladies' Home Journal* (November 1913), p. 103; L. D. Hall, 'Better Meat for Less Money', *Good Housekeeping*, October (1912), pp. 553–6.

56. For more on rationing in the United States during World War II, see A. Bentley, *Eating for Victory: Food Rationing and the Politics of Domesticity* (Urbana, IL: University of Illinois Press, 1998).

57. C. A. Heller and M. C. Pfund, 'Meals with and without Meat' (Ithaca, NY: New York State College of Home Economics, 1942).

58. 'Make a Little Meat Go a Long Way', advertisement, *Journal of Home Economics*, 34:3 (1943), p. 14.

59. P. Prudence, *Coupon Cookery* (Hollywood, CA: Murray and Gee, 1943).

60. See, for example, Gardner, 'Value of Meat in the Diet'; 'Variety Meats: They Are Good, Abundant, Highly Nutritious', *Life* 11 January 1943, p. 62.

61. 'Meat Shortage Ills Are Traced to Booming Purchasing Power', *Newsweek*, 31 August 1942, pp. 46, 48.

62. M. Jacobs, '"How About Some Meat?" The Office of Price Administration, Consumption Politics, and State Building from the Bottom up, 1941–1946', *Journal of American History* 84:3 (1997), pp. 931–3; H. Levenstein, *Paradox of Plenty: A Social History of Eating in Modern America* (New York: Oxford University Press, 1993), pp. 86–7.

63. Barrows, 'Making a Little Meat Go a Long Way'; F. M. Crawford, 'Eat High on Low-Cost Meat Cuts', *American Home* (September 1972), pp. 80–1; 'Here's How to Eat Well and Save on the Meat Bill', *Woman's Home Companion* (November 1951), pp. 84–5; 'How to Select Meat', *Good Housekeeping* (November 1914), pp. 647–9; H. Wiley, 'Meat Substitutes', *Good Housekeeping* (November 1918), pp. 46, 126–9.

64. For example, M. Pollan, *The Omnivore's Dilemma: A Natural History of Four Meals* (New York: Penguin, 2006, 2007); E. Schlosser, 'Bad Meat: The Scandal of Our Food Safety System', *Nation* (16 September 2002), pp. 6–7; E. Schlosser, *Fast Food Nation* (Boston, MA: Houghton Mifflin, 2001); E. Schlosser, 'Order the Fish', *Vanity Fair* (November 2004), pp. 240, 243–6, 255–7; M. L. Sifry, 'Food Money', *Nation*, 27 December 1999, p. 20.

65. T. Egan, 'A Year Later, Raw Meat Still Lacks Labels', *New York Times*, 20 December 1993; N. Fox, 'The Case of the Deadly Hamburger', *Ladies' Home Journal* (July 1997), pp. 36, 42, 44–5; 'The Meat Industry's Bad Beef', *New York Times*, 20 November 1994; P. Weintraub and M. Teich, 'Fatal Food: How to Protect Your Family', *Redbook* (July 1994), pp. 134, 136–7.

66. M. Krantz, 'An Inedible Beef Stew', *Time* (1 September 1997), p. 34; Schlosser, 'Bad Meat'; Schlosser, *Fast Food Nation;* Schlosser, 'Order the Fish'.

67. 'Chicken: What You Don't Know Can Hurt You', *Consumer Reports*, March 1998, pp. 12–18; 'Dirty Birds: Even "Premium" Chickens Harbor Dangerous Bacteria', *Consumer Reports* 72:1 (2007), pp. 20–3; C. Law, 'America's Looming Food Safety Crisis', *USA Today*, November 1992; E. Licking and J. Carey, 'How to Head Off the Next Tainted-Food Disaster', *Business Week*, 1 March 1999, p. 34.

68. P. Lyons, 'How Safe Is Your Supermarket?' *Ladies' Home Journal* (October 1993), pp. 70, 78–9. See also, K. Wallace, 'A Plateful of Trouble', *Readers' Digest* (August 2004), pp. 110–12., B. Holcomb, 'How Safe Is Your Dinner?', *Good Housekeeping* (May 2000), pp. 75–6; Law, 'America's Looming Food Safety Crisis'; Weintraub and Teich, 'Fatal Food: How to Protect Your Family'; B. Yeoman, 'Dangerous Food: The Shocking Truth That Puts Your Family at Risk', *Redbook* (August 2000), pp. 110–11, 123–4.

69. 'Chicken: What You Don't Know Can Hurt You'.

70. For some background on the history of vegetarianism, see J. Gregerson, *Vegetarianism: A History* (Fremont, CA: Jain Publishing Company, 1994); Iacobbo and Iacobbo, *Vegetarian America: A History;* J. C. Whorton, '"Tempest in a Flesh-Pot": The Formulation of a Physiological Rationale for Vegetarianism', *Journal of the History of Medicine and Allied Sciences*, 32:2 (1977), pp. 115–39.

71. For example, Schlosser, *Fast Food Nation*.

72. J. Schwartz, 'PETA's Latest Tactic: $1 Million for Fake Meat', *New York Times*, 21 April 2008.

73. The changing circumstances also introduced a wider appreciation of the impact of the ideology of meat on the planet. The fear of contaminated meat crossing national borders was but one marker of this transformation. In addition, there was growing concern over the world's food supply, coupled with worries over the impact of global warming on food production. T. J. Allen, 'As Hunger Rises, Chew on This', *In These Times* (May 2008), p. 45; M. Bittman, 'Rethinking the Meat-Guzzler', *New York Times*, 27 January 2008. For an earlier exposé of the deleterious effects of extensive meat production, see J. Robbins, *Diet for a New America* (Walpole, NH: Stillpoint, 1987), esp. ch. 12, 'All things considered', which discussed the relationship between meat and energy, fossil fuels, rain forests, species extinction, US deforestation, water pollution, water use, and even world peace. Even in the 1980s, commentators analyzed the connection between meat-eating, food scarcity, and the subsequent fear that can promote war over insufficient resources.

74. A helpful chronology can be found at Kansas State University Agricultural Experiment Station and Cooperative Extension, *The Economic Impact of BSE on the US Beef Industry: Product Value Losses, Regulatory Costs, and Consumer Reactions* (Kansas Department of Agriculture, [2004]).

75. http://www.cjdfoundation.org/staff.html. L. Belkin, 'Two Women against Mad Cow', *Good Housekeeping* (November 2001), pp. 70–2, 76, 78.

76. A. M. Gallup, Frank Newport, and Gallup Organization, *The Gallup Public Opinion – Google Books Results* (2006). url: books.google.con/books?isbn=-742551385, accessed 24 July 2008.

77. J. Adler, 'Madcow: What's Safe Now?' *Newsweek*, 12 January 2004, pp. 42–8; S. Brink and N. Shute, 'Is It Safe?' *US News and World Report*, 12 January 2004, pp. 16–21; D. Grady et al., 'US Issues Safety Rules to Protect Food against Mad Cow Disease', *New York Times*, 31 December 2003; '"Mad-Cow Disease": Where Do We Go from Here?', *Consumer Reports*, 66:5 (2001), p. 6.

78. F. Kuchler and A. Tegene, 'Did BSE Announcements Reduce Beef Purchases?' (Washington, DC: US Department of Agriculture, Economic Research Service, 2006), p. iii. See also Extension, *The Economic Impact of BSE on the US Beef Industry: Product Value Losses, Regulatory Costs, and Consumer Reactions;* F. Kuchler and A. Tegene, 'US Consumers Had Short-Term Response to First BSE Announcements', *Amber Waves*, 5:4 (2007), pp. 24–9.

79. A. P. Rimal, 'Factors Affecting Meat Preference among American Consumers', *Family Economics and Nutrition Review* (2002).

80. 'Is It Time to Stop Eating Meat?' *Harvard Health Letter* 26:11 (2001), pp. 6–7.

8 Thoms, Vegetarianism, Meat, and Life Reform in Early Twentieth-Century Germany and their Fate in the 'Third Reich'

1. A. Speer, *Erinnerungen* (Frankfurt: Ullstein, 1993), pp. 53, 110, 133, a list of references in R. N. Proctor, *The Nazi War on Cancer* (Princeton, NJ: Princeton University Press, 1999), pp. 134ff; E. G. Schenck, *Patient Hitler: Eine medizinische Biographie* (Düsseldorf: Droste, 1989), pp. 34ff.

2. H. Picker, *Hitlers Tischgespräche im Führerhauptquartier* (Frankfurt: Ullstein, 1989), p. 242.

3. Speer, *Erinnerungen*, p. 177. Time and again, authors polemically cite now-familiar quotations asking with irony whether liver dumplings, caviar and ham should also be counted as vegetarian dishes; D. Driscoll, 'What Sort of Vegetarian was Hitler?', October 1998, http://www.geocities.com/CapitolHill/Lobby/6423/hv.tx (last accessed on 13 October 2007) and 'Hitler was a Vegetarian', http://www.geocities.com/hitlerwasavegetarian (last accessed on 27 October 2007). Anyone interested in the history of critiques of meat consumption and vegetarianism during the first half of the twentieth Century will soon encounter references to the debate on whether Hitler was a vegetarian, both on Internet sites of vegetarian associations and especially in the American literature. R. Berry, *Hitler, Neither Vegetarian nor Animal Lover* (New York: Pythagorean, 2004); T. Stuart, *The Bloodless Revolution: A Cultural History of Vegetarianism from 1600 to Modern Times* (New York and London: W.W. Norton and Company, 2007); C. Spencer, *The Heretic's Feast: A History of Vegetarianism* (Hanover, NH: University Press of New England 1996), pp. 306ff.

4. H.-J. Teuteberg, 'Der Verzehr von Nahrungsmitteln in Deutschland pro Kopf und Jahr seit Beginn der Industrialisierung (1850–1975). Versuch einer quantitativen Langzeitanalyse', in H.-J. Teuteberg and G. Wiegelmann (eds), *Unsere tägliche Kost. Geschichte und regionale Prägung* (Münster: Coppenrath Verlag, 1986), pp. 225–79, esp. pp. 240–1.

5. See A. Roerkohl, *Hungerblockade und Heimatfront: Die kommunale Lebensmittelversorgung in Westfalen während des Ersten Weltkrieges* (Stuttgart: Franz Steiner Verlag, 1991); L. Burchardt, 'Die Auswirkungen der Kriegswirtschaft auf die deutsche Zivilbevölkerung im Ersten und im Zweiten Weltkrieg', *Militärgeschichtliche Mitteilungen*, 15 (1974), pp. 65–97.

6. Compare C. von Tyszka, *Ernährung und Lebenshaltung des Deutschen Volkes. Ein Beitrag zur Erkenntnis des Gesundheitszustandes des Deutschen Volkes* (Berlin: Springer, 1934), especially p. 76 and the references given there.

7. Compare U. Thoms, *Anstaltskost im Rationalisierungsprozess. Die Ernährung in Krankenhäusern und Gefängnissen im 18. und 19. Jahrhundert* (Stuttgart: Franz Steiner Verlag, 2005), p. 304ff, and K. J. Carpenter, *Protein and Energy: A Study of Changing Ideas in Nutrition* (Cambridge: Cambridge University Press, 1994).

8. Thoms, *Amstaltskost*, pp. 351ff.

9. The increasing number of young men being unfit for service and their poor bodily state was explained with their bad nutrition and explained with the missing meat see: C. A. Meinert, *Armee- und Volksernährung. Ein Versuch Professor C. von Voit's Ernährungstheorie für die Praxis zu verwerthen*, vol. 1 (Berlin: Mittler and Sohn, 1880).

10. On the diet of workers and the role of meat within see D. Stockhaus, '"Aber mir sind trotzdem satt wordn mit unserer Suppn": Nürnberger Arbeiterkost um die Jahrhundertwende', *Mitteilungen des Vereins für Geschichte der Stadt Nürnberg*, 81 (1994), pp. 243–72; U. Spiekermann, 'Die Ernährung städtischer Arbeiter in Baden an der Wende vom 19. zum 20. Jahrhundert', in *Internationale wissenschaftliche Korrespondenz zur Geschichte der Deutschen Arbeiterbewegung*, 32 (1996), pp. 453–83.

11. See U. Frevert, '"Fürsorgliche Belagerung": Hygienebewegung und Arbeiterfrauen im 19. und frühen 20. Jahrhundert', *Geschichte und Gesellschaft*, 11 (1985), pp. 420–46.

12. Thoms, *Anstaltskost*, p. 597ff.

13. H. Karmasin, *Die geheime Botschaft unserer Speisen. Was Essen über uns aussagt* (Munich: Bastei-Lübbe, 1999), p. 26.

14. With further bibliographic references: A. Wirtz and E. Meyer-Renschhausen, 'Dietetics, Health Reform and Social Order: Vegetarianism as a Moral Physiology: The Example of Maximilian Bircher-Benner', *Medical History*, 43 (1999), pp. 323–341; A. Schwab, *Monte Verità – Sanatorium der Sehnsucht* (Zürich: Orell Füssli, 2003); J. Melzer, *Vollwerternährung. Diätetik, Naturheilkunde, Nationalsozialismus, sozialer Anspruch* (Stuttgart: Franz Steiner Verlag, 2003); F. Fritzen, *Gesünder leben: Die Lebensreformbewegung im 20. Jahrhundert* (Stuttgart: Franz Steiner Verlag, 2006). Today the scope and extent of the Anglo-American literature on the topic is enormous. See: N. Fiddes, *Meat: A Natural Symbol* (London: Routledge, 1991); Spencer, *The Heretic's Feast*; E. Crook, *Vegetarianism in Australia – 1788 to 1948: A Cultural and Social History* (S.I.: Huntingdon Press, 2006); K. S. Walters and L. Portmess, *Ethical Vegetarianism: From Pythagoras to Peter Singer* (New York: State University of New York Press, 1999); C. P. Vaclavik, *The Vegetarianism of Jesus Christ: The Pacifism, Communalism and Vegetarianism of Primitive Christianity* (Three Rivers, CA: Kaweah Pub. Co, 1986); S. J. Rosen, G. Cerquetti and J. Greene, *Diet for Transcendence: Vegetarianism and the World Religions* (Badger, CA: Torchlight Publishing, 1997); J. Gregory, *Of Victorians and Vegetarians. The Vegetarian*

Movement in Nineteenth-Century Britain (London: Tauris Academic Studies, 2007); M. Iacobbo, *Vegetarian America: A History* (Westport, CT: Praeger, 2004).

15. J. Baumgartner, 'Die Entstehung der vegetarischen Vereine: Entwicklung des Vereineswesens bis 1945', *Der Vegetarier*, 3 (1992), pp. 99–104; E. Barlösius, *Naturgemässe Lebensführung: Zur Geschichte der Lebensreform um die Jahrhundertwende* (Frankfurt a.M.: Campuss 1997), pp. 174ff.

16. H. J. Teuteberg, 'Zur Sozialgeschichte des Vegetarismus', *Vierteljahrschrift für Sozial- und Wirtschaftsgeschichte* 81 (1994), pp. 33–65.

17. *Vegetarische Warte*, January 1896, p. 3ff.

18. F. Steger, 'Antike Diätetik – Lebensweise und Medizin', *N.T.M. Internationale Zeitschrift für Geschichte und Ethik der Naturwissenschaften, Technik und Medizin*, 12 (2004), pp. 146–60; Thoms, *Amstaltskost*, pp. 275f.

19. M. J. Metzger, 'Warum ißt man Fleisch?' *Die Vegetarische Presse*, 23 (1940), p. 19.

20. See N. Mellinger, *Fleisch: Ursprung und Wandel einer Lust* (Frankfurt: Campus Verlag, 2000), p. 29.

21. Mellinger, *Fleisch*, p. 69; M. Schwantje, *Tiermord und Massenmord: Vegetarismus und Pazifismus* (Berlin: Bund für radikale Ethik, 1919); C. Spencer, *Vegetarianism: A History* (New York and London: Four Walls Eight Windows, 2002), pp. 69ff.

22. I. Munk and C. A. Ewald, *Ernährung des gesunden und kranken Menschen* (Wien/Leipzig: Urban and Schwarzenberg, 1895), pp. 195–9.

23. Munk and Ewald, *Ernährung des gesunden und kranken Menschen*, p. 199.

24. This argument is similarly made today by vegetarian activists who argue that the fact of hunger in many regions of the world makes the consumption of meat both an ethical and an animal rights matter H. F. Kaplan, *Philosophie des Vegetarismus. Kritische Würdigung und Weiterführung von Peter Singers Ansatz* (Frankfurt a.M.: Lang, 1988); D. Jamieson (ed.), *Singer and His Critics* (Oxford: Blackwell, 1999).

25. J. Baumgartner, 'Die Anfänge der Obstbau-Kolonie 'Eden' E.G.M.B.H. in Oranienburg (1893–1914)', *Zeitschrift für Unternehmensgeschichte*, 35 (1990), pp. 154–65.

26. On the most famous one see Schwab, *Monte Verità*.

27. J. Baumgartner, 'Reformwaren und Markennamen in der DDR und der Bundesrepublik Deutschland. Eden Reformwarenprodukte – Traditionsunternehmen und Genossenschaft', in C. Kleinschmidt and F. Triebel (eds): *Marketing. Historische Aspekte der Wettbewerbs- und Absatzpolitik* (Essen: Klartext Verlag, 2004), pp. 221–46.

28. Barlösius, *Lebensführung*, p. 8.

29. Ibid. pp. 278–83.

30. J. Baumgartner, *Ernährungsreform – Antwort auf Industrialisierung und Ernährungswandel. Ernährungsreform als Teil der Lebensreformbewegung am Beispiel der Siedlung und des Unternehmens Eden seit 1893* (Frankfurt/M. u.a.: Peter Lang Verlag, 1992).

31. Hampke (1939), cited according to Melzer, *Vollwerternährung*, p. 145.

32. H. Vahle, *Zielskizze der Freikörperkultur. Ein Leitfaden für Leibeszucht und gesundes Leben* (Wallen: Polverlag, 1933), p. 9.

33. Fritzen, *Gesünder leben*, p. 227.

34. Stuart, *The Bloodless Revolution: A Cultural History of Vegetarianism from 1600 to Modern Times*, pp. 435, 443.

35. Melzer, *Vollwerternährung*, p. 147, Fritzen, *Gesünder leben*, p. 226, D. Bothe, *Neue Deutsche Heilkunde 1933–1945. Dargestellt anhand der Zeitschrift, Hippokrates' und der Entwicklung der volksheilkundlichen Laienbewegung* (Husum: Matthiesen Verlag, 1991), p. 217.

36. H. G. Müller, 'Neue Form gestaltet sich', *Leib und Leben*, 7 (1939), pp. 1–3.
37. Cited in Baumgartner, *Lebensreformbewegung*, p. 104.
38. See 'Die Satzung der Deutschen Gesellschaft für Lebensreform e.V.', *Leib und Leben*, 4 (1935), pp. 250–1.
39. *Hippokrates*, 9 (1938), p. 853.
40. H. G. Müller, 'Absage an diesen Vegetarismus!', *Leib und Leben*, 3 (1935), pp. 291–3.
41. Ibid., p. 292.
42. H. Helmel, 'Lebensreform als heroische Lebensgestaltung', *Leib und Leben*, 3 (1935), p. 59.
43. Ibid.
44. H. G. Müller, 'Neue Form gestaltet sich', *Leib und Leben*, 7 (1939), pp. 1–3.
45. Lecture of Prof. Dr Otto Flößner, 16 September 1940 on the relationship between diet reform and nutritional science, in Federal Archives, Berlin, R86/3526 (hereafter Federal Archives, Berlin).
46. U. Thoms, '"Ernährung ist so wichtig wie Munition". Die Verpflegung der deutschen Wehrmacht 1933–1945', in W. U. Eckart und A. Neumann (eds), *Medizin im Zweiten Weltkrieg. Militärmedizinische Praxis und medizinische Wissenschaft im 'Totalen Krieg'* (Paderborn: Schöningh Verlag, 2006), pp. 207–30.
47. M. Baidinger, 'Vegetarier, Abstinenten, Lebensreformer – kleine und große Unterschiede!', *Leib und Leben*, 3 (1935), p. 31.
48. Vegetarians got 600g of cereals, 360g of butter and 500g of quark per month instead of their meat ration, see 'Versorgungsregelung für Vegetarier', *Deutsches Ärzteblatt*, 69 (1939), p. 658.
49. 'Richtlinien für Ernährung', *Reichsgesundheitsblatt*, 10 (1935), pp. 729–30.
50. Müller, 'Neue Form gestaltet sich', pp. 1–3.
51. H. G. Müller, 'Richtlinien für Ernährung', *Leib und Leben*, 4 (1935), p. 276.
52. See the pictures at the exhibition of the 'Obstbaukolonie Eden' at Oranienburg and from the 8th International Vegetarian Congress in: http://www.eden-eg.de/chronik.htm (last accessed 25 August 2009).
53. Scheunert presented his findings in a talk at a meeting of the Working Group for Scientific Preserve Research (Arbeitsgemeinschaft für wissenschaftliche Konserven-Forschung (Awiko)), see the paper: 'Konserven als Vitaminquellen. Interessante wissenschaftliche Untersuchungen', *Hamburger Nachrichten* 18 November 1930, in Archiv der Brandenburgischen Akademie der Wissenschaften, Nachlaß Scheunert, Nr. 65.
54. P. Schenk, 'Die Verpflegung von 4700 Wettkämpfern aus 42 Nationen im Olympischen Dorf während der XI. Olympischen Spiele 1936 zu Berlin', *Münchener Medizinische Wochenschrift*, 83 (1936), pp. 1535–1539.
55. K. Lang, and W. Grab, 'Kälteresistenz und Ernährung', *Klinische Wochenschrift*, 23 (1944), pp. 226–30, for the trials on forced labourers with different food rations see D. Eichholtz, *Geschichte der deutschen Kriegswirtschaft*, Bd. III 1943–1945 (München: Saur, 1996), pp. 246–66 and U. Thoms, 'Einbruch, Aufbruch, Durchbruch? Strukturen und Netzwerke der deutschen Ernährungsforschung vor und nach 1945', in R. v. Bruch and U. Gerhardt (eds), *Kontinuitäten und Diskontinuitäten in der Wissenschaftsgeschichte* (Stuttgart: Franz Steiner Verlag, 2006), pp. 111–30.
56. Tyszka, *Die Ernährung*, p. 97.
57. J. Drews, 'Die 'Gleichschaltung im Stullenverzehr.' Ernährungspsychologie im 'Dritten Reich', – zwei Fundstücke', *WerkstattGeschichte*, 32 (2002), pp. 82–92.
58. See the regulations in: Federal Archives, Berlin, NS 3/499.

59. H. Bottenberg, 'Leidet die Potenz bei fleischfreier Ernährung?', *Hippokrates*, 8 (1943), p. 67.

60. E.-G. Schenck, *1945: Als Arzt in Hitlers Reichskanzlei* (Stockach: Verlag Bavarian Connection, 1985), pp. 18–9.

61. E.-G. Schenck, Ein Tätigkeitsbericht, in Federal Archive/Military Archive Freiburg, MSG 23/2970 and Thoms, 'Ernährung ist so wichtig', p. 225.

62. Steinwehr, 'Warum sollen wir – warum müssen wir Vegetarier sein?', *Vegetarische Presse*, 23 (1940), pp. 29–30.

63. Proctor, *Nazi War*.

64. See e.g. Himmler's opinion on this, which fits quite well in Drew's picture, Felix Kersten, *Totenkopf und Treue. Heinrich Himmler ohne Uniform. Aus den Tagebuchblättern des finnischen Medizinalrats Felix Kersten* (Hamburg: Mölich, o.J. [1952]), pp. 49–50.

9 Waddington, 'Mad and Coughing Cows'

1. M. Ferriares, *Sacred Cow, Mad Cow: A History of Food Fears* trans. J. Gladding (New York: Columbia University Press, 2006) has suggested a longer history. She argues that virtually all foods have been called into question between the Middle Ages and the twentieth century.

2. J. Burnett, *Plenty and Want: A Social History of Diet in England from 1815 to the present day* (London: Routledge, 1966), pp. 222–30.

3. See M. French and J. Phillips, *Cheated Not Poisoned? Food Regulation in the United Kingdom, 1875–1938* (Manchester: Manchester University Press, 2000); J. R. Fisher, 'Cattle Plagues Past and Present', *Journal of Contemporary History*, 33 (1998), pp. 215–28.

4. P. J. Atkins, 'White Poison: The Social Consequences of Milk Consumption, 1850–1930', *Social History of Medicine*, 5 (1992), pp. 216–18; S. D. Jones, 'Mapping a Zoonotic Disease: Anglo-American Efforts to Control Bovine Tuberculosis', *Osiris*, 19 (2004), pp. 133–48; B. G. Rosenkrantz, 'The Trouble with Bovine Tuberculosis', *Bulletin of the History of Medicine*, 59 (1985), pp. 155–75.

5. G. Wells et al., 'A novel progressive Spongiform Encephalopathy in Cattle', *Veterinary Record*, 121 (1987), pp. 419–20.

6. *The BSE Inquiry: Volume 1: Findings and Conclusions* (London: HMSO, 2000).

7. *Lancet*, 346 (1995), p. 1155; *British Medical Journal*, 311 (1995), pp. 1415–21.

8. R. Will et al., 'A new variant of Creutzfeldt– Jakob disease in the UK', *Lancet*, 347 (1996), pp. 921–5.

9. *Transactions of the British Congress on Tuberculosis*, 4 (London, 1901), p. 44.

10. *Bibby's Book on Milk*. Section IV. *Bovine Tuberculosis* (Liverpool: J. Bibby, 1911), p. 185.

11. L. Bryder, *Below the Magic Mountain: A Social History of Tuberculosis in Twentieth-century Britain* (Oxford: Clarendon Press, 1988), p. 1; G. Leighton and L. Douglas, *The Meat Industry and Meat Inspection*, 5 vols (London: Educational Book Company, 1910), vol. 3, p. 890.

12. W. Savage, *Milk and the Public Health* (London: Macmillan, 1912), p. 149; *British Journal of Tuberculosis*, 1 (1907), p. 250.

13. *Journal of State Medicine*, 10 (1902), pp. 595; 692.

14. *The Times*, 18 May 1990.

15. A. Hardy, 'Animals, Disease and Man: Making Connections', *Perspectives in Biology and Medicine*, 46 (2003), pp. 210–11.

16. *Guardian*, 15 November 1988.
17. See S. Hinchliffe, 'Indeterminacy In-decisions: Science, Policy and Politics in the BSE Crisis', *Transactions of the Institute of British Geographers*, 26 (2001), pp. 190–2.
18. *Lancet Neurological*, 5 (2006), pp. 393–8.
19. Hardy, 'Animals, Disease and Man', p. 205.
20. Savage, *Milk and the Public Health*, p. 125.
21. *Journal of Preventive Medicine*, 13 (1905), p. 492.
22. *Field*, 5 October 1901, p. 566.
23. *Sanitary Record*, 8 August 1901, p. 126.
24. *Evening Standard*, 12 February 2001, p. 13.
25. *Lancet*, 341 (1993), p. 642.
26. *Nutritional Review*, 54 (1996), p. 208.
27. Local Government Board, *Report* (London: HMSO, 1912/13), p. lvi.
28. *Veterinary Record*, 16 December 1899, p. 341.
29. *Veterinary Record*, 19 August 1905, p. 139.
30. *Journal of the Sanitary Institute*, 17 (1896), p. 429.
31. R. Edelmann, *Text-Book of Meat Hygiene* (Washington, DC: G. E. Howard Press, 1908), p. 266.
32. *Veterinary Record*, 6 March 1906, p. 599.
33. Such reassurances about the value of cooking were designed to encourage consumers, and in particular working-class consumers, to properly prepare and cook meat as part of an attempt to reform manners and the perceived unhygienic behaviours of the 'ignorant and unwashed': A. Hardy, 'Food, Hygiene and the Laboratory: A Brief History of Food Poisoning in Britain, *c.* 1850–1950', *Social History of Medicine*, 12 (1999), pp. 293–311.
34. A. Hardy, 'Pioneers in the Victorian Provinces: Veterinarians, Public Health and the Urban Animal Economy', *Urban History*, 29 (2002), p. 380.
35. *Veterinary Record*, 12 August 1905, pp. 115–18.
36. *Practitioner*, September 1889, p. 228.
37. *Second Interim Report of the Royal Commission to Inquire into the Effect of Food Derived from Tuberculous Animals*, PP (1907) 57, part II, appendix, vol. 3, pp. 221–4.
38. *Select Committee on the Tuberculosis (Animals) Compensation Bill* (London: HMSO, 1904), p. iii.
39. *Report of the Working Party on Bovine Spongiform Encephalopathy* (London: MAFF, 1989); *Guardian*, 11 February 1989, p. 1.
40. *The BSE Inquiry.*
41. *Nature*, 19 July 1990, p. 211; *Guardian*, 23 March 1995, p. 23.
42. *Nature*, 26 October 2000, p. 932.
43. S. Dealler, *Fatal Legacy. BSE, the Search for the Truth* (London: Corgi, 1996), pp. 60–4.
44. *Report of the Medical Officer of the Local Government Board* (London: HMSO, 1903), p. xxix.
45. 'The Transmission of Consumption by Animals to Man', *Cowkeeper and Dairyman's Journal*, March 1907, p. 193.
46. E. Willoughby, *Milk: Its Production and Uses* (London: Charles Griffin, 1903), p. 170.
47. *Final Report of the Royal Commission appointed into the relations of Human and Animal Tuberculosis*, PP (1911), pp. 4–29, 35, 36–7, 40–1.
48. *Nature*, 19 July 1990, p. 211.

49. *Annual Report of the Veterinary Department of the Privy Council Office for the Year 1878* (London: HMSO, 1879), p. 4.
50. *The Times*, 4 November 1895, p. 4.
51. *The BSE Inquiry.*
52. See M. Beck, D. Asenova and G. Dickson, 'Public Administration, Science, and Risk Assessment', *Public Administration Review*, 65 (2005), pp. 403–4.
53. I. Taylor, 'Policy on the Hoof: The Handling of the Foot and Mouth Disease Outbreak in the UK 2001', *Policy and Politics*, 31 (2003), p. 535.
54. Hinchliffe, 'Indeterminacy In-decisions', p. 196.
55. MAFF, *BSE in Great Britain. A Progress Report* (London: HMSO, 1995), appendix 3.
56. *Nature*, 9 April 1998, p. 533.
57. Report of the Medical Officer of Health on Meat Inspection of the Central Meat Market, 29 November 1906, PH/159, Corporation of London Record Office (hereafter CLRO), Guildhall, London.
58. Report of the City Solicitor and Medical Officer of Health on Importation and Inspection of Foreign Meat, June. 1905, PH/140, CLRO.
59. Report of the Veterinary Surgeon for 1904–5, C2/1/6, Glasgow City Archive, Mitchell Library, Glasgow.

10 Gaudillière, 'Food, Drug and Consumer Regulation'

1. 'DES Livestock Implants Are Prohibited by FDA Because of Cancer Link', *Wall Street Journal*, 26 April 1973.
2. R. J. Apfel and S. M. Fisher, *To Do No Harm, DES and the Dilemmas of Modern Medicine* (New Haven, CT: Yale University Press, 1984). R. Meyers, *DES: The Bitter Pill* (New York: Putnam, 1986). D. B. Dutton, *Worse Than Disease: Pitfalls of Medical Progress* (Cambridge: Cambridge University Press, 1988). N. Pfeffer, 'Lessons from History: The Salutary Tale of Stilboestrol', in P. Alderson (ed.) *Consent to Health Treatment and Research: Differing Perspectives* (Report of the Social Science Research Unit Conference, 1992).
3. S. Bell, 'The Synthetic Compound DES, 1938–1941: The Social Construction of a Medical Treatment' (PhD thesis, Brandeis University, 1980). L. Marks, *Sexual Chemistry: A History of the Contraceptive Pill* (New Haven, CT: Yale University Press, 2001). S. Morgen, *In Our Own Hands: The Women's Health Movement in the United States* (New Brunswick, NJ: Rutgers University Press, 2002).
4. O. Shell, *Modern Meat* (New York: Random House, 1984). J. Rifkin, *Beyond Beef: The Rise and Fall of the Cattle Culture* (New York: Dutton, 1992). A. I. Marcus, *Cancer from Beef: DES, Federal Food Regulation and Consumer Confidence* (Baltimore, MD: Johns Hopkins University Press, 1986). J. Rodrick, 'FDA's Ban of the Use of DES in Meat Production a Case Study', *Agriculture and Human Values*, 3 (1986), pp. 10–25.
5. J-P Gaudillière, *La médecine et les sciences* (Paris: La Découverte, 2006).
6. On the early history of DES see Bell, 'The Synthetic Compound DES'. J-P Gaudillière, 'Hormones at Risk: Cancer and the Medical Uses of Industrially Produced Sex Steroids in Germany, 1930–1960', in T. Schlich and U. Tröhler (eds), *Risk and Safety in Medical Innovation* (London: Routledge, 2004), pp. 148–69.
7. Bell, 'The Synthetic Compound DES'.
8. A.I. Marcus, *Cancer from Beef*, ch. 1 and 2. For the expertise conducted during this first phase, see the NAS report: Committee on Animal Nutrition, Subcommittee on Hor-

mones, *Hormonal Relationship and Applications in the Production of Meats, Milk, and Eggs* (Washington DC: National Academy of Science, NRC, 1959).

9.   'Hormones and Cancer', *New York Times*, 29 January 1956.

10. N. Silber, *Test and Protest: The Influence of Consumers Union* (New York: Random House, 1983).

11. A. I. Marcus, *Cancer from Beef*.

12. 'Bill on Food Additives Gains', *New York Times*, 14 August 1958; 'An Act to Protect the Public Health by Amending the Federal Food, Drug, and Cosmetic Act to Prohibit the Use in Food of Additives Which Have Not Been Adequately Tested to Establish Their Safety', *US Statutes*, 1958, pp. 1784–9.

13. For more on this aspect see, in addition to Marcus, *Cancer from Beef*, T. R. Dunlap, *DDT: Scientists, Citizens, and Public Policy* (Princeton, NJ: Princeton University Press, 1981). S. P. Hays, *Beauty, Health and Permanence: Environmental Politics in the United States, 1955–1985* (Cambridge: Cambridge University Press, 1987). B. Gillespie, D. Eva, R. Johnson, 'Carcinogenic Risk Assessment in the United States and Great Britain: The Case of Aldrin/Dieldrin', *Social Studies of Science*, 14 (1984), pp. 265–301. R. Brickman, S. Jasanoff, T. Ilgen, *Controlling Chemicals: The Politics of Regulation in Europe and in the United States* (Ithaca, NY: Cornell University Press, 1985).

14. On the 1962 Act in general, see P. Temin, *Taking Your Medicine: Drug Regulation in the United States* (Cambridge, MA: Harvard University Press, 1980). A. Daemmrich, *Pharmacopolitics: Drug Regulation in the United States and Germany* (Chapel Hill, NC: University of North Carolina Press, 2004). On the amended clause, see *Congressional Record*, 87th Congress, II, p. 12713.

15. R. Carson, *Silent Spring* (Boston, MA: Houghton Mifflin, 1962). W. Longgood, *The Poisons in Your Food* (New York: Simon and Schuster, 1960). J. S. Turner, *The Chemical Feast: Ralph Nader's Study Group Report on the Food and Drug Administration* (New York: Grossman Publishers, 1970).

16. R. Nader, *Unsafe at Any Speed: The Designed-in Dangers of the American Automobile* (New York: Grossman Publishers, 1965).

17. B. Seaman, *The Doctors' Case against the Pill* (New York: P. H. Wyden, 1969).

18. In addition to the above-mentioned literature on the DES medical crisis: C. Bonah, J-P Gaudillière, 'Faute, accident ou risque iatrogène? La régulation des évènements indésirables du médicament à l'aune des affaires Stalinon et Distilbène', *Revue Française des Affaires Sociales*, 3–4 (2007), pp. 123–51.

19. A.L. Herbst, H. Ulefelder, D.C. Poskanzer, 'Adenocarcinoma of the Vagina: Association of Maternal Stilbestrol Therapy with Tumor Appearance in Young Women', *New England Journal of Medicine*, 284 (1971), pp. 878–81.

20. P. Greenwald *et al.*, 'Vaginal Cancer after Maternal Treatment with Synthetic Estrogens', *New England Journal of Medicine*, 285 (1971), pp. 390–2.

21. J-P Gaudillière, 'Better Prepared than Synthesized: Adolf Butenandt, Schering AG and the Transformation of Sex Steroids into Drugs', *Studies in History and Philosophy of the Biological and the Biomedical Sciences*, 36 (2005), pp. 612–44.

22. Gaudillière, 'Hormones at Risk'.

23. Many of these letters emanated from citizens with no apparent engagement in consumer or environmental groups. Thus, a certain Mrs. Hutchinson from Greensborough (NC) simply wrote in September 1972: 'I appreciate your concern about Hexachlorophene by taking it off the market. But why overlook DES? I realize you have taken it off the market to animals, but why leave it for human consumption?', RG 88, Box 4662, National Archives, College Park, Maryland (hereafter National Archives).

24. Answering a certain Ronald Riba from Arlington, Illinois, about the fate of the drug, the Bureau of Drugs and the Bureau of Veterinary Medicine, for instance, wrote separate answers, respectively focusing on the redefinition of therapeutic indications and on the imminent withdrawal of DES implants in application of the Delaney clause. Both letters nonetheless needed to refer to the interventions of the other bureau. RG 88, Box 4876, National Archives,

25. One unexpected text of this sort was a devastating article by the editorialist of *Science*, by N. Wade, written in 1972. N. Wade, 'DES. A Case Study of Regulatory Abdication', *Science*, 177 (1972), pp. 335–7.

26. S. Jasanoff, *The Fifth Branch. Science Advisors as Policy Makers* (Cambridge: Harvard University Press, 1990). S. Jasanoff, 'Science, Politics and the Renegotiation of Expertise at EPA', *Osiris*, 2nd series, 7 (1992), pp. 195–217.

27. W. Halffman, 'Boundaries of Regulatory Science. Eco/toxicology and Aquatic Hazards of Chemicals in the US, England and the Netherlands, 1970–1995' (PhD Thesis, University of Amsterdam, 2003).

28. For instance, Dieckmann's study: W. J. Dieckmann *et al.*, 'Does the Administration of Diethylstilbestrol During Pregnancy have Therapeutic Value?', *American Journal of Obstetrics and Gynecology*, 66 (1953), pp. 1062–81.

29. NDA 4038-DES Lilly, Report of the National Academy of Sciences, 1969, Federal Drug Administration archives, Twinbrook, Maryland (hereafter FDA archives).

30. US Congress, House of Representatives, Intergovernmental Relations Subcommittee of the Committee on Government Operations, *Regulation of DES. It's Uses as a Drug for Humans and in Animal Feeds*, Hearings of 11 November 1971. Testimony of Dr Arthur Herbst (Washington DC: Government Printing Office, 1971), p. 8.

31. Committee on Government Operations, House of Representatives, Hearings held on 11 November 1971, *Regulation of DES*, Testimony of C. Edwards, Commissioner FDA (Washington, DC: Government Printing Office, 1972), pp. 49–54 and 76–84.

32. A. Gross to L. Friedmann, Director of Toxicology, Bureau of Foods, 'Carcinogenicity of DES: Estimation of Safe Levels in Diet', 5 December 1971. US Congress, House, Regulation of Diethylstilbestrol (DES) in Its Use as a Drug for Humans and in Animal Feeds (Part 2), December 13, 1971 (Washington, DC: Government Printing Office, 1972), pp. 115–18.

33. Congress, 1971, p. 118.

34. P. Lehmann, Director of the Division of Nutritional Sciences to C. D. Van Houweling, 'Comments in reference to the memo of December 5, 1971 from Dr Adrian Gross', in Congress, 1971, pp. 124–7. L. Friedman to V. O. Wodicka, Bureau of Food, 'Mathematical Models in Safety Evaluation', 21 December 1971, Congress 1971, pp. 123–4. For Gross's reply, see pp. 128–34 and pp. 137–43.

35. Congress 1971, p. 127.

36. See for instance, L. Friedmann, Director of Toxicology to Rep. Fountain, February 15, 1972, pp. 170–3.

37. Committee on Labor and Public Welfare, Senate Hearings held on July 20, 1972, *Regulation of DES*, Testimony of C. Edwards, FDA Commissioner (Washington DC, Government Printing Office, 1975), pp. 206–11.

38. 76N002, 2 November 1977, FDA Archives.

39. R. Proctor, *Cancer Wars: How Politics Shape What We Know and Don't Know About Cancer* (New York: Basic Books, 1995).

INDEX

Printed and bound by CPI Group (UK) Ltd, Croydon, CR0 4YY

22/10/2024

01777623-0014